Percutaneous Transluminal Angioplasty

Technique, Early and Late Results

Edited by
C.T. Dotter A.R. Grüntzig W. Schoop
E. Zeitler

With 179 Figures

Springer-Verlag Berlin Heidelberg New York Tokyo 1983

Charles T. Dotter, M. D., University of Oregon, Health Sciences Center, Department of Diagnostic Radiology, Portland, Oregon 97201, USA

Professor Dr. Andreas R. Grüntzig, Emory University School of Medicine, Department of Medicine, 1364 Clifton Road, N.E., Atlanta, Georgia 30322 USA

Professor Dr. Werner Schoop, Aggertalklinik, D-5250 Engelskirchen

Professor Dr. Eberhard Zeitler, Klinikum Nürnberg, Radiologisches Zentrum, Flurstr. 17, D-8500 Nürnberg

ISBN-13: 978-3-540-12654-6 e-ISBN-13: 978-3-642-69278-9
DOI: 10.1007/978-3-642-69278-9

Library of Congress Cataloging in Publication Data. Main entry under title: Percutaneous transluminal angioplasty. Bibliography: p. Includes index. 1. Transluminal angioplasty – Addresses, essays, lectures. I. Dotter, Charles T. [DNLM: 1. Angioplasty, Transluminal – Congresses. WG 300 P429 1982] RD598.5.P47 1983 617'.413 83-19581

Typesetting, printing, and bookbinding: v. Starck'sche Druckereigesellschaft m.b.H., 6200 Wiesbaden
2127/3130–543210.

Preface

In the past ten years, there have been significant advances in the diagnosis and therapy of arterial vascular disease. While long-term morbidity can only be improved by changing the patient's life-style and removing any risk factors that may be present (hypertension, hyperlipidemia, obesity, diabetes mellitus, nicotine abuse), symptomatic relief may be obtained by various procedures. Besides conservative treatment of arterial occlusive disease (physical therapy, medical treatment) and surgical vascular interventions (thromboendarterectomy, bypass procedures), balloon catheters introduced percutaneously under local anesthesia have found increased application in virtually all areas for the dilatation and recanalization of obstructive lesions in the past few years.

The technique of balloon dilatation, as introduced by Grüntzig as a further development of the percutaneous interventions by Dotter and Judkins, is no longer the decisive issue. The main objective of present clinical research is to determine the proper indications and patient selection for this procedure, which has found its place between conservative treatment and surgery.

The contents of this Symposium should provide some guidelines for the indications and postprocedural therapy for the referring physician, the angiologist, and for the radiologist and cardiologist performing the dilatation.

We owe our thanks to all the specialists involved, who have provided us with the benefits of their experience. Mrs. H. Beilmann and Dr. M. Wojtowycz contributed substantially to the preparation of the text. I would like to thank them and the staff of Springer-Verlag for their conscientious work in the interest of composition and publication quality.

The large number of patients suffering peripheral vascular and coronary arterial disease who could be helped objectively and subjectively by percutaneous transluminal angioplasty (PTA) underscores the special value of this mode of treatment. In addition, PTA also shows that close interdisciplinary communication and cooperation serves the best interests of the patient.

E. Zeitler

Contents

V. Primary Results: Leg Arteries

VI. Percutaneous Transluminal Angioplasty in Combination With Fibrinolysis

VII. Complications

VIII. Percutaneous Transluminal Angioplasty: Late Results in Leg Arteries

IX. Percutaneous Transluminal Angioplasty of Coronary Arteries

X. Percutaneous Transluminal Angioplasty for Supra-aortic Stenoses

XI. Percutaneous Transluminal Angioplasty of Renal Arteries

XII. Indications for Percutaneous Transluminal Angioplasty

XIII. Percutaneous Transluminal Angioplasty Today and in the Future

Appendix

List of Collaborators

J. E. ABELE	MEDI-TECH INC. 480 Pleasant St., P.O.B. 7407, Watertown, MA 02172 USA
K. AMPLATZ	Department of Radiology, University of Minnesota Hospitals, 420 Delaware Street S.E., Minneapolis, MN 55455 USA
K. BACHMANN	Medizinische Poliklinik, Universität Erlangen-Nürnberg, D-8520 Erlangen
C. F. BARKER	Department of Surgery, Hospital of the University of Pennsylvania, 4 Silverstein, Philadelphia, PA 19104 USA
H. BAUMRUCK	Physikalisch-technische Prüfanstalt für Radiologie und Elektromedizin. Allgemeines Krankenhaus, Alserstr. 4, A-1190 Wien
G. BERGER	Neurologisch-psychiatrische Klinik, Neurophysiologische Abteilung, Klinikum Nürnberg, Flurstr. 17, D-8500 Nürnberg
H. D. BERKOWITZ	Hospital of the University of Pennsylvania, 4th Floor Silverstein Pavilion, 3400 Spruce Street, Philadelphia. Pa. 19104 USA
W. BLÄTTLER	Praxis für Gefäßerkrankungen, Eisengasse 2, CH-8008 Zürich
GISELA BOLLE	Radiologisches Zentrum, Diagnostische Abteilung, Klinikum Nürnberg, Flurstr. 17, D-8500 Nürnberg 91
A. BOLLINGER	Department für Innere Medizin, Poliklinik, Angiologische Abteilung, Universitätsspital, Rämistr. 100, CH-8091 Zürich
U. BRUNNER	Abteilung für Periphere Vaskuläre Chirurgie, Chirurgie B, Universitätsspital, Rämistr. 100, CH-8091 Zürich
W.-D. BUSSMANN	Zentrum der Inneren Medizin, Abteilung für Kardiologie, Klinikum der J. W. Goethe-Universität, Theodor-Stern-Kai 7, D-6000 Frankfurt/M. 70
GABRIELE CAPPIUS	Aggertalklinik, D-5250 Engelskirchen
W. R. CASTANEDA-ZUNGIA	Department of Radiology, University of Minnesota Hospitals, 420 Delaware Street S.E., Minneapolis, MN 55455 USA
R. F. COLAPINTO	Toronto General Hospitals, 101 College Street, Toronto, Ont. M5G 1L7 Canada
CORNELIA DEMMER	Aggertalklinik, D-5250 Engelskirchen
H. DENCK	Krankenhaus der Stadt Wien-Lainz, I. Chirurgische Abteilung, Wolkersbergenstr. 1, A-1130 Wien
G. DILBAT	Radiologisches Zentrum, Diagnostische Abteilung, Klinikum Nürnberg, Flurstr. 17, D-8500 Nürnberg 91
C. T. DOTTER	University of Oregon, Health Sciences Center, Department of Diagnostic Radiology, Portland, Oregon 97201 USA

S. DOWINSKY — Zentrum der inneren Medizin, Abteilung für Kardiologie, Klinikum der J. W. Goethe-Universität, Theodor-Stern-Kai 7, D-6000 Frankfurt/M. 70

MARIANNE ERNSTING — Radiologisches Zentrum, Diagnostische Abteilung, Klinikum Nürnberg, Flurstr. 17, D-8500 Nürnberg 91

W. FASSBINDER — Zentrum der Inneren Medizin, Abteilung für Kardiologie, Klinikum der J. W. Goethe-Universität, Theodor-Stern-Kai 7, D-6000 Frankfurt/M. 70

K. FENDLER — Radiologische Klinik, H-7643 Pécs

B. J. O. FIEBACH — Zentrale Strahlendiagnostik und Neuroradiologie, Städtische Kliniken Duisburg, Zu den Rehwiesen 9, D-4100 Duisburg 1

E. FINGERHUT — Aggertalklinik, D-5250 Engelskirchen

N. FOULLON — Aggertalklinik für Gefäßkrankheiten, D-5250 Engelskirchen

D. B. FREIMANN — Department of Radiology, Presbyterian-University of Pennsylvania, Medical Center, 51 North 39th Street, Philadelphia, PA 19104 USA

H. GAILER — Radiologisches Zentrum, Abt. Diagnostik, Klinikum Nürnberg, Flurstr. 17, D-8500 Nürnberg

A. GALLINO — Medizinische Universitätsklinik, Inselspital, CH-3010 Bern

G. G. GEYSKES — Department of Nefrology, University Hospital, Catharijnesingel 101, NL-3500 CG Utrecht

R. GHISLA — Universitätskinderklinik, Inselspital, CH-3010 Bern

Z. GLÜCK — Medizinische Universitätsklinik, Inselspital, CH-3010 Bern

T. GODULA — Städtische Kliniken Duisburg, Geriatrische Klinik, Zu den Rehwiesen 9, D-4100 Duisburg 1

R. GROSSE-VORHOLT — Radiologisches Zentrum, Diagnostische Abteilung, Klinikum Nürnberg, Flurstr. 17, D-8500 Nürnberg 91

A. R. GRÜNTZIG — Emory University School of Medicine, Department of Medicine, 1364 Clifton Road, N.E., Atlanta, Georgia 30322 USA

P. GRÜTZMACHER — Zentrum der Inneren Medizin, Abteilung für Kardiologie, Klinikum der J. W. Goethe-Universität, Theodor-Stern-Kai 7, D-6000 Frankfurt/M. 70

M. HAERTEL — Institut für Radiologie, Kantonsspital, CH-9000 St. Gallen

H. HARTJES — Röntgendiagnostisches Zentralinstitut, Universitäts-Klinikum Essen, Hufelandstr. 55, D-4300 Essen 1

C. R. HATCHER — Emory University School of Medicine, Department of Medicine, 1364 Clifton Road, N.E., Atlanta, Georgia 30322 USA

H. HESS — Medizinische Poliklinik der Universität München, Pettenkoferstr. 8a, D-8000 München 2

R. HOPF — Zentrum der inneren Medizin, Abteilung für Kardiologie, Klinikum der J. W. Goethe-Universität, Theodor-Stern-Kai 7, D-6000 Frankfurt/M. 70

L. HORVÁTH — Radiologische Klinik, H-7643 Pécs

J. W. HURST — Emory University School of Medicine, Department of Medicine, 1364 Clifton Road, N.E., Atlanta, Georgia 30322 USA

I. ILLÉS — Radiologische Klinik, H-7643 Pécs

H. INGRISCH — Radiologische Klinik und Poliklinik der Universität München, Poliklinik, Pettenkoferstr. 8a, 8000 München 2

K. W. JOHNSTON	Department of Surgery, Toronto General Hospital, Toronto, Ont. M5G 1L7 Canada
M. KALTENBACH	Zentrum der Inneren Medizin, Abteilung für Kardiologie, Klinikum der J. W. Goethe-Universität, Theodor-Stern-Kai 7, D-6000 Frankfurt/M. 70
J. W. KEIFER	St. Anne's Hospital, 4950 W Thomas Street, Chicago, IL 60651, USA
G. KOBER	Zentrum der Inneren Medizin, Abteilung für Kardiologie, Klinikum der J. W. Goethe-Universität, Theodor-Stern-Kai 7, D-6000 Frankfurt/M. 70
M. KÖHLER	Aggertalklinik, D-5250 Engelskirchen
A. KRNETA	Chirurgische Abteilung, Tiefenauspital, CH-3004 Bern
E. KRÖNERT	Radiologisches Zentrum, Klinikum Nürnberg, Abteilung Nuklearmedizin, Flurstr. 17, D-8500 Nürnberg
G. KÜFFER	Radiologische Klinik und Poliklinik der Universität München, im Klinikum Großhadern, Marchioninistr. 15, 8000 München 70
U. KUHLMANN	Angiologische Abteilung des Departments für Innere Medizin, Poliklinik, Universitätsspital, Rämistr. 100, CH-8091 Zürich
H. J. LEU	Institut für Pathologie der Universität Zürich, Kantonsspital, Schmelzbergstr. 12, CH-8091 Zürich
E. LÖHR	Röntgendiagnostisches Zentralinstitut des Klinikums der Universität Essen, Hufelandstr. 55, D- 4300 Essen 1
E. LUX	4. Medizinische Klinik des Klinikums Nürnberg, Institut für Nephrologie an der Universität Erlangen-Nürnberg, Kontumazgarten 14–18, D-8500 Nürnberg
F. MAHLER	Medizinische Universitätsklinik, Inselspital Bern, CH-3010 Bern
W. P. T. MALI	Department of Röntgendiagnosis, University Hospital, Catharijnesingel 101, NL-3500 CG Utrecht
M. MARTIN	Städtische Kliniken Duisburg, Geriatrische Klinik, Zu den Rehwiesen 9, D-4100 Duisburg 1
G. MCLEAN	Department of Radiology, University of Pennsylvania Hospital, Philadelphia, Pennsylvania 19104, USA
A. MOTARJEME	St. Anne's Hospital, 4950 W. Thomas Street, Chicago, IL 60651 USA
N. MUZIKA	Röntgenstation der I. Chirurgischen Abteilung des Krankenhauses der Stadt Wien-Lainz, Wolkersbergenstr. 1, A-1130 Wien
P. NABAVI	St. Anne's Hospital, 4950 W. Thomas Street, Chicago, IL 60651 USA
B. NACHBUR	Klinik für Thorax-, Herz- und Gefäßchirurgie, Inselspital, CH-3010 Bern
M. NELL	Physikalisch-technische Prüfanstalt für Radiologie und Elektromedizin, Allgemeines Krankenhaus, Alserstr. 4, A-1090 Wien
O. OETLIKER	Universitäts-Kinderklinik, Inselspital, CH-3010 Bern
F. OLBERT	Krankenhaus der Stadt Wien-Lainz, Röntgenstation, Wolkersbergenstr. 1, A-1130 Wien
W. OSTHEIM-DZEROWYCZ	Röntgen-Abteilung Hochrheinklinik, Bergseestr. 57, D-7880 Bad Säckingen
T. PALDEN	Aggertalklinik, D-5250 Engelskirchen

G. Pouliadis	Röntgendiagnostisches Zentralinstitut, Universitätsspital, Rämistr. 100, CH-8091 Zürich
P. Probst	Radiologische Abteilung, Bürgerspital, CH-4500 Solothurn
C. B. A. J. Puijlaert	Department of Röntgendiagnosis, University Hospital, Catharijnesingel 101, NL-3500 CG Utrecht
G. Raab	Medizinische Poliklinik, Universität Erlangen-Nürnberg, 8520 Erlangen
Eva-Iris Richter	Radiologisches Zentrum, Klinikum Nürnberg, Flurstr. 17, 8500 Nürnberg
H. Rieger	Aggertalklinik, D-5250 Engelskirchen
E. Ring	Department of Radiology, University of California, San Francisco, California, USA
B. Roberts	Department of Surgery, Hospital of the University of Pennsylvania, 4 Silverstein, Philadelphia, PA 19104 USA
E. Rossi	Universitäts-Kinderklinik, Inselspital, CH-3010 Bern
F.-J. Roth	Aggertalklinik, D-5250 Engelskirchen
Enid J. Ruble	University of Oregon, Health Science Center, 3181 S.W. Sam Jackson Park Road, Portland, Oregon 97201 USA
J. H. J. Ruijs	Department of Röntgendiagnosis, University Hospital, Catharijnesingel 101, NL-3500 CG Utrecht
R. Ruminsky	Zentrum der Inneren Medizin, Abteilung für Kardiologie, Klinikum der J. W. Goethe-Universität, Theodor-Stern-Kai 7, D-6000 Frankfurt/M. 70
D. Rummel	Zentrum der Inneren Medizin, Abteilung für Kardiologie, Klinikum der J. W. Goethe-Universität, Theodor-Stern-Kai 7, D-6000 Frankfurt/M. 70
N. D. Scherer	Zentrum der inneren Medizin, Abteilung für Kardiologie, Klinikum der J. W. Goethe-Universität, Theodor-Stern-Kai 7, D-6000 Frankfurt/M. 70
M. Schlumpf	Angiologische Abteilung des Departments für Innere Medizin, Poliklinik, Universitätsspital, Rämistr. 100, CH-8091 Zürich
Ingeborg Schmidtke	Aggertalklinik, D-5250 Engelskirchen
R. Schmitt-Rüth	2. Med. Klinik, Klinikum Nürnberg, Flurstr. 17, D-8500 Nürnberg
E. Schneider	Department für Innere Medizin, Universitätsspital, Rämistr. 100, CH-8091 Zürich
W. Schoeppe	Zentrum der Inneren Medizin, Abt. für Kardiologie, Klinikum der J. W. Goethe-Universität, Theodor-Stern-Kai 7, D-6000 Frankfurt/M. 70
W. Schoop	Aggertalklinik, D-5250 Engelskirchen
A. Schrijvers	Röntgendiagnostisches Zentralinstitut, Universitätsklinikum Essen, Hufelandstr. 55, D-4300 Essen 1
F. Seuter	BAYER AG, Institut für Pharmakologie, Aprather Weg 18a, D-5600 Wuppertal 1
D. Seybold	4. Med. Klinik des Klinikums Nürnberg, Institut für Nephrologie an der Universität Erlangen-Nürnberg, Kontumazgarten 14–18, D- 8500 Nürnberg
W. Seyferth	Radiologisches Zentrum, Diagnostische Abteilung, Klinikum Nürnberg, Flurstr. 17, D-8500 Nürnberg 91

D. SINAPIUS	Pathologisches Institut der Universität Göttingen, Robert-Koch-Str. 40, D-3400 Göttingen
R. K. SPENCE	Department of Surgery, Cooper Medical Center, One Cooper Plaza, Camden, NJ 08103 USA
C. TORRES	Angiologische Abteilung des Departments für Innere Medizin, Universitätsspital, Poliklinik, Rämistr. 100, CH-8091 Zürich
M. WEGENER	Aggertalklinik, D-5250 Engelskirchen
C. WEICHERT	Rötgendiagnostisches Zentralinstitut, Universitäts-Klinikum Essen, Hufelandstr. 55, D-4300 Essen 1
P. WEIDMANN	Medizinische Universitätsklinik, Poliklinik, Inselspital, CH-3010 Bern
H. P. J. WÜSTEFELD	Department of Röntgendiagnosis, St. Franciscus Hospital, Boerhaavelaan 25, NL-4708 AE Roosendaal
E. ZEITLER	Radiologisches Zentrum, Klinikum Nürnberg, Flurstr. 17, D-8500 Nürnberg
C. L. ZOLLIKOFER	Röntgendiagnostisches Zentralinstitut der Universität Zürich, Rämistr. 100, CH-8091 Zürich
A. ZUSKA	St. Anne's Hospital, 4950 W. Thomas Street, Chicago, IL 60651 USA

1. Transluminal Angioplasty: Method, Indications, and Role in Therapy

C. T. Dotter

As physicians, we are all agreed upon the need to treat vascular obstructions in our patients, but we hold a variety of differing opinions as to how and by whom this is best done.

Transluminal angioplasty is indicated wherever it is anatomically feasible and clinically desirable. Mild claudication brings the patient to his doctor and it should be treated. Advanced gangrene, heart failure, diabetes, and prior myocardial infarction need not be considered contraindications to catheter therapy. If prevention is the best form of therapy, it seems reasonable to treat "silent" stenoses discovered during noninvasive or arteriographic appraisal. For the present, at least, most iliac and long femoropopliteal occlusions are best treated by appropriate bypass surgery. Though the success of angioplasty reflects the circumstances, in nearly all patients in whom amputation would otherwise be necessary, catheter salvage should be attempted, since at least one patient in ten will keep the leg and one in five will lose less of it. Lacking a remnant native arterial pathway of promise, patients with organized thrombosis of bypass grafts are not candidates for transluminal angioplasty. The reverse situation is somewhat happier, since the failure of angioplasty rarely compromises the outlook for surgical treatment. The worst outcome is usually failure of the procedure; death (0.15%) and complications requiring surgery (1.5%–3%) are rare with angioplasty as compared to vascular reconstruction, where published mortality figures for iliac bypass performed by skilled hands run between 3% and 5%. Amputation for atherosclerotic ischemia bears a mortality of 5%–20%. Following initially successful transluminal angioplasty, delayed recurrences (20% in the 1st year, rarely thereafter) promptly acted upon are readily and more permanently relieved by repeat angioplasty. Saphenous veins are not lost to limit further therapy in patients whose femoropopliteal, iliac, or renal artery stenoses are treated by transluminal angioplasty. We now have evidence that 5- and 10-year patency rates rival those obtained surgically. If angioplasty is done first and bypass becomes necessary at a later time, additive palliation can be achieved (not so if surgery is done first). Whatever the form of treatment, its outcome will reflect individual circumstances – anatomic, technical, and professional. The socioeconomic and psychological advantages of transluminal angioplasty are, after 15 years, at last receiving serious consideration from referring physicians, informed patients, and health care providers. Among its advantages is the ability of angioplasty to restore, rather than jeopardize, sexual potency in certain instances of aortoiliac disease.

Percutaneous Transluminal Angioplasty
(ed. by C. T. Dotter, A. Grüntzig, W. Schoop, E. Zeitler)

Techniques for percutaneous transluminal angioplasty vary considerably, as do those for invasive vascular reconstruction. Ideally, diagnostic arteriography and, if indicated, angioplasty are done as a single procedure and require only 1 or 2 days of hospitalization. While strategic approaches vary, retrograde femoroaortic catheterization and contrast visualization will disclose all treatable lesions and, in most cases, indicate the appropriate therapeutic strategy.

Iliac dilation can be carried out on the same and/or opposite side by replacing diagnostic with dilating catheter over a guide passed through an entry side stenosis or over the bifurcation and down through a contralateral lesion. While the latter is usually the best way to attack a contralateral common or deep femoral lesion and requires only the initial arterial puncture, for contralateral iliac stenoses it may not be the best way to go. These are probably better attacked by separate retrograde catheterization from below. Fluoroscopy during the hand injection of a few milliliters of dilute contrast agent through the already positioned diagnostic catheter in the aorta simplifies the second arterial puncture, and by visualizing the path facilitates swift, nontraumatic catheter placement through the stenosis. The added visibility of this approach virtually eliminates the traumatic subatheromatous catheter pathways usually responsible for immediate thrombosis or early restenosis. Subatheromatous dissection is doubly undesirable, since it is the sine qua non of iliac perforation – a complication I cannot recall causing in any of about 250 cases that I have treated.

Predilation pressure gradients, especially during reactive hyperemia, are nice to have, but not at the risk of failure due to the loss of a desirable transstenotic pathway. Once the arterial lesion to be dilated has been traversed – whether iliac, femoropopliteal, aortic, renal, splanchnic, coronary, or brachiocephalic, an anatomically appropriate dilating catheter is passed over the guide, the stenosis dilated, blood pressures checked to ensure that no significant residual gradient remains, a postangioplasty arteriogram made, and the catheter(s) removed.

Skillfully managed, a 95% iliac stenosis can usually be removed in much less time than it has taken to write and revise this brief account of how it is done. An adequate description of various tools, techniques, and strategies would run to many pages and, however carefully prepared, could never substitute for the direct observation and hard-won experience of arterial catheterization which are essential to any professionally responsible attempt at angioplasty.

Schwarten, who has done nearly 1,000 transluminal angioplasty procedures (including 200 renal) without a death, has said that a critical essential is the availability of a cooperative vascular surgeon to deal with possible serious complications. To quibble: however desirable the surgeon's cooperative attitude, it is his skilled services rather than his approval which must be available.

During the past 18 years, my experience has grown from nil to about 800 cases. Inevitably, especially at the beginning, there were complications and, though less frequently, there will be more. That thus far I have only encountered medical complications, not legal ones, I gladly credit to backup surgical support which, when needed, was given promptly and skillfully, if not always gracefully!

To look at the matter both ways: for today's vascular surgeon to recommend aortofemoral surgery for a local iliac narrowing which could be more safely, surely, and swiftly disposed of by catheter dilatation must reflect either a lack of knowledge or a lack of principles, at least in my opinion. For him to push surgery without informing his patient about available alternatives would be to invite a malpractice action.

I hope the foregoing will neither be counted offensive nor discounted as uninformed or unduly biased. As a radiologist, I hope transluminal angioplasty will remain a referral practice in the hands of skilled angiographers. For practical reasons evidenced by the many surgeons attending this symposium and the creative, participative interest of surgeons such as Fogarty, this may not turn out to be the case. In any event, if my fellow angiographers prove unwilling or unable to accept the clinical responsibilities attendant on transluminal angioplasty, they will become expensive plumbers facing forfeiture of territorial rights based solely on imaging equipment that others can obtain and skill that others can learn.

I. Diagnosis

2. Noninvasive Diagnosis and Natural Course of Arteriovascular Obstruction

W. Schoop

The following report cannot deal with the entire peripheral arterial system. I should like to attempt to give some indications and data on those obliterations of the arteries of the extremities that are of interest to us with regard to percutaneous transluminal angioplasty (PTA). Primarily, these are:

1. Stenoses in
   a) The large pelvic arteries.
   b) The femoropopliteal region.
   c) The deep femoral artery.
2. Occlusions in the femoropopliteal region.

Noninvasive Diagnosis

The presence of a hemodynamically significant obstruction in a large extremity artery can be objectively determined with a great degree of certainty by means of pulse-registering methods and comparative measurement of blood pressure (usually with the aid of the Doppler ultrasonic technique). The question as to whether the prerequisite conditions for a successful PTA probably exist can also frequently be answered without an angiogram [1, 2, 3].

Stenoses, as is well known, usually cause circulatory murmurs from the localization and character of which important information can be derived. Murmurs above the popliteal artery and the distal femoral artery especially are of great importance as signs of a clinically meaningful stenosis.

Substantial stenoses above the groin can best be objectified and judged by means of oscillography after exercise if they represent the only blockage in the vascular system of the leg. The question as to whether there is also an iliac stenosis present in patients with a femoral occlusion is usually more difficult to answer. The weakening of the groin pulse is sometimes not a significant finding, e.g., in cases of obesity or when the possibility of comparison is lacking (occlusion or stenosis on the other side). In these cases the measurements of the oscillogram on the proximal thigh and the Doppler sonographic groin flow curve are a help.

The probability of obliterations in the distal femoral artery and proximal popliteal artery region can be determined by means of clinical findings (one knee warmer, collateral pulses at the knee) and segmentally applied pulse-registering methods. In addition, in such cases the pulse of the femoral artery from the groin to the middle of the thigh can often be followed by hand; this is especially so in the case of slender patients. Occlusions of the middle and distal popliteal artery

Percutaneous Transluminal Angioplasty
(ed. by C. T. Dotter, A. Grüntzig, W. Schoop, E. Zeitler)

can be recognized through the combination of the palpable popliteal pulse with a strongly pathological lower leg oscillogram (at rest and after exercise).

Spontaneous Development

The decision whether to carry out a therapeutic procedure expected to bring a more lasting improvement is facilitated by a knowledge of the spontaneous development and natural course of vascular occlusive lesions. Interesting from a prognostic point of view are the life expectancy, which is generally not altered by PTA, and the assumed spontaneous development of the obliteration, which is changed by PTA.

Life expectancy is reduced in persons with peripheral occlusive vascular disease – for younger patients, especially those under 50 years of age relatively more than for older patients. Factors having an unfavorable effect are: previously present symptoms of a coronary sclerosis; high blood pressure; and, in smokers, failure to give up cigarettes. Moreover, a 10-year study of our own on more than 600 patients with occlusive vascular disease has shown the great prognostic importance of the localization of the occlusion [4]. The death rate is highest among patients with the so-called pelvic type; among those with the thigh type it is not quite so high, but still clearly above average; in cases where the occlusions are limited to the lower leg arteries, the death rate is hardly higher than the average for the same age group. The spontaneous development of the stenoses and occlusions which are often treated by PTA is interesting. Our own systematic observations of the development of stenoses in the femoropopliteal region have indicated a relatively strong tendency toward occlusion for hemodynamically effective femoral stenosis. Without prophylactic measures an occlusion rate of about 80% within 4–5 years must be expected. With consistent prophylactic treatment with acetylsalicylic acid, however, these values are significantly lower. The tendency toward complete occlusion in the large pelvic arteries is apparently less than in the femoropopliteal region. In our own examinations of patients with femoral occlusions plus iliac stenosis the occlusion rate was 7%–8% per year.

Occlusions in the femoropopliteal region have a good prognosis with regard to amputation; such an operation threatens to be necessary within 10 years in about 10% of cases. The frequency of progression toward the proximal in the sense of an iliac occlusion within 4–5 years is as follows, depending upon the clinical and angiological finding: in cases of clinically free pelvic blood flow, 5%; with the presence of circulatory murmurs in the groin and/or proximal to it, 10%; with a proven hemodynamically meaningful iliac stenosis, 30%.

References

1. Bollinger A (1980) Ultraschall-Doppler-Diagnostik bei peripheren arteriellen Durchblutungsstörungen. Ultraschall in der Medizin. Band 1, Heft 3, 1980, p 208–216
2. Heberer G, Rau G, Schoop W (1974) Angiologie. Thieme, Stuttgart
3. Kappert A (1976) Lehrbuch und Atlas der Angiologie, 8. Aufl. H. Huber, Bern
4. Schoop W, Indikationen und Langzeitergebnisse der konservativen Behandlung peripherer arterieller Durchblutungsstörungen. Hämostaseologie. Heft 3, Juni 1981, 1. Jahrg., F. K. Schattauer, Stuttgart-New York

3. Ultrasound Techniques for Follow-up of Hemodynamic Changes After Peripheral Transluminal Angioplasty

A. Bollinger

In recent years, the success of methods aiming at the reopening of stenosed or occluded vascular segments has been routinely estimated by measurements of distal blood pressure. The difference between systolic arm and ankle blood pressure (Δp) approximates to the systolic pressure gradient from aorta to ankle. Even more sensitive than measurements at rest are determinations after exercise. The work load may be standardized by means of foot or treadmill ergometers.

The standard technique for assessing limb blood flow in the vascular laboratory is venous occlusion plethysmography. Easier to perform are flow velocity tracings using Doppler ultrasound [10, 11, 21]. In addition, with pulsed techniques the flow profiles can be defined in larger vessels [5] and the pulsatile flow computed [8, 9], which indicates impaired vascular dynamics earlier than does mean blood flow. Reactive hyperemia after arterial occlusion or after exercise gives additional information on the degree of ischemia [9].

Distal Blood Pressure

Different methods are currently available for measuring distal blood pressure – mercury strain gauges [14], Doppler ultrasound [1, 2, 4, 6, 7, 11, 17, 19–23], photoelectric devices [15], and clearance techniques [18]. All these techniques are indirect, since they require the inflation of blood pressure cuffs. Direct micromanometry [3] has not yet been applied to routine measurements, but it is a promising tool which permits evaluation of indirect procedures. The correlation between directly and indirectly measured blood pressure in the dorsal artery of the foot and the posterior tibial artery shows good general agreement, with the exception of cases with marked edema and Mönckeberg's mediasclerosis [3], both of which exclude accurate measurements by indirect methods.

In our laboratory Doppler ultrasound is preferred for measurements of systolic blood pressure at the ankle and the strain gauge technique for determining pressure at the fingers. Systolic blood pressure at rest (p) and the systolic pressure gradient between arm and ankle (Δp) are ideal tools for evaluation of long-term results, since they require a minimum of time. An increase in absolute pressure or in the arm to ankle pressure ratio and a decrease in Δp means improvement in the hemodynamic situation. Normally the systolic

Percutaneous Transluminal Angioplasty
(ed. by C. T. Dotter, A. Grüntzig, W. Schoop, E. Zeitler)

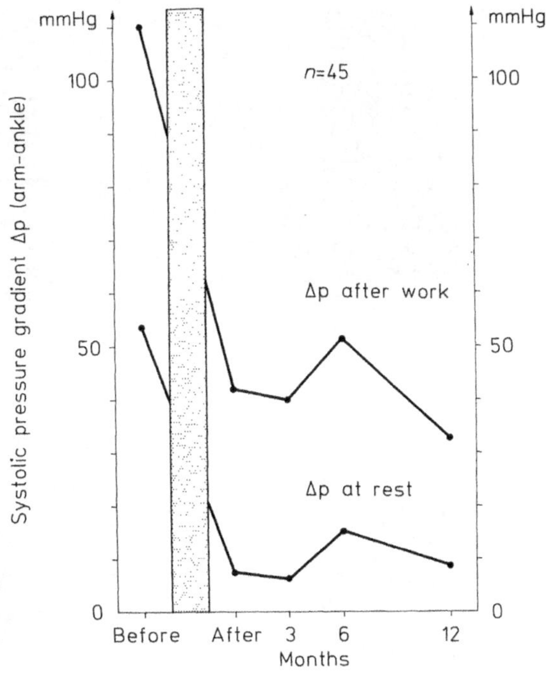

Fig. 1. Mean systolic pressure difference between arm and ankle arteries before and after PTA in 45 consecutive patients. The differences are given at rest and 1 min after treadmill exercise (100 m with a speed of 3.2 km/h and an inclination of 12.5°)

pressure at the ankle is at least as high as the systolic arm pressure. In healthy volunteers the mean values for Δp are in the negative range (−23.7 mm Hg [6], −15.5 mm Hg [1]). The normal values at rest vary between +5 and −30 mm Hg.

Successful percutaneous transluminal angioplasty (PTA) induces significant improvement in Δp or of the arm to ankle pressure ratio. In 45 consecutive patients treated in the femoropopliteal segment, mean Δp dropped from 53.8 mm Hg to 7.4 mm Hg (Fig. 1). As a rule it may be stated that improvement in Δp by 20 mm Hg or more indicates successful PTA. This may not be true for cases with distal occlusions remaining in situ. A typical example is the dilatation of an iliac artery stenosis in the presence of an additional femoral artery occlusion not suited for PTA. In this situation the early improvement in Δp may be by less than 20 mm Hg. The flow velocity tracings of the femoral artery in the groin then reflect the hemodynamic improvement better. An alternative method is multilevel systolic pressure measurement with application of a tourniquet at the thigh [11, 17].

As mentioned, measurements of poststenotic systolic pressures after exercise are more sensitive than determinations at rest [2, 6, 17, 19, 21]. Normally, 1 min after exercise (100 m on a treadmill with a speed of 3.2 km/h and an inclination of 12.5° or 30 toe-tippings) the ankle pressure reaches at least 90% of the resting values [19]. Lower values document significant stenoses. In the group of patients included in Fig. 1, mean Δp before PTA was 110.1 mm Hg, after PTA 42.0 mm Hg. An example for ankle pressure measurements at rest and after treadmill

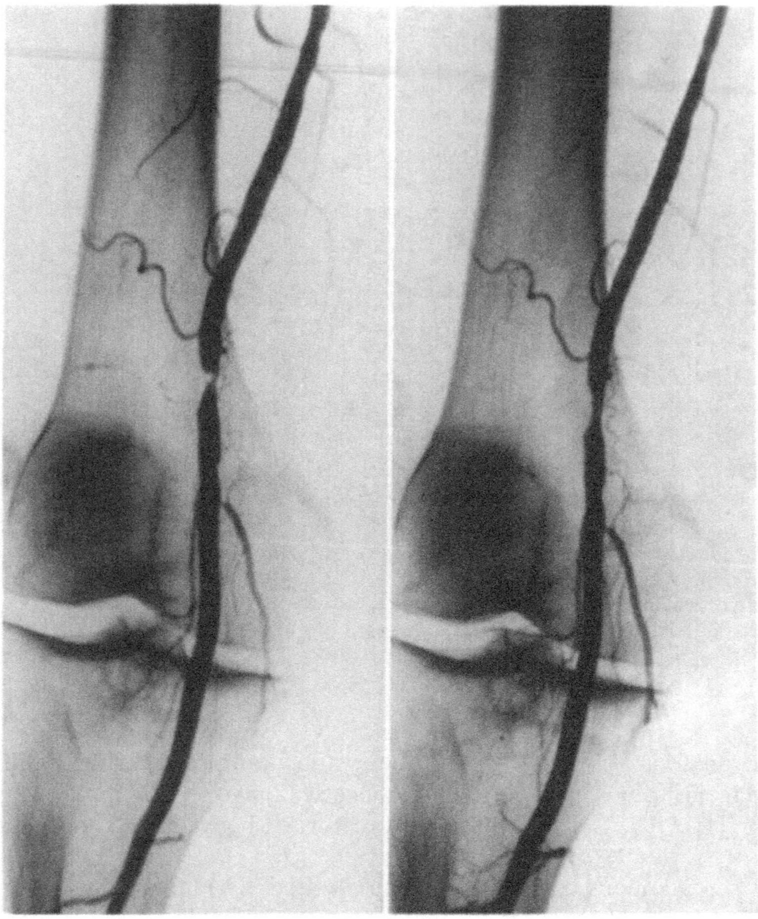

a b

Fig. 2. a Arteriography before PTA by means of the original Dotter method, showing subtotal stenosis of the superficial femoral artery. **b** After PTA: remaining stenosis to about 50% of the original diameter of the vessel. **c** Systolic ankle pressure response to treadmill exercise before and after PTA in the same patient. **d** Systolic pressure difference after treadmill exercise before and after PTA

exercise in a single case is given in Fig. 2. The pathological hemodynamic response before treatment was normalized after PTA. Despite a remaining lesion stenosing the superficial femoral artery to about 50% of its normal diameter, Δp 1 min after the end of exercise was in the negative range. During the first months after PTA a tendency to a further improvement is noted, especially in cases with favorable long-term results. This tendency is reflected by the mean values given in Fig. 1. Between the 3rd and the 6th months a deterioration was observed in this group, indicating reocclusion in some of these patients. The values at 12 months are again better because the patients with relapses have been excluded at this later time (second PTA, operation).

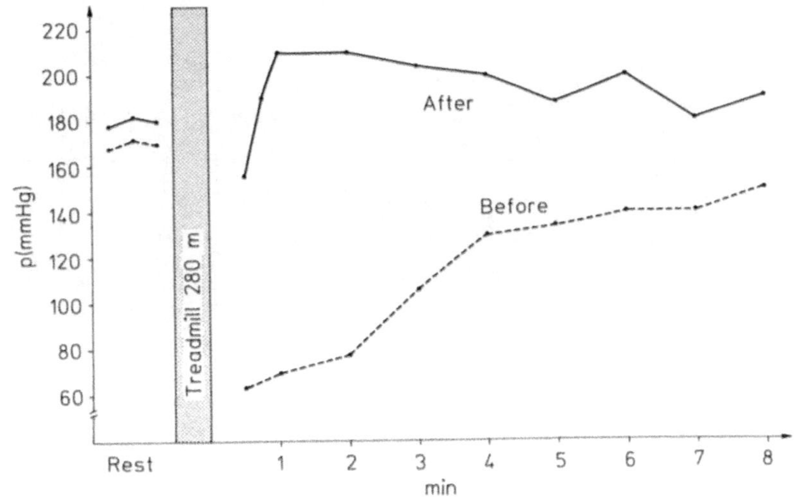

Fig. 2c

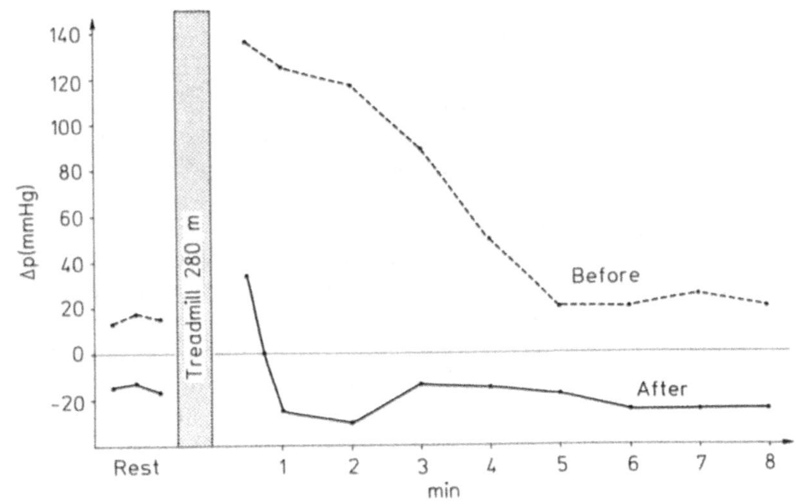

Fig. 2d

Pulsatile Flow or Flow Velocity

Velocity [10, 11] or flow [8, 9] tracings obtained percutaneously by Doppler ultrasound are sensitive enough to detect the hemodynamic changes induced by transluminal recanalization. In the femoral, popliteal, and posterior tibial arteries the flow curves at rest are characterized by a reflux in early diastole. This type of tracing contrasts with pulsatile flow found in the carotid artery, which normally exhibits forward flow during the whole systole and diastole [8].

The negative backflow wave is abolished distal to stenoses in the aortoiliac segment (Fig. 3a) [4, 5, 10, 21]. As in the normal carotid artery, positive flow is

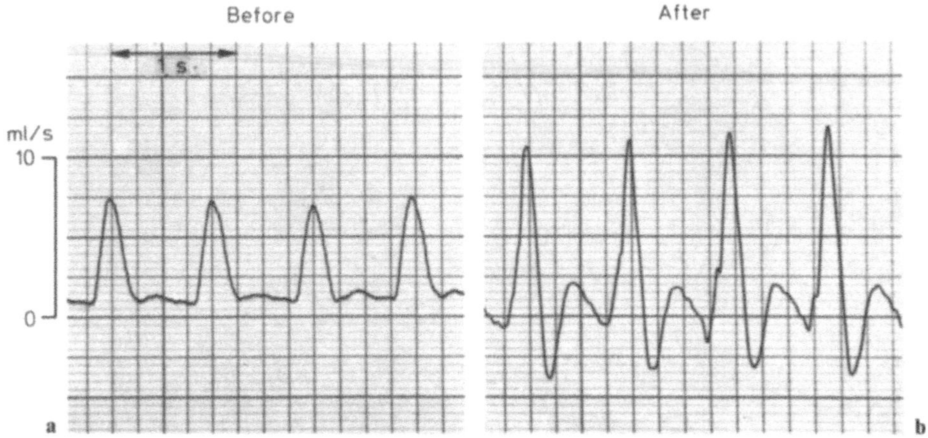

Fig. 3. a Before PTA in a case of subtotal stenosis of the common iliac artery: the flow curves of the femoral artery, obtained by a pulsed Doppler device, show reduced amplitudes and continuous positive diastolic flow. **b** After PTA the characteristic backflow in early diastole has reappeared

present during the whole diastolic period; the pulsation of flow is decreased. Reduced peak systolic flow is compensated for, at least in part, by increased diastolic flow. This explains why pulsatile flow measurements are more sensitive for evaluating stenosing lesions than determinations of mean flow. Mean volume flow evaluated by clearance technique or venous occlusion plethysmography is maintained until severe ischemia develops. Pulsatile velocity or flow measurements in single vessels are of special interest when multilevel disease is present. The comparison of values in the femoral and popliteal arteries may assess the effect of an iliac dilating procedure in the presence of additional lesions in the superficial femoral artery.

After successful transluminal dilatation, normal pulsatile flow is restored (Fig. 3b), although some compressed thrombotic material is still seen in the follow-up aortography. In the femoral artery the following normal values were obtained for the various parameters describing pulsatile flow tracings: maximal systolic flow (n = 12) 23.1 ± 10.3 ml/s, minimal diastolic flow (backflow wave) −6.9 ± 4.1 ml/s, and mean flow 3.7 ± 1.5 ml/s [8]. In the example of Fig. 3, clearly decreased values were measured before the procedure. After dilatation the values lay at the lower limit of the normal range.

A period of arterial occlusion lasting 3–5 min induces reactive hyperemia, which is often used to quantify ischemic disease [1, 5, 10]. In normals, the backflow wave typical for the femoral artery disappears during reactive hyperemia. The minimal diastolic flow increases after 3 min circulatory arrest to +6.2 ± 3.8 ml/s, the maximal systolic flow to 32.2 ± 9.0 ml/s (n = 10 [8]). Mean reactive hyperemia flow averages 17.0 ± 6.6 ml/s [8]. Figure 4 illustrates the course of reactive hyperemia in the patient of Fig. 3. The delayed and decreased reaction to arterial occlusion typical for iliac stenosis contrasts with the finding after dilatation. Again the posttreatment values are in the lower range of the normal values.

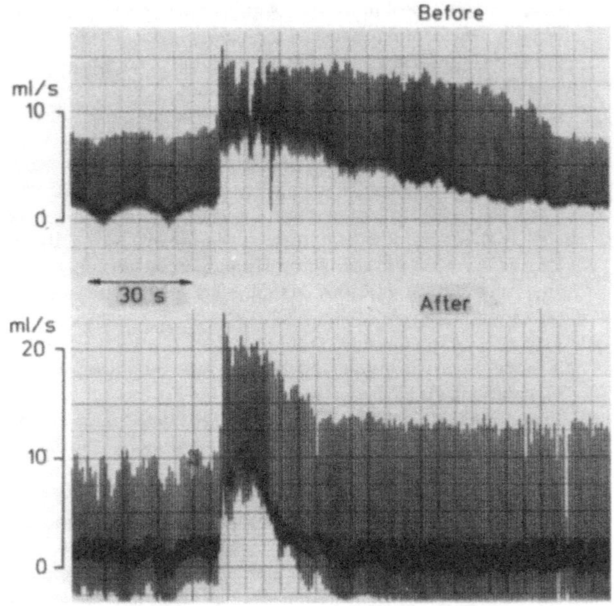

Fig. 4. Reactive hyperemia after 3 min of circulatory arrest before and after PTA of the common iliac artery (same patient as Fig. 3)

Conclusions

Doppler ultrasound is suitable for checking the hemodynamic changes induced by transluminal recanalization. The ankle blood pressure data at rest (p and Δp), which are easy to obtain, are of prognostic significance during the long-term follow-up and permit differentiation of the hemodynamic results in the iliac and in the femoral region. Borderline stenoses require exercise tests sensitive enough to detect stenoses limiting the inner vessel diameter to less than 75%. Additional information is given by the registration of pulsatile flow velocity or volume flow measurements using continuous wave or pulsed Doppler ultrasound.

References

1. Bollinger A, Mahler F, Grüntzig A (1971) Peripheral hemodynamics in patients with coarctation, normotensive and hypertensive arteriosclerosis obliterans of the lower limbs. Angiology 22: 354
2. Bollinger A, Schlumpf M, Butti P, Grüntzig A (1973) Measurement of systolic ankle blood pressure with Doppler ultrasound at rest and after exercise in patients with leg artery occlusion. Scand J Clin Lab Invest [Suppl 128] 31: 123
3. Bollinger A, Barras JP, Mahler F (1976) Measurement of foot artery blood pressure by micromanometry in normal subjects and in patients with arterial occlusive disease. Circulation 53: 506
4. Bollinger A (1979) Funktionelle Angiologie. Thieme, Stuttgart

5. Brunner HH, Bollinger A, Anliker M, Zweifel HJ, Rutishauser W (1974) Bestimmung instantaner Strömungsgeschwindigkeitsprofile in der A. femoralis communis mit gepulstem Doppler-Ultraschall bei Stenosen und Verschlüssen der Beckenarterien. Dtsch Med Wochenschr 99: 3
6. Carter SA (1972) Response of ankle systolic pressure to leg exercise in mild or questionable arterial disease. N Engl J Med 287: 578
7. Carter SA (1978) Role of pressure measurements in vascular disease. In: Bernstein EF (ed) Noninvasive diagnostic techniques in vascular disease. Mosby, St. Louis, p 261
8. Casty M (1976) Perkutane atraumatische Flußmessung in großen hautnahen Gefäßen mit einem vielkanaligen gepulsten Ultraschall-Doppler-Gerät. Dissertation, Zürich
9. Doriot PA, Casty M, Milakara B, Anliker M, Bollinger A, Siegenthaler W (1975) Quantitative analysis of flow conditions in simulated vessels and large human arteries and veins by means of ultrasound. Excerpta Med 363: 160
10. Fronek A, Johansen K, Dilley RB, Bernstein EF (1973) Ultrasonographically monitored postocclusive reactive hyperemia in the diagnosis of peripheral arterial occlusive disease. Circulation 48: 149
11. Fronek AM, Coel EF, Bernstein EF (1978) The importance of combined multisegmental pressure and Doppler flow velocity studies in the diagnosis of peripheral arterial occlusive disease. Surgery 84: 840
12. Grüntzig A, Brunner U, Meier W, Bollinger A (1971) Die Veränderungen der systolischen Knöchelarteriendrucke nach Gefäßoperationen, gemessen mit Doppler-Ultraschall. Schweiz Med Wochenschr 101: 905
13. Grüntzig A (1976) Die perkutane Rekanalisation chronischer arterieller Verschlüsse (Dotter-Prinzip) mit einem neuen doppellumigen Dilatationskatheter. ROEFO 124: 80
14. Gundersen J (1972) Segmental measurements of systolic blood pressure in the extremities including the thumb and the great toe. Acta Chir Scand [Suppl] 426
15. Gyntelberg F, Nielsen PE, Lönsmann-Poulsen H (1974) Skin blood pressure in hypertensive subjects measured by photoelectric technique. Scand J Clin Lab Invest 33: 45
16. Köhler M, Hinger HU, Schoop W (1970) Vergleichende Messungen der Durchblutung (Venenverschlußplethysmographie) und des Blutdruckes (Ultraschall-Dopplermethode) an durchblutungsgestörten Extremitäten. Verh Dtsch Ges Inn Med 76: 200
17. Kriessmann A, Bollinger A, Keller H (ed) (1982) Praxis der Doppler-Sonographie. Thieme, Stuttgart
18. Lassen NA, Holstein P (1974) Use of radioisotopes in assessment of distal blood flow and distal blood pressure in arterial insufficiency. Surg Clin North Am 54: 39
19. Lomazzi F, Mahler F (1980) Wirkung verschiedener Belastungsarten auf den Knöchelarteriendruck bei Patienten mit arteriellen Durchblutungsstörungen. Schweiz Med Wochenschr 110: 1925
20. Raines JK, Darling RC, Buth J, Brewster DC, Austen WG (1976) Vascular laboratory criteria for the management of peripheral vascular disease of the lower extremities. Surgery 79: 21
21. Strandness DE, Sumner DS (1975) Ultrasonic techniques in angiology. Huber, Bern
22. Thulesius O, Gjöres JE (1971) Use of Doppler shift detection for determining peripheral arterial blood pressure. Angiology 22: 594
23. Yao ST, Needham TN, Gourmoos C, Irvine WT (1972) A comparative study of strain-gauge plethysmography and Doppler ultrasound in the assessment of occlusive arterial disease of the lower extremities. Surgery 71: 4

4. Digital Subtraction Angiography – A Method of Following Percutaneous Transluminal Angioplasty

W. Seyferth, G. Dilbat, E. Zeitler, and G. Bolle

Introduction

Follow-up after percutaneous angioplasty has, up to now, generally consisted of assessment of the clinical course and measurement of physical parameters related to the vascular system, such as pulse status, vascular auscultation, and rest and stress oscillogram [2, 4]. In the past few years objective determinations of ankle arterial blood pressure have been made possible by Doppler ultrasound. However, in cases of deterioration of the clinical condition or physical findings, renewed arterial angiography has stood alone as a procedure for morphological evaluation.

Following the introduction of intravenous digital subtraction angiography (DSA), one can now for the first time evaluate the morphological substrate without potential damage to the arterial system.

We have so far investigated more than 160 patients after percutaneous transluminal angioplasty (PTA). Analysis of the results underscores the value of DSA in the follow-up care of patients after therapeutic vascular procedures.

Method

The examinations were performed with the Angiotron, the DSA unit manufactured by Siemens. Technical specifications and performance are described elsewhere [5, 6]. The largest image intensifier field, 25 cm in diameter, was used for subtraction fluoroscopy of the peripheral vascular system. In cases of suspected renal artery stenosis a field of 17 cm diameter, with its additional magnification, proved advantageous.

In order to compensate for density differences in the region of the abdomen and pelvis, as well as in examinations of the peripheral vessels of the arms and legs, a special motorized filter could be brought into position, providing a considerable improvement in the image [7]. In the abdomen contrast was improved by reducing the body diameter using balloon compression. This may to some extent also help to reduce artifacts caused by displacement of bowel gas. In any case, the medication Buscopan® is employed in the examination of abdominal vessels, in order to counter intestinal movement. The site of contrast medium application is adjusted to the particular situation of patients treated with

Percutaneous Transluminal Angioplasty
(ed. by C. T. Dotter, A. Grüntzig, W. Schoop, E. Zeitler)

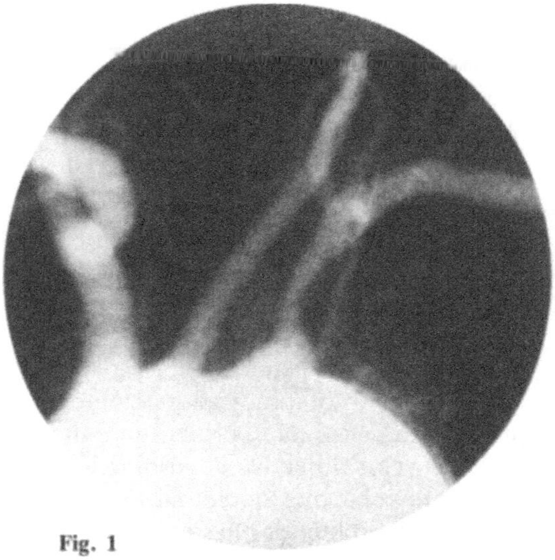

Fig. 1

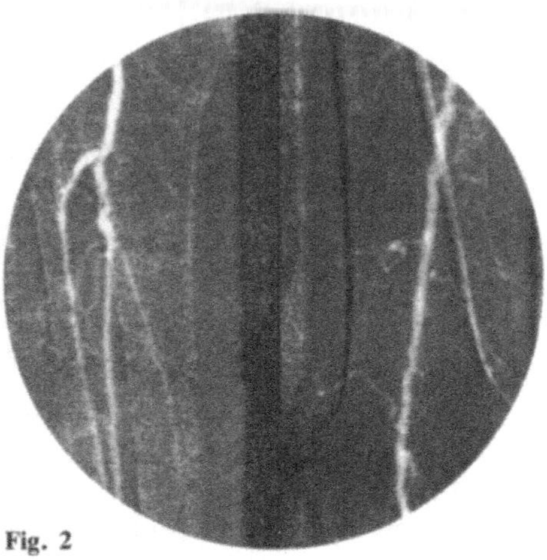

Fig. 2

Fig. 1. Arterial control angiogram (30 ml, flow rate 12 ml/s) after percutaneous transluminal dilatation of a left subclavian stenosis with the Grüntzig balloon catheter

Fig. 2. Control angiogram 6 months after percutaneous transluminal recanalization of a distal occlusion in the superficial femoral artery (*right*). Recognizable stenosis at the trifurcation of the tibiofibular trunk (*left*)

angioplasty. In order to spare the region of the groin for a possible second interventional procedure, the antecubital approach for catheter introduction into the superior vena cava (pigtail F-7) was preferred. It is possible to inject contrast medium through a short cannula (1.4-mm diameter, 17-gauge lying in an antecubital vein, provided that the patient has good cardiac output and is of normal weight, and that the vascular area in question is in the trunk.

In every case 40 ml contrast agent (300–370 mg iodine per milliliter) was injected at a rate of 17 ml/s for central venous catheters and 12–15 ml/s for peripherally lying cannulas. In cases where the latter mode was employed, an additional 20 ml 0.9% saline was injected immediately afterward to flush the bolus. The risks involved in the use of the contrast medium correspond to those attending intravenous urography.

A special advantage presented by DSA is that control angiography can be performed directly through the balloon dilatation catheter after dilatation of renal artery stenoses or subclavian stenoses (Fig. 1). With a reduction of the flow rate and of the amount of contrast agent needed to only 30% of that used in conventional arterial studies, arteriography can be performed safely even through the relatively stiff Grüntzig balloon catheter, which has only an end hole.

The continuous mode represents a real time procedure, and one can decide immediately afterward whether additional projections are necessary. In "postprocessing," two different areas can be examined after a single injection when a step-motion table is employed [7].

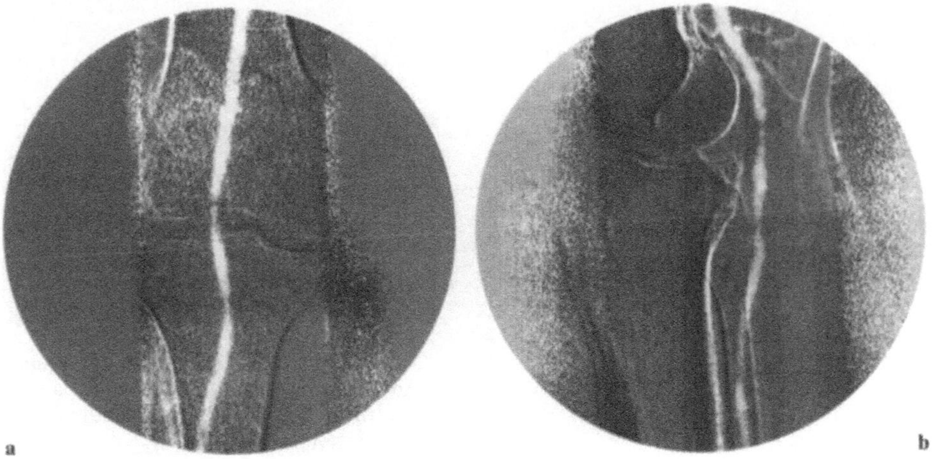

a b

Fig. 3. a Control angiogram after percutaneous transluminal recanalization of an occlusion in the right popliteal artery with two residual stenoses. **b** Residual stenoses can better be evaluated in lateral projection, since bone masking does then not interfere

Results

Digital subtraction angiography qualifies as a reliable method of following PTA in areas of special interest, such as the kidneys and pelvis. Unequivocal diagnostic information about the vessel in question can be obtained in 90%–95% of studies.

In the lower extremities, equally good results can be obtained down to the level of the trifurcation (Fig. 2).

One source of possible error exists in areas where a vessel crosses the margin of a bone. Vascular stenoses at such points can be hidden by slight movement artifacts. Such errors can be avoided by correcting for movement by "remasking" or by reexamining the same level with a second injection and a different projection (Fig. 3a, b). Obviously, just as in conventional angiography, small mural lesions can be missed if they are not precisely tangential to the axial beam.

Renal Arteries

Digital subtraction angiography is the procedure of choice for the initial evaluation of suspected renal artery stenoses (Fig. 4). It should also be used following percutaneous dilatations of renal artery stenoses when blood pressure fails to normalize or rises after a normotensive interval (Fig. 5a, b).

Among 27 patients followed up, we found 14 angiographically normal renal arteries. In the remaining 13, mural changes were seen in the renal arteries. The question whether these changes required retreatment has up to now been decided only after direct arterial pre- and poststenotic blood pressure measurements.

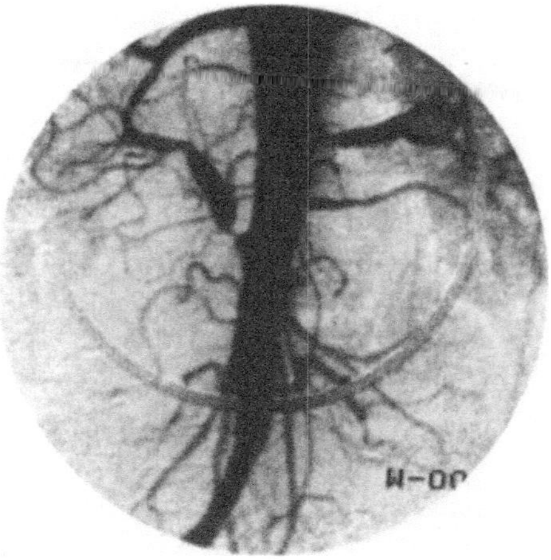

Fig. 4. Intravenous DSA of the abdominal aorta. Stenosis in an aortorenal bypass on the *right*. Left renal artery stenosis. Pelvic artery occlusion on the *left*

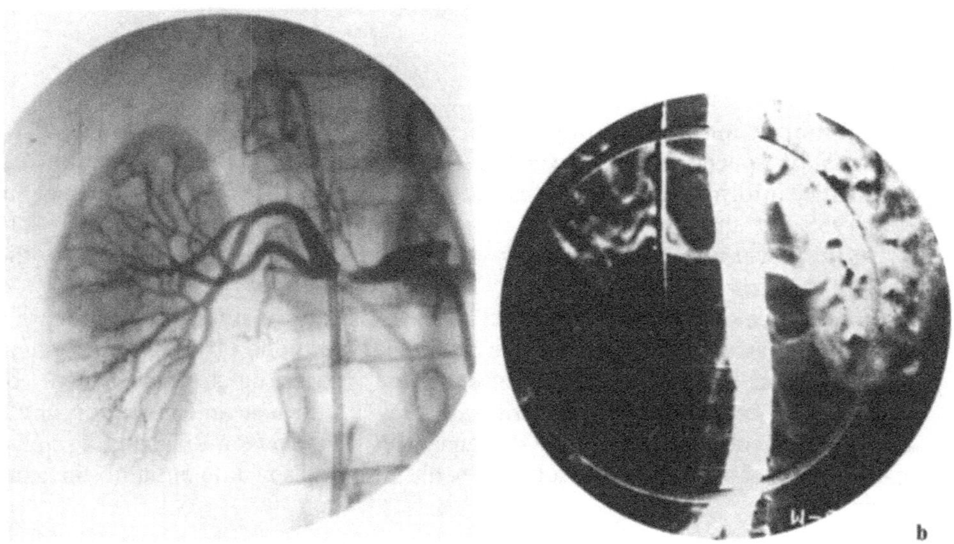

a b

Fig. 5. a Conventional renovasogram of a right renal artery stenosis immediately before percutaneous transluminal dilatation. **b** Control angiogram taken by intravenous DSA 4 months after dilatation

Pelvic Arteries

Intravenous substraction angiography is employed as the preliminary radiographic investigation in those patients where the clinical findings (groin pulse, arterial auscultation, and Doppler ultrasound) lead one to presume unilateral or bilateral pathological vascular changes in the pelvic arteries. After successful

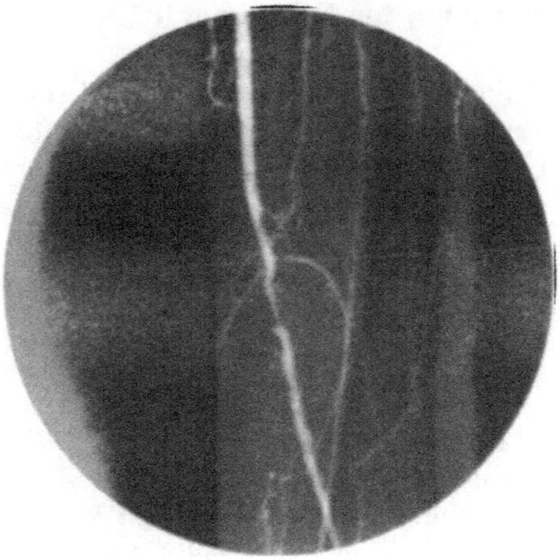

Fig. 6. Restenosis 5 months after percutaneous transluminal dilatation of a stenosis in the left superficial femoral artery in the mid-adductor canal

localization of pelvic arterial stenoses, vascular therapeutic measures can be planned with the least vascular trauma possible. Of 25 patients investigated after angioplasty we had 10 with normal findings, 13 with a stenosis, and 2 demonstrating wall dissection.

Arteries of the Lower Extremities

The use of DSA as a primary investigative procedure is limited by the number of injections necessary to evaluate the vessels of the lower extremity completely. However, direct investigations of areas in question can be performed simply. Therapy can then be planned using the results of DSA. In 57 patients examined after PTA, we have so far found 18 cases with stenotic irregularities, 13 cases with vascular occlusion both at the site of the obliteration and at other sites, and one case of aneurysm formation at the puncture site (Fig. 6).

Carotid and Vertebral Arteries

Digital subtraction angiography is employed as a primary means of investigation of the arteries of the neck. In accordance with the literature [3, 4, 9], we experienced a very low complication rate. With the exception of a patient suffering an allergic contrast medium reaction with pulmonary edema and cerebral hypoxia, we have observed no cases of stroke in over 1,000 patients examined [1]. After dilatation of a subclavian stenosis, DSA can serve as a postprocedural control or can be used to evaluate recurrent blood pressure differential or arterial bruit.

Indication for DSA after PTA

After percutaneous transluminal dilatation, the following are typical applications arranged in order of time interval after PTA:

1. In the immediate post-PTA phase DSA can serve to elucidate the course of an acute deterioration in clinical status. DSA can detect thromboembolic material in such cases, while the area of recanalization remains freely patent. Thus indications for local or generalized streptokinase therapy can be confirmed.
2. The success or failure of thrombolytic therapy can be checked by means of repeated DSA.
3. Immediate treatment complications, such as vascular perforation with possible proximally extending vascular thrombosis, can be definitively diagnosed. False aneurysm formation at the site of puncture and catheter introduction or vascular perforation elsewhere resulting from catheter or guide wire can also be diagnosed.
4. Early DSA after PTA helps in deciding on further therapy in cases with questionable primary results. When it concerns a decision about possible bypass (femoro-crural bypass), the runoff can be best demonstrated by use of the third memory, a special feature of the equipment used.
5. Follow-up investigations of the treated vessel are still possible in the absence of clinical deterioration if the patient returns to the study with another problem. For example, the peripheral vessel can be reinvestigated in a patient who has returned for confirmation of a suspected carotid stenosis.

However, the patient most often returns because of renewed clinical deterioration and further therapy must be planned. This underscores the negative selection of the collective studied by us to date. Having determined the morphological-pathological substrate one can decide among the various options: repeated PTA, an operative procedure, or conservative therapy in those with general worsening of the underlying disease.

Summary

With adequate indications, the minimal risks of intravenous digital video subtraction angiography (DSA) allow broad indications to be drawn for the follow-up study of PTA patients. The morphological control studies made possible by DSA do not, as a rule, endanger the pathologically affected arterial vessel. The method helps in the planning of further directed therapy. The increased use of DSA in the early phases after PTA may contribute to the knowledge of the mechanism of the procedure and the patient's prognosis. In cases of clinical deterioration DSA can elucidate whether the patient's symptoms are due to recurrence at the treated site or to a new obstructive lesion in another area of the same vessel.

References

1. Berger C, Sprügel W, Seyferth W (1983) Diagnostik extrakranieller Carotiserkrankungen. Dtsch Med Wochenschr 108: 86–93
2. Bollinger A (1979) Funktionelle Angiologie. Lehrbuch und Atlas. Thieme, Stuttgart
3. Buonocore E, Meaney TF, Borkowski GP et al. (1981) Digital subtraction angiography of the abdominal aorta and renal arteries. Radiology 139: 281
4. Chilcote WA, Modic MT, Pavlicek W et al. (1981) Digital subtraction angiography of the carotid arteries: a comparative study in 100 patients. Radiology 139: 287
5. Seyferth W, Marhoff P, Zeitler E (1982) Transvenöse und arterielle digitale Videosubtraktionsangiographie (DVSA). ROEFO 136: 301–309
6. Seyferth W, Marhoff P, Zeitler E (1982) Digital subtraction angiography (DSA): diagnostic importance and risk. Electromedica 2/82: 60–68
7. Seyferth W, Dilbat G, Herde R et al. (1982) Digitale Subtraktionsangiographie (DSA) an einem konventionellen Röntgen-Durchleuchtungsgerät. Electromedica 4: 120
8. Schoop W (1967) Angiologie-Fibel. Thieme, Stuttgart
9. Stieghorst MF, Strother C, Mistretta CA, Crummy AB et al. (1981) Digital subtraction angiography – a clinical overview. Appl Radiol p. 43

5. Evaluation of Peripheral Transluminal Angioplasty by a Score System Applied to Routine Arteriographic Images

A. Bollinger, E. Schneider, G. Pouliadis, C. Torres, and M. Schlumpf

The success of therapy in reopening occluded artery segments may be objectively assessed by hemodynamic measurements or by arteriography. Recently, a score system has been developed for evaluation of routine angiographic images [1]. The system consists of a vectorial score coding the pattern of occlusions, stenoses, and plaques, and of an additive score describing the severity of the lesions visualized. The technique is suitable for computerized data analysis. In the present study 40 consecutive patients were examined before and after percutaneous transluminal angioplasty (PTA) of the superficial femoral or popliteal artery. The additive scores obtained were compared to those in a group of patients subjected to surgical endarterectomy [4].

Patients and Methods

Successful PTA was performed in 40 consecutive patients (43 legs) with femoropopliteal artery stenoses or short occlusions (less than 10 cm in length). The mean age of the patients was 62.8 years. In 37 the indication for PTA was limiting intermittent claudication, in 3 rest pain or incipient gangrene. In all cases the dilatation catheter described by Grüntzig [2] was used with local anesthesia. The number of treated segments was 47. The superficial femoral artery was reopened 39 times, the popliteal artery 6 times, and the initial segments of the calf arteries twice. All the patients were taking part in a prospective study which was designed to investigate a possible reduction in the rate of reocclusions by antiplatelet drugs.

In every patient arteriographies before and immediately after successful PTA were performed and evaluated by the score system described previously [1]. The following arterial segments were coded: the deep femoral artery, the popliteal artery including the tibiofibular trunk, and the proximal parts of the anterior tibial, posterior tibial, and fibular arteries.

The additive score [1] was used to describe and quantify the morphological changes induced by PTA. Coding before and after the intervention gives two numbers. The difference between the two characterizes improvement. An example is given in Fig. 1. Plaques, stenoses, and occlusions were also coded in the untreated segments in order to express the severity of disease in these segments of the arterial system.

Percutaneous Transluminal Angioplasty
(ed. by C. T. Dotter, A. Grüntzig, W. Schoop, E. Zeitler)

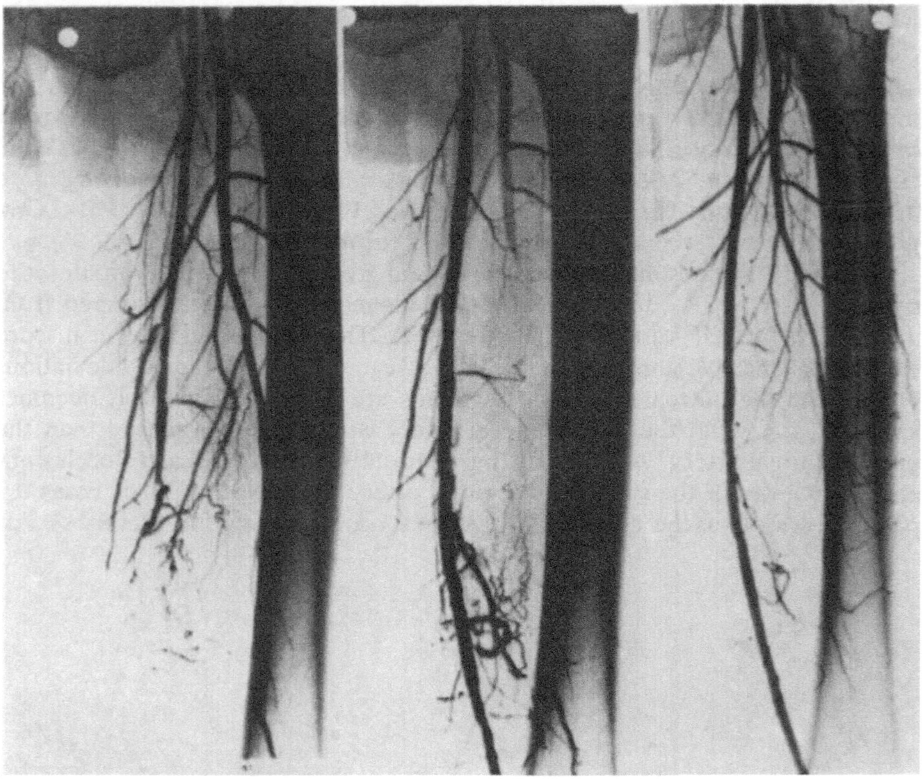

a

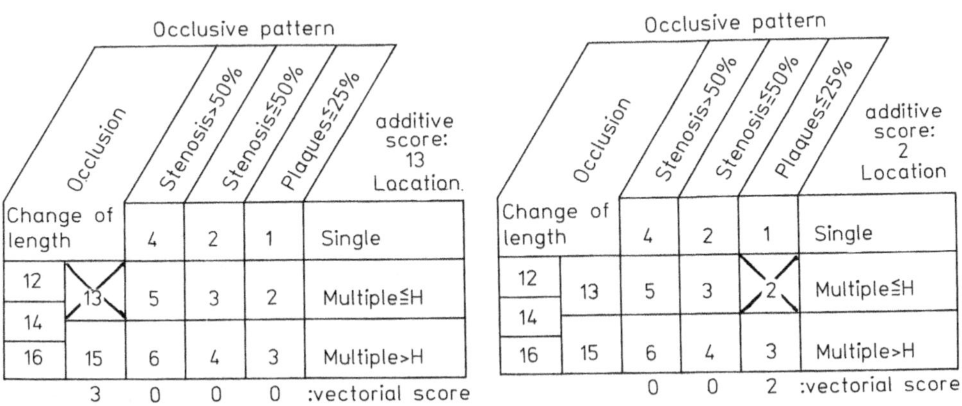

b

Fig. 1. a Arteriography before, immediately after, and 1 year after PTA of the superficial femoral artery. **b** Score evaluation of arteriography in the femoropopliteal segment before PTA. *Above* the severity of the lesion is indicated, *at the right* the extension of the lesion in the segment defined. **c** Score evaluation 1 year after PTA. H = half the length of the segment

Results

In Fig. 1 a typical example of a score evaluation is given. Before PTA the vectorial score of the superficial femoral artery was 3,000. This number designs a complete occlusion of less than half the length of the segment. After PTA the number changed to 003, which corresponds to multiple plaques involving more than half the length. The additive score reached 13 before and 3 after PTA. One year after therapy there was even a small further decrease to 2.

Figure 2 illustrates the results in the patient group ($n = 45$ dilatation sites; the two calf artery PTA, are excluded). The mean additive score dropped from 9.4 ± 3.2 before PTA to 4.0 ± 1.8 after PTA. This decrease in the mean score value is statistically significant ($p < 0.001$). Mean values and standard deviations obtained in the untreated arterial segments are given in Table 1. It becomes apparent, e.g., that the deep femoral artery is less severely altered than the posterior tibial artery. Analysis of the vectorial score shows that 17 occlusions and 22 stenoses of the superficial femoral artery were treated. In six cases the popliteal artery was the site of PTA (two short occlusions and four stenoses). For

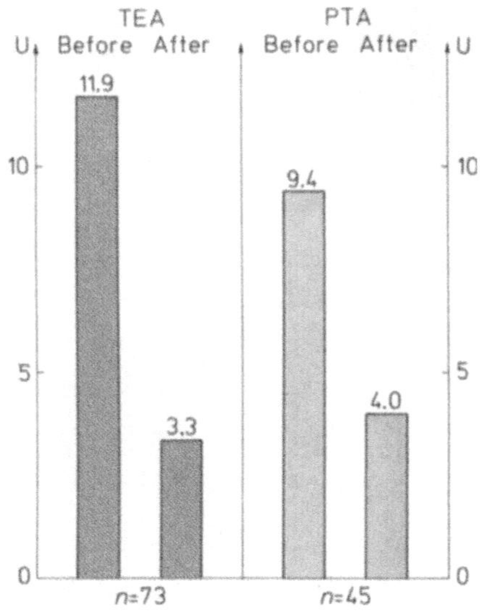

Fig. 2. Mean additive scores in 73 patients before and after femoropopliteal thromboendarterectomy (*TEA*) and in 45 consecutive patients before and after PTA in the femoropopliteal region. U = score units or numbers

Table 1. Mean values and standard deviation of the additive score in the segments not treated by PTA ($n = 43$ legs)

Deep femoral artery ($n = 43$)	1.2 ± 2.5
Superficial femoral artery ($n = 4$)	4.0 ± 2.0
Popliteal artery ($n = 37$)	3.0 ± 3.9
Anterior tibial artery ($n = 42$)	2.1 ± 4.0
Fibular artery ($n = 42$)	2.2 ± 3.9
Posterior tibial artery ($n = 43$)	3.5 ± 3.8

comparison the mean systolic pressure difference between arm and ankle arteries is indicated. Before treatment the value was 39.9 ± 21.8 mm Hg, after PTA 5.5 ± 22.6 mm Hg ($p < 0.001$).

Discussion

The present results show that the score system described [1] is suitable for evaluation of the success of PTA. Difficulties arise only in patients with remaining thrombi partially occluding the arterial lumen. In these cases single-plane arteriography does not allow an accurate measurement of the degree of stenosis. However, the increasing use of combined PTA and local thrombolysis should diminish the number of remaining mural thrombi. There is no score number for intimal ruptures. These events have to be marked separately.

In Fig. 2 the additive score before and after PTA is compared to that in a group of patients having been subjected to surgical endarterectomy. Before the operative treatment the mean additive score was 11.9 ± 3.4 (PTA: 9.4 ± 3.2), after operation 3.3 ± 1.4 (PTA: 4.0 ± 1.8). The difference between the mean values before endarterectomy and before PTA is statistically significant ($p < 0.001$). Endarterectomy was performed mostly on long occlusions, whereas in the PTA group stenoses and short occlusions predominated. After surgical intervention, however, the mean additive scores were only slightly better than after PTA ($p < 0.02$).

The method does not replace hemodynamic measurements, but adds a possibility of semiquantitative coding of anatomic lesions.

References

1. Bollinger A, Breddin K, Hess H, Heystraten FMJ, Kollath J, Konttila A, Pouliadis G, Marshall M, Mey T, Mietaschk A, Roth FJ, Schoop W (1981) Semiquantitative assessment of lower limb atherosclerosis from routine angiographic images. Atherosclerosis 38: 339
2. Grüntzig A (1977) Die perkutane transluminale Rekanalisation chronischer Arterienverschlüsse mit einer neuen Dilatationstechnik. Witzstrock, Baden-Baden
3. Hess H, Specker R, Mietaschk A, Ingrisch A (1981) Niedrig dosierte thrombolytische Therapie bei arteriellen Verschlüssen. Vasa 10: 97
4. Lohner D, Bollinger A, Schneider E, Pouliadis G, Brunner U (1981) Langzeitverlauf nach femoro-poplitealer Endarteriektomie, beurteilt durch ein computer-fähiges Code-System. Vasa 10: 102

6. Exposure of Physicians and Patients to Radiation During Transluminal Dilatation and Recanalization According to Dotter

F. Olbert, M. Nell, and H. Baumruck

Transluminal dilatation and recanalization of stenosed pelvic arteries and of femoral arteries with stenoses and short obstructions has gained considerable importance in recent years. Here our method for the determination of the exposure of physicians and patients to radiation is described.

We determined the exposure of patients to radiation in terms of the mean gonadal dose by means of thermoluminescence detectors. Measurements were made by means of lithium fluoride crystals approximately 6 × 6 × 1 mm or 3 × 3 × 1 mm large. The exposure of the physician to radiation was determined by two methods:

1. A thermoluminescence dosimeter was affixed to the physician's forehead, and two ring dosimeters to his right and left ring fingers.
2. The trunk radiation exposure was measured by means of a specially developed film dosimetry process. High-speed X-ray films (15× 30 cm) were placed between two highly intensifying films (calcium tungstate) and slipped into flexible plastic sleeves with light-impermeable closing flaps. Five such sleeves were stuck onto the outside of the protective apron by means of adhesive tape, covering it almost completely except for lateral strips about 10 cm wide. A sixth sleeve was worn on the middle of the back. The sensitivity of this combination was very high, the limit of detection being approximately 0.1 mR.

In the course of transluminal dilatation according to Dotter, 4 mR per examination was measured on the right ring finger and 10 mR on the left ring finger. The dose to the lens of the eye was 2.3 mR per examination and the gonadal dose measured on the patient 44 mR. Since the maximum permissible dose to the lens is 288 mR/week, the physician may perform up to 125 examinations per week.

The average screening time is 12 min. Since the maximum permissible daily dose on the hand is 250 mR, 25 examinations per day would be possible, a figure

Table 1. Radiation doses involved in transluminal dilatation (recanalization according to Dotter)

Measured dose of radiation per examination (mR)		Maximum permissible dose
Right ring finger	4	1,250 mR/week
Left ring finger	10	1,250 mR/week
Lens dose (Forehead)	2.3	288 mR/week
Gonadal dose (patient)	44	25 rad (genetically harmful)

Percutaneous Transluminal Angioplasty
(ed. by C. T. Dotter, A. Grüntzig, W. Schoop, E. Zeitler)

never reached in practice. The radiation measured on the physician's trunk behind the protective apron shows no significant exposure.

The patient is subjected to a gonadal dose of 44 mR per examination. In terms of the genetically harmful dose this would mean a permissible number of 568 examinations, again a figure never reached in practice. Note should also be taken of the angiography preceding the intervention as well as of a possible follow-up angiography 3–6 months after the intervention, which increase the gonadal dose more than twofold. Since our patients average 60 years, this does not constitute a major problem. By way of summary we can say that the mean gonadal dose to which the patient is exposed during the three radiological procedures in question remains so much below the genetically harmful dose that no serious problem arises.

The exposure of the physician to radiation (in terms of the values measured on the trunk shielded by the protective apron) is not alarming either.

References

1. Messerschmidt O, Olbert F (1980) Strahlenschutz in Forschung und Praxis, vol XX. Thieme, Stuttgart

II. Percutaneous Transluminal Angioplasty: Instrumentation and Technique

7. Single Teflon Catheters

E. Zeitler

Rigid Teflon catheters have long been used for percutaneous angiography by the Seldinger technique. Teflon catheters with various preformed tips have been used in preference to the soft Dacron catheters because of their firmness. For the same reason Dotter and Judkins [1, 2] have employed Teflon in their coaxial catheter dilating set for the treatment of femoropopliteal obstructions. In consideration of the large wall defect induced at the puncture site by the outer catheter of 12 Charrière, Staple [12] referred to his employment of a simple catheter. Several groups have used simple Oedman catheters and had unsatisfactory results. In 1968, we reported on our first experiences in percutaneous transluminal angioplasty with the Gensini catheter [14]. This catheter had been developed for thoracic aortography. The shape of the tip was mildly preformed and four side holes were placed behind the tip. Prior to the development of the Grüntzig balloon catheter [6], we employed the coaxial dilating set of Dotter and the Gensini catheter with either straight or bowed tip in the 7-F and 8-F sizes. With the additional employment of a stiff inner metal cannula for introduction, even long femoral arterial occlusions could be recanalized with the Dotter or special Gensini catheters without increased risk of bleeding at the puncture site after the procedure. The visit of van Andel and Puijlaert to our institution led to the development of the "van Andel catheter system" (Fig. 1).

Seventy-nine cases of femoral artery occlusion in stage II were followed up for more than 10 years, demonstrating patency and clinical success over this period. We still occasionally employ this same longitudinally stabilizing metal cannula in procedures with the Grüntzig catheter.

Since that time a new situation has arisen, since not only embolic complications [5, 7] and puncture site bleeding but also rethrombosis rates within 6 months were shown to be significantly higher with coaxial catheter systems than with single Teflon catheters [13, 13] and/or Grüntzig balloon catheters [3, 4, 8, 9].

We usually begin our percutaneous transluminal angioplasties of the femoropopliteal arteries with a 7–9-F-catheter with a tip tapered to 5-F (Fig. 2). Most of the femoropopliteal occlusions are in the middle to distal third of the superficial femoral artery.

In these cases we utilize a catheter with a long tapered tip that widens from 5 to 7 F. Several side holes are placed 10–12 cm proximal to the tip. A 0.38 guide wire occludes the end hole exactly, so that there is no step-off capable of causing

Percutaneous Transluminal Angioplasty
(ed. by C. T. Dotter, A. Grüntzig, W. Schoop, E. Zeitler)

1 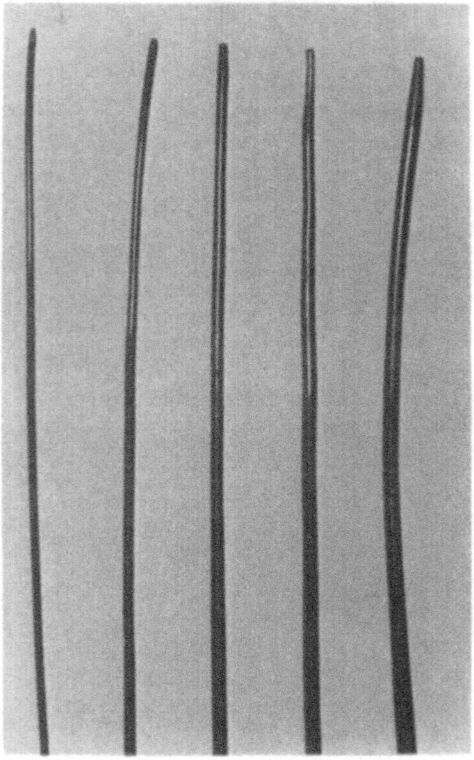

2 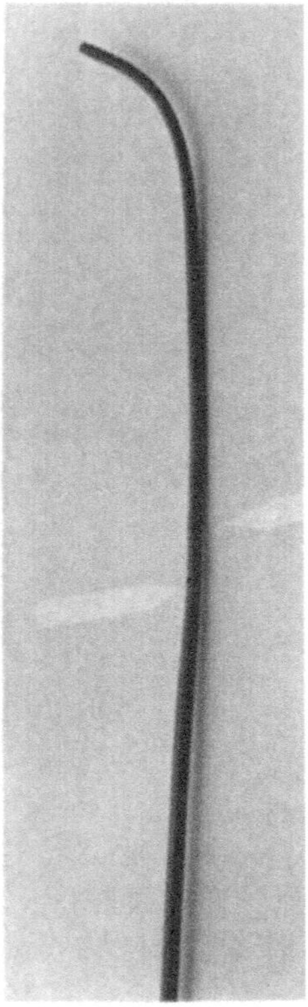

Fig. 1. Single Teflon van Andel catheters

Fig. 2. Single Teflon catheter with proximal side holes and preshaped catheter tip

a "snowball phenomenon" as so often cited from Staple's coaxial catheter experience.

After a diagnostic angiogram has been obtained through the Teflon catheter, the guide wire, which does not have to be removed, is directed through the stenosis under fluoroscopic control. Through a Y-connector 35% iodinated contrast solution can be injected during the guide wire advancement. In such fashion intraluminal passage of the wire can be guaranteed and perforation prevented. In addition, direction of the guide wire and the catheter into a collateral vessel can immediately be recognized. Only after the secure placement of the guide wire intraarterially past the obliteration is the Teflon catheter advanced into the region of the obliteration or obstruction. At this point, with fluoroscopy and additional contrast medium injections, one can determine whether there are further significant obstructions in the region of the popliteal artery or proximal trifurcation vessels. If such obstructions exist, either as high-grade stenoses or short occlusions, they may immediately be opened by advancing the Teflon catheter with its tapered tip (Figs. 2 and 3).

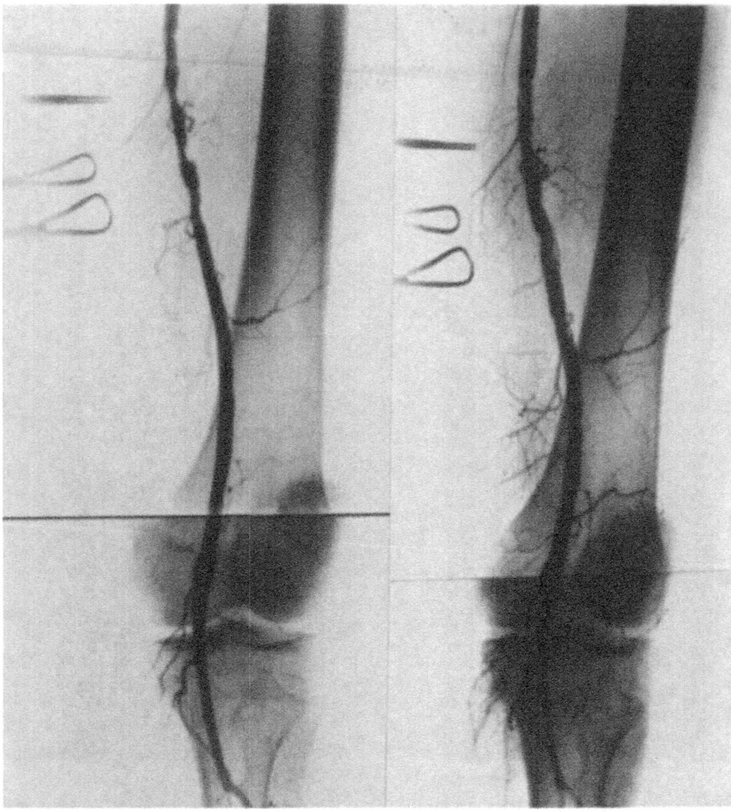

a b

Fig. 3a, b. Multiple femoral stenoses and occlusion of the tibiofibular trunk in a 59-year-old woman with diabetes and hypertension. **a** Pretherapeutic angiogram. The stenosis was passed with a single Teflon catheter and the tibiofibular trunk recanalized. Additional segmental dilatation was performed in the areas of the marked femoral stenoses. **b** Follow-up angiogram after PTA. Intimal tears apparent in the region of the femoral stenoses as well as signs of overdistention. The tibiofibular trunk is wideopen, its diameter correponding to that of the Teflon catheter tip

When the results in the region of the knee and upper calf have been checked, the Teflon catheter is exchanged for a Grüntzig balloon catheter. Thus the vascular obstruction can be dilated at the correct level with the appropriate Grüntzig or Olbert balloon catheter [10].

A second indication for the use of a single Teflon catheter is when, in patients with extensive obliterations and gangrene or rest pain, general or local circumstances contraindicate operative treatment. In these instances, a single passage of the Teflon catheter through a long obliteration may suffice to improve the arterial perfusion, at least temporarily. In the more favorable cases a local balloon catheter dilatation can follow immediately (Fig. 4). In other cases additional dilatation may be performed at another time, if the patient no longer suffers from rest pain. In such cases the dilatation of long stretches can proceed by use of the van Andel catheters.

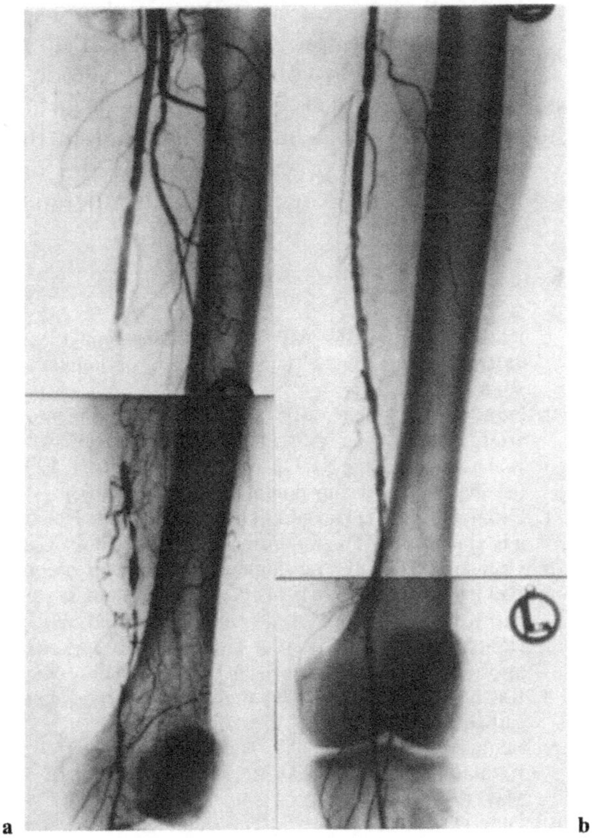

Fig. 4a, b. A 73-year-old woman with diabetic macro- and microangiopathy and gangrene involving the second to fourth toes. **a** Pretherapeutic angiogram demonstrating proximal femoral stenoses, segmental occlusion of the superficial femoral artery, and multiple high-grade long stenoses of the distal superficial femoral artery. **b** Recanalization and dilatation performed with single Teflon catheters. Passage first achieved with a catheter with proximal side holes; additional dilatation performed with a Teflon catheter of 10 F

While Teflon catheters with additional side holes are useful for peripheral femoropopliteal dilatations, they are not appropriate in proximal obliterations. In these cases one can use a catheter with side holes immediately behind the tip, such as the Oedman or Gensini catheters.

Teflon catheters with preformed tips are useful in the selective catheterization of the anterior tibial artery or the deep femoral artery. They may also be employed in procedures with contralateral access, such as the treatment of iliac artery stenoses, where the initial passage of the stenosis may be easier with such catheters than with a sidewinder catheter.

The Teflon coaxial dilating set of Dotter and Judkins and the combined Teflon catheter and instrumentation of Porstmann [11] for the occlusion of Botalli's duct, as well as the caged balloon catheter, laid the foundations for interventional cardiovascular radiology. From this basis the balloon catheter systems were developed and are today most decidedly the instruments of choice. Teflon catheters maintain their importance in special types of obstruction, especially in the lower leg, and in their advantages for ensuring the safe intraluminal passage of wire and catheter beyond obstructions. In obstructions of the proximal calf arteries, or in long obstructions, the disadvantages of large puncture defects and limited dilatation capabilities do not apply. In our considerable experience, the simple Teflon catheters have never led to "overstretching," in contrast to the balloon catheter systems. In high-grade stenoses tapered Teflon catheters provide an advantage in the first passage of the stenosis, just as does the lead catheter in the coronary system.

Therefore, for practical purposes the exclusive employment of balloon catheters appears to me to limit the therapeutic possibilities.

References

1. Dotter CT, Judkins MP (1964) Transluminal treatment of arteriosclerotic obstruction: description of a new technic and a preliminary report of its application. Circulation 30: 654–670
2. Dotter CT, Judkins MP, Rösch J (1968) Nichtoperative transluminale Behandlung der arteriosklerotischen Verschlußaffektionen. ROEFO 109: 125–133
3. Freimann DB, Ring EJ, Oleago JA, Berkowitz H, Roberts B (1979) Transluminal angioplasty of the iliac, femoral and popliteal arteries. Radiology 132: 285–288
4. Grüntzig A (1977) Die perkutane transluminale Rekanalisation chronischer Arterienverschlüsse mit einer neuen Dilatationstechnik. Witzstrock, Baden-Baden
5. Grüntzig A (1978) Transluminal dilatation of coronary artery stenoses. Lancet I: 263
6. Grüntzig A, Hopff H (1974) Perkutane Rekanalisation chronischer arterieller Verschlüsse mit einem neuen Dilatationskatheter. Dtsch Med Wochenschr 99: 2502–2505
7. Höhn P, Wagner R, Zeitler E (1975) Histologische Befunde nach der Katheterbehandlung arterieller Obliterationen nach Dotter und ihre Bedeutung. Herz:Kreisl 7: 13–23
8. Katzen BT, Chang J (1979) Percutaneous transluminal angioplasty with the Grüntzig balloon catheter. Radiology 130: 623–626
9. Mathias K, Schlosser V, Heiss HW, Staiger J (1980) Erfahrungen mit mehr als 350 Katheterangioplastiken der Becken-Beinarterien. Deutscher Röntgenkongreß, Cologne, 15–17 May 1980
10. Olbert F, Hanecka L (1978) Transluminal vascular dilatation with a modified dilatation catheter. In: Zeitler G, Grüntzig A, Schoop W (eds) Percutaneous vascular recanalization. Springer, Berlin Heidelberg New York, pp 32–38
11. Porstmann W (1973) Ein neuer Korsett-Balloon-Katheter zur transluminalen Rekanalisation nach Dotter unter besonderer Berücksichtigung von Obliterationen an den Beckenarterien. Radiol Diagn (Berl) 14: 239–244
12. Staple TW (1968) Modified catheter for percutaneous transluminal treatment of arteriosclerotic obstructions. Radiology 91: 1041
13. van Andel GJ (1976) Percutaneous transluminal angioplasty. Excerpta Medica, Amsterdam
14. Zeitler E, Müller R (1969) Erste Ergebnisse mit der Katheterrekanalisation nach Dotter bei arterieller Verschlußkrankheit. ROEFO 111: 345–352
15. Zeitler E, Schmidtke I, Schoop W, Giessler R, Dembski J, Mansjoer H (1976) Ergebnisse nach perkutaner transluminaler Angioplastik bei über 700 Behandlungen. Röntgenpraxis 294: 7887
16. Zeitler E, Grüntzig A, Schoop W (eds) (1978) Percutaneous vascular recanalization. Springer, Berlin Heidelberg New York

8. Basic Technology of Balloon Catheters

J. E. Abele

It is now almost 20 years since Dotter first published on percutaneous transluminal angioplasty, and almost 10 years since Grüntzig made improvements to the technique which remain the standard of practice today. A lot has been learned about the technique, the devices, and the principles but a lot more has to be learned and many improvements can still be made.

The objectives of dilatation are relatively simple:

1. To enlarge the vessel lumen (increase blood flow)
2. To keep the vessel open
3. To provide a smooth inner surface
4. To prevent distal debris
5. To assure minimal interruption or disruption of the vessel wall structure.

Although it is not clear whether it is better to remove the obstructing material or simply move it to the side, it is certainly easier to do the latter.

Ironically, if one were to chose an ideal material for a percutaneous vascular prosthesis, arteriosclerotic plaque (at least some types) would have to be one of the possible choices. It remodels quite well, it holds the vessel open, and it appears to be quite biocompatible.

Nevertheless, research projects with the objective of removing the blocking substance abound:

1. Laser [1]. A number of different investigators are experimenting with different wavelengths of light which can be used to destroy plaque without damaging the intima. Handling the heat and the combustion by-products produced remains a problem. Wavelengths which affect only plaque are still elusive.

2. Ultrasonic Emulsification (P. M. Platzmann, personal communication). This technique has been used to break up plaque, but solving the problem of the debris is a major difficulty.

3. Miniature Augers (I. Hawkins, personal communication). These tools have been used by a number of investigators and a project is in progress which has the aim of making this technique more feasible.

4. Biochemical Techniques. Discovering the universal plaque solvent would probably win a Nobel prize for the inventor. Different drugs are being used, sometimes in combination with external radiation to accelerate the process.

Percutaneous Transluminal Angioplasty
(ed. by C. T. Dotter, A. Grüntzig, W. Schoop, E. Zeitler)

Other techniques, such as hydraulic drills and trained bacteria, have been tried or are being investigated, but do not seem practicable at this point. The purpose of this discussion is to review the basic technology of balloon catheters and their application in the hope that a better understanding will lead to improved clinical technique and better product design.

To perform its job well, a balloon dilatation catheter should be able to reach the lesion, pass it, open it, and be removed, all with minimum trauma. The catheter may also aid in providing diagnostic information about the lesion and the optimum end point. Preliminary research results on this possibility are discussed in Chap. 12.

These objectives require a series of unique and sometimes conflicting design characteristics. Some of these factors are common to angiographic catheters; for example, the need for flexibility (the catheter must be soft enough to follow a guide wire, but stiff enough to advance through a lesion) and the need for a large lumen and relatively small outside diameter.

The unique characteristics of dilating catheters relate to inflation and deflation, profile, and dilating force.

Inflation and Deflation

Although most users are aware that syringes with smaller cross sections produce greater pressures, there seems to be some confusion about the best technique for rapid evacuation of the balloon. The amount of suction is proportionate to the syringe volume. Employing a pump to withdraw a 10-ml syringe quickly is far less effective than using a 50-ml syringe on a two-way shopcock. This is particularly important with large-volume balloons.

Profile

It is a common problem to be unable to advance the balloon catheter through the lesion even though the guide wire has already traversed it. Numerous improvements in lower profiles have been made on many catheters but there is probably not a universal design. Different lesions will require a different tip taper length and folded balloon profile. In some tight lesions or total obstructions, it is necessary to use multiple catheters.

Dilating Force

Dilating force is a result of two factors: (a) the hydrostatic force produced by the inflation fluid, and (b) the radial force vector produced when the circumference of the balloon becomes taut and tries to assume its unconstrained shape. This latter phenomenon, called "hoop stress" and also known as Laplace's law, is the tendency of the circumference of the balloon to become taut as pressure in the

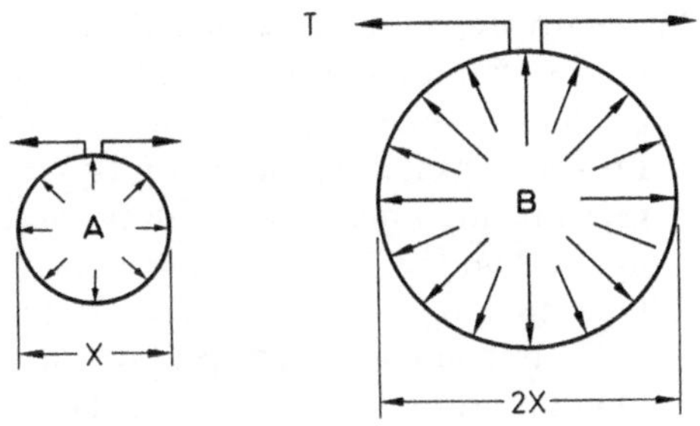

Fig. 1. Hoop stress (Laplace's law) (*T*). T is a function of pressure × radius and is therefore greater in *B* than in *A*

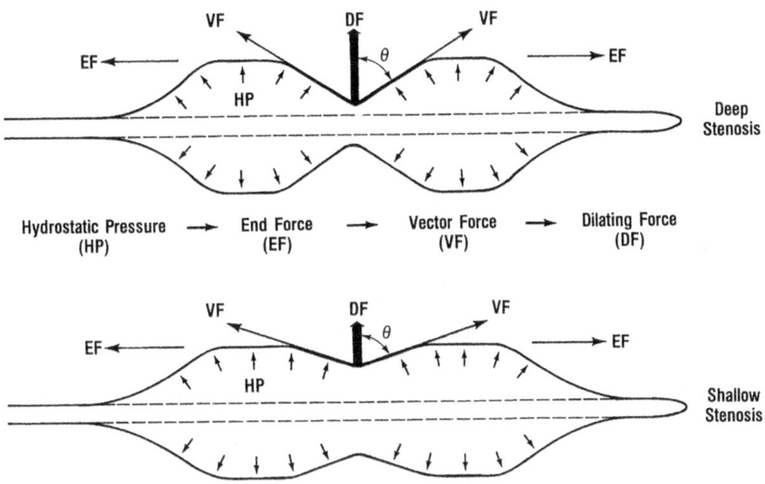

Fig. 2. Clothesline effect force: dilating force occurring as a result of hoop stress

balloon is increased. Because a balloon of larger diameter has more inside surface area, the hoop stress, T, which is a function of pressure × radius, is greater in the larger balloon. This is why larger balloons as well as larger catheters or larger arteries of the same wall thickness rupture at lower pressures than small ones (see Fig. 1).

Dilating force which occurs as a result of hoop stress may be called "clothesline effect" force. It is a resultant force which is perpendicular to the surface of the balloon. When the balloon surface is depressed by a lesion, the end forces produce vector forces, whose resultant is the dilating force. It is like trying to lift a weight in the center of a clothesline by pulling on one end. This force is greatest when the depression is deepest, since the vector forces are more perpendicular (see Fig. 2).

In a lesion of large area, the hydrostatic force is the more important. For the shorter, focal lesions, the clothesline effect force is the more important.

There are a number of different techniques which may be employed to measure dilating force. One can create a "standardized stenosis" out of rubber or clay and measure the pressure necessary to produce a predetermined change.

Alternatively, one can use one of various types of force-measuring devices which will sense that force produced by the balloon directly. We have used all of these techniques to make the following observations.

1. Pressure vs dilating force: for a given stenosis size, a given balloon size, and a given balloon material, dilating force is directly proportional to the pressure in the balloon.
2. Dilating force vs stenosis area: dilating force increases with increased stenosis area, but not in direct proportion to that area.
3. Dilating force vs balloon size: larger balloon catheters will produce greater dilating force in a lesion with the same diameter. Conversely, a balloon of the same size will produce more dilating force in a smaller lesion than in a large one.
4. Balloon diameter vs pressure: diameter vs pressure curves for balloon catheters are a very important indication of how the device will perform. The curve describes the stretch or compliance characteristics of the balloon. A nonstretch balloon has a flat curve [2].

Because all balloon materials will stretch a small amount, and to varying degrees, the balloon diameter will increase with pressure. These diameter vs pressure curves vary according to material and also according to temperature and sometimes degree of use. If the "yield" strength (the force that causes permanent deformation of the material) is very close to the "ultimate tensile strength" (the force required to break the material), then the diameter will change very little with pressure.

The advantages of chosing the balloon with the least stretch (lowest compliance) include:

1. More dilating force: Balloons with the same dimensions will produce considerably greater dilating force at the same pressure if the balloon material does not stretch. If the balloon stretches or deforms under pressure, it prevents a concentration of force at the stenosis. The balloon stretches around the lesion rather than exerting force on it. For maximum dilating force, one should chose a balloon with the smallest amount of stretch. In addition, it is easier to maintain a dilating force over a period of time since the nonstretch balloon does not deform.
2. A more predictable diameter, a better feel of the lesion, a retained cylindrical profile, and a safer failure mode.
3. Dilating force vs balloon length: with a balloon material that has some stretch to it, a short balloon will produce considerably more force than a long balloon. With a nonstretch balloon, however, there is relatively little difference in dilating force, regardless of the balloon length. In an eccentric lesion, where the side of the vessel opposite the lesion is elastic, a longer balloon can be more effective because the increased surface area in contact with the flexible portion of the vessel provides more support to push against.

Some interventional radiologists, particularly the pioneers, suggest that it is not necessary to measure balloon pressure or even pressure gradients across lesion before and after the procedure. They suggest that clinical results are what is important and that the skill and experience of the good physician will provide the information necessary to achieve a good result. I strongly disagree.

In an evolving technique like angioplasty, where indications are changing, the procedure is being modified, and the devices are changing substantially, it is especially important to keep good quantitative records, even when some of the data appear to be irrelevant at the time. These records will be important for the patient, should additional procedures be required, and are even more important for the procedure, since they improve the ability of these users to compare devices, techniques, and results.

Controversy still exists over the best technique for inflation. Should there be one quick inflation or multiple inflations; should the pressure gradually be increased; or should combinations of these techniques be used? One conclusion of the Registry on Coronary Angioplasty was that there was a greater chance of initial success if there were more than four inflations and a pressure greater than 4 atm was employed [3]. I submit that it is not the number of inflations that is important but the time of inflation. Anecdotal observations by a number of clinicians suggest that sustained pressure on plaque will produce a better and more permanent remodeling than short squeezes.

Therefore, the longer one can hold the balloon inflated without starving the artery beyond, the more likely it is that the stenosis will hold its new and enlarged shape. Perhaps it would be best to increase the pressure slowly to minimize large cracks, and to hold the balloon inflated for longer (10-min?) periods. It may be necessary to reconsider distal perfusion or at least a technique for providing continued circulation during such a long-term angioplasty procedure. Although this is conjecture at this point, it certainly warrants further study.

Controversy also exists over the appropriate amount of dilatation. In a tight stenosis, a very small difference in size could mean a very large difference in flow. Although flow depends on peripheral resistance, turbulence, compliance, and rheological factors, Poisseuille's law states that the flow in a 70% stenosis could be more than five times the flow in an 80% stenosis (a difference in caliber that is difficult or impossible to observe on radiography). The radiological measurement of stenosis is not very accurate, not only because of the poor resolution, but also because of the unlikely assumption that the vessel cross section is round.

Nevertheless, it is important to understand that reduction in flow is not linear with the reduction in diameter. The effect on flow produced not only by the degree but also by the shape and number of stenoses is hard to determine. By smoothing a rough stenosis and changing turbulent flow to laminar, it is possible to improve flow without any change in diameter [4].

In conclusion, significant improvements in clinical effectiveness have occurred as a result of improved understanding of the technique and improved devices. Additional improvements will occur as we learn more, as when noninvasive imaging techniques are applied to follow-up studies as well as when improved direct imaging techniques such as vascular endoscopy are applied to pre- and postprocedural situations. It is an exciting field and I look forward to participating in its continued development.

References

1. Abela GS et al. (1982) The effect of laser radiation on atheromatous plaques: A preliminary report. Presented at the American College of Cardiology, 31st Annual Scientific Session, April 28, 1982
2. Abele J (1980) Balloon Catheters and Transluminal Dilatation: Technical Considerations. Am J Roentgenol 135: 901–906
3. Faxon DP et al. (1982) Determinants of a successful percutaneous transluminal coronary angioplasty. American College of Cardiology, 31st Annual Scientific Session, April 26, 1982
4. Robbins SL, Bentov I (1967) The kinetics of viscous flow in a model vessel: effect of stenoses of varying size, shape and length. Lab Invest, vol 16, No 6

9. Dilatation and the Expanding Balloon Catheter. Advantages of the Expanding Balloon Catheter

F. Olbert and N. Muzika

The expanding balloon catheter was first presented by our group in 1977 [1–4] and has been commercially available for 6 months (Surgimed, Copenhagen). The major differences between this new catheter and that ones used so far are the following:

1. The fluid contained in the balloon is subjected to considerably higher pressure (8–12 atm); accordingly, the balloon is harder.
2. Once the balloon is filled an increase in pressure will not lead to a change in size or shape because it is not elastic in the direction of the diameter.
3. The balloon has only a longitudinal elasticity. When the catheter is introduced into the vessel the dilatation segment has the same transverse diameter as the tube. Folding – a major problem with other catheters – can thus be prevented (Figs. 1–3).

The catheter consists of an inner tube with a small lumen for the introduction of the guide wire, heparin, and the radiopaque substance, and a concentrically arranged outer catheter and the balloon. The space between the two radiopaque Teflon tubes is designed for the transport of the pressure fluid (30% Urographin). The polyurethane balloon is firmly attached to the distal end of the outer tube by means of an adhesive.

The major advantages of this balloon catheter are: (a) the outer diameter of the balloon in the noninflated state is practically identical with the diameter of the rest of the catheter, and (b) the balloon does not develop any folds, and thus allows smooth introduction into as well as smooth retraction from the skin and subcutaneous tissue. The catheter can also be introduced through one of the commercially available guide tube systems, permitting it to be painlessly exchanged for another one with a different lumen or for a balloon with a different length or width. Even at maximum pressure the balloon does not show any annular fold in the narrowest part of the stenosis.

So far we have used this catheter to treat 100 patients, 58 males and 42 females. The age distribution is shown in Table 1. Table 2 shows the localization of the stenoses and occlusions and Fig. 4 shows the effect of recanalization in terms of changes in the Doppler index. The blood flow in the lower leg was completely blocked in 6 patients, 4 patients had one patent vessel, and 20 patients had two patent vessels. The stages of disease before and after transluminal dilatation are shown in Table 3. Table 4 is a documentation of improvement of Dopplerindices in the different treated areas.

Percutaneous Transluminal Angioplasty
(ed. by C. T. Dotter, A. Grüntzig, W. Schoop, E. Zeitler)

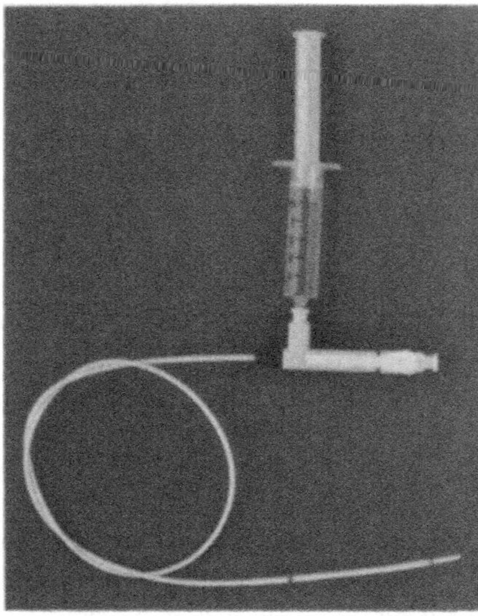

1

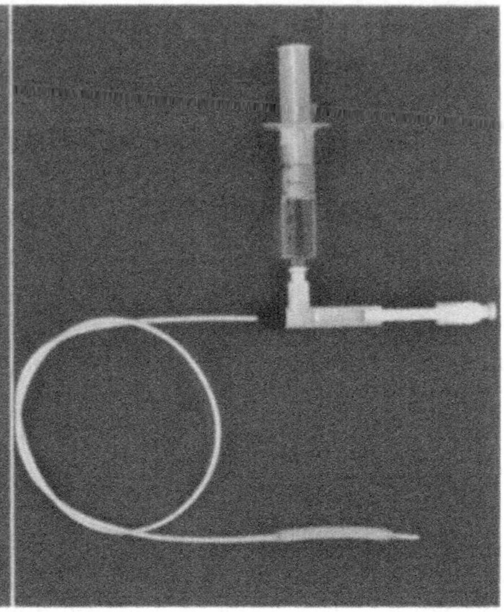

2

Fig. 1. The catheter-system in its uninflated state

Fig. 2. The catheter-system in its inflated state

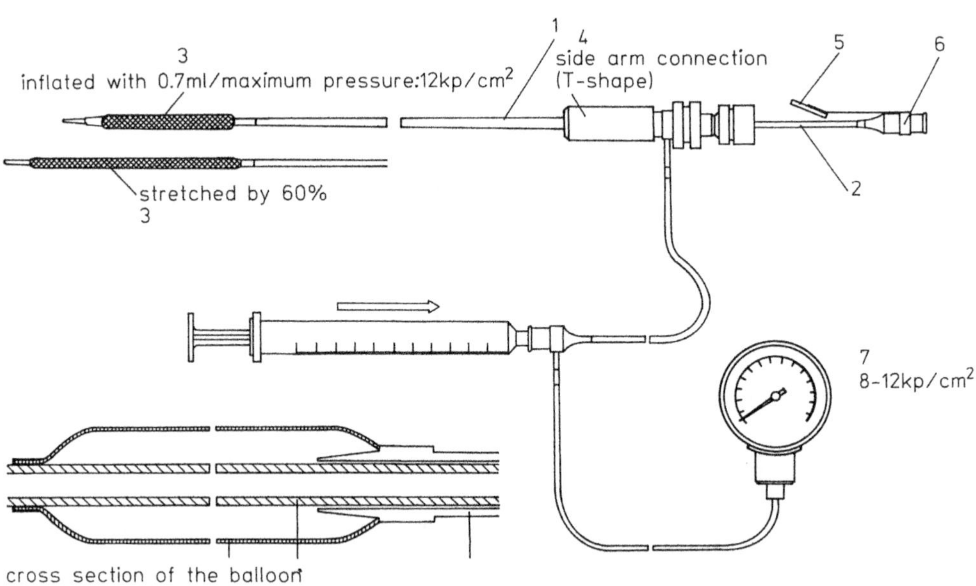

Fig. 3. The primarely component drawing shows the cross-section of the balloon

Table 1. Age distribution of our patients

Age					
30–40	41–50	51–60	61–70	71–80	81–90
5	12	27	30	24	2

58 ♂ + 42 ♀

Table 2. Localization of the stenosis and of the occlusion

Localization		
Distal Aorta		1
Iliac occlusion		0
Iliac stenosis		14
Femoral occlusion	≤ 3 cm	8
	≥ 3–10 cm	17
	> 10 cm	14
Femoral stenosis	≤ 3 cm	12
	≤ 8 cm	25
Popliteal stenosis		5
Subclavian stenosis		4
Total		100

Table 3. Efficiency of angioplasty in relation to the clinical stage before and after treatment

Before treatment	IIa	7			
	IIb		50		
	III			24	
	IV				13
After treatment	I	4	0	0	0
	IIa	3	31	7	3
	IIb	0	19	15	5
	III	0	0	2	3
	IV	0	0	0	2

Table 4. Documentation of the improvement of Dopplerindex according to the anatomical localization. Transluminal dilatation and recanalization (August 1st 1981–March 31st 1982); Olbert-catheter-system N-100

Doppler index	Stenosis of distal aorta	Iliac stenosis	Femoral occlusion >3 (>10) cm	Femoral occlusion ≤ 3 cm	Femoral stenosis ≤ 3 cm	Femoral stenosis ≤ 3 cm	Popliteal stenosis	Subclavian stenosis
− 0.2	–	–	1	–	1	–	–	–
− 0.1	–	–	1	–	–	–	–	–
0	–	1	4	–	1	–	1	–
0.1	–	2	4	–	3	2	2	–
0.2	–	2	5	2	4	2	1	–
0.3	–	3	5	1	2	2	–	–
0.4	–	4	5	1	5	1	–	–
0.5	1	2	2	1	4	3	1	2
0.6	–	–	2	3	4	2	–	2
0.7	–	–	2	–	1	–	–	–
Total	1	14	31	8	25	12	5	4

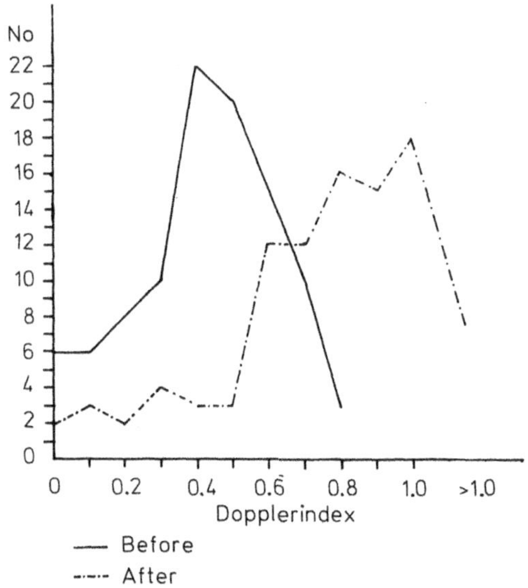

Fig. 4. Development of Dopplerindex before and after treatment

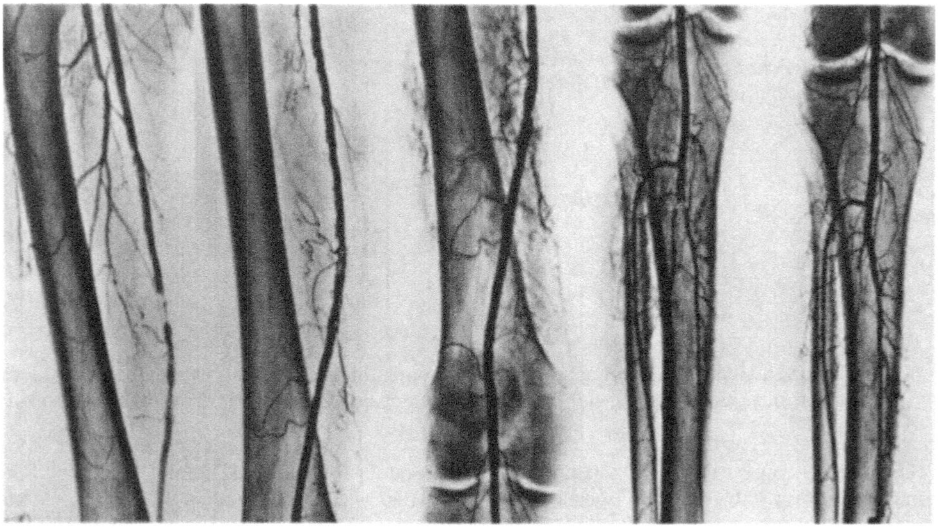

Fig. 5a–d. Angiography of a short stenosis in the right femoral artery **a.** After angioplasty there are severe irregularities visible at the vessel wall **b.** 14 days later these irregularities are no more visible **c.** But now a stenosis in the proximal part of the tibial artery appeared **d.** which could be dilated successfully

Case Reports

Following transluminal dilatation for a stenosis in the left iliac artery in 1976, in April 1981 the patient (now aged 60) returned to our out-patient department complaining of a sudden shortening of his walking distance to 50–100 m (stage II b) (Fig. 5). Attempted conservative treatment proved unsuccessful, and

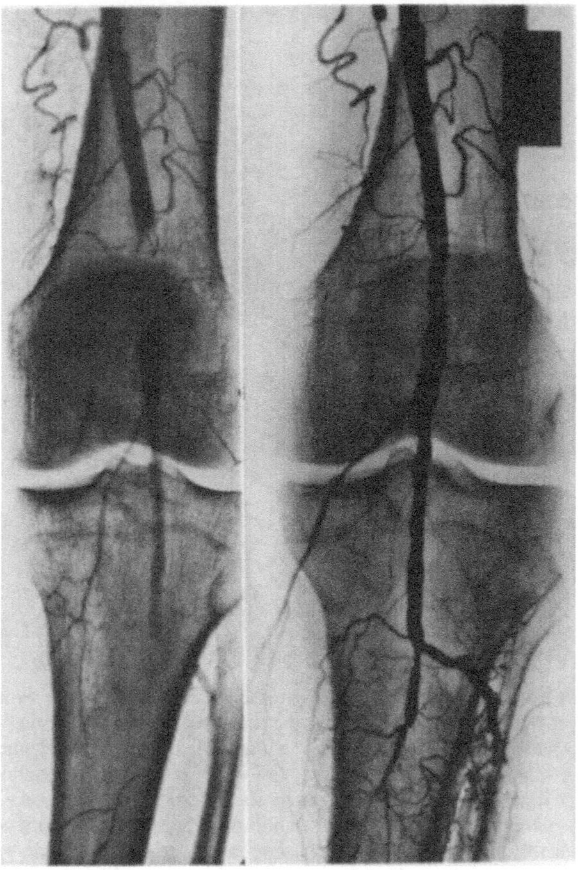

Fig. 6. Acute occlusion in the proximal part of the popliteal artery. The 5 cm long occlusion is primarily treated with 30,000 IU. Streptokinase and in further consequence the reststenosis is successfully dilated

angiography performed on 31. August 1981 revealed an approximately 1,5 cm long stenosis of the right femoral artery, which was dilated transluminally 2 weeks later. Upon follow-up angiography, the dilated portion showed marked irregularities of the vascular wall, suggesting reocclusion of this segment. The patient was free from symptoms for 2 weeks, but then aortography had to be performed because of severe pain at rest in the left lower leg. Surprisingly, the dilated segment of the femoral artery was now seen to be completely smooth and patent. This time however, a partial obstruction of the trifurcation was found, which was dilated with an Olbert catheter. Since then the patient has been completely free from symptoms. The patient shows a merked pulse in the region of the dorsal artery of the foot and of the retromalleolar artery. At the patient's request anticoagulation therapy (Marcoumar) was prescribed (the patient's profession as a sculptor involving frequent risk of injury).

A 67-year-old male patient was referred to our department with a diagnosis of acute vascular obstruction in the area of the left popliteal artery (Doppler index: 0) (Fig. 6). The angiogramm showed a complete occlusion of the left popliteal artery some 3 cm above the interarticular space of the knee.

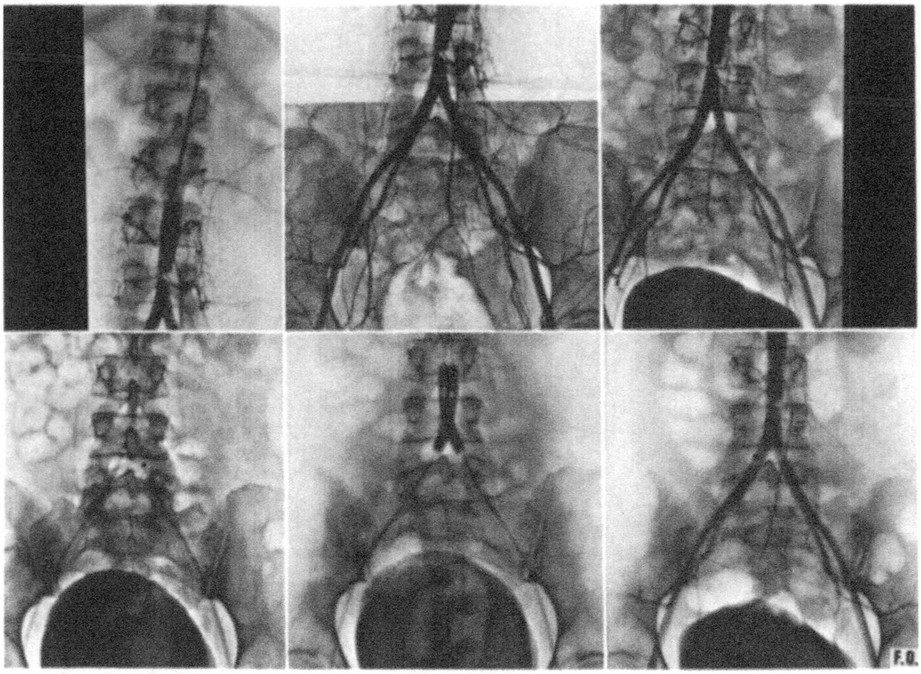

a–c

d–f

Fig. 7a–f. Transaxillary angiography in a 45-year-old woman with a walking distance of 300 m revealed a stenosis reducing the lumen of the distal portion of the aorta to the diameter of a knitting needle **a.** As a first step the stenosis was dilated by the transaxillary route by means of an 8-mm-balloon **b, c.** Following this intervention the inguinal pulse was palpable on both sides, so that it was now possible to puncture the common femoral artery in the inguinal region by the Seldinger technique in order to insert an 8-mm-balloon both from the left and from the right common femoral artery into the distal aorta after introduction of a guide wire **d, e.** In this way the stenosis was removed except for minor plaque formations **f**

Transluminal recanalization was carried out immediately. After local application of streptokinase the vessel was mechanically recanalized. The postoperative Doppler index of 0.8 proves the excellent result of the intervention. With the exception of minor parestesia in the area of the left forefoot, the patient was free from symptoms immediately after dilatation, with an almost unlimited walking distance. Postoperative anticoagulation therapy with Marcoumar was prescribed.

In a 45-year-old female patient with severe circulatory impairment in both legs (walking distance 300 m), a major stenosis of the distal abdominal aorta was found (Fig. 7). The Dopplerindex was 0.5. Bilaterally, no pulse was palpable in the inguinal region. The distal stenosis of the abdominal aorta was visualized by means of the transaxillary catheterization technique. Subsequently, the Olbert catheter system was introduced via the transaxillary route by the guide tube technique, and the distal stenosis of the abdominal aorta was first dilated with an 8-mm-balloon. The inguinal pulse was now palpable on either side. Then the femoral artery was punctured bilaterally in the inguinal region and an 8-mm-

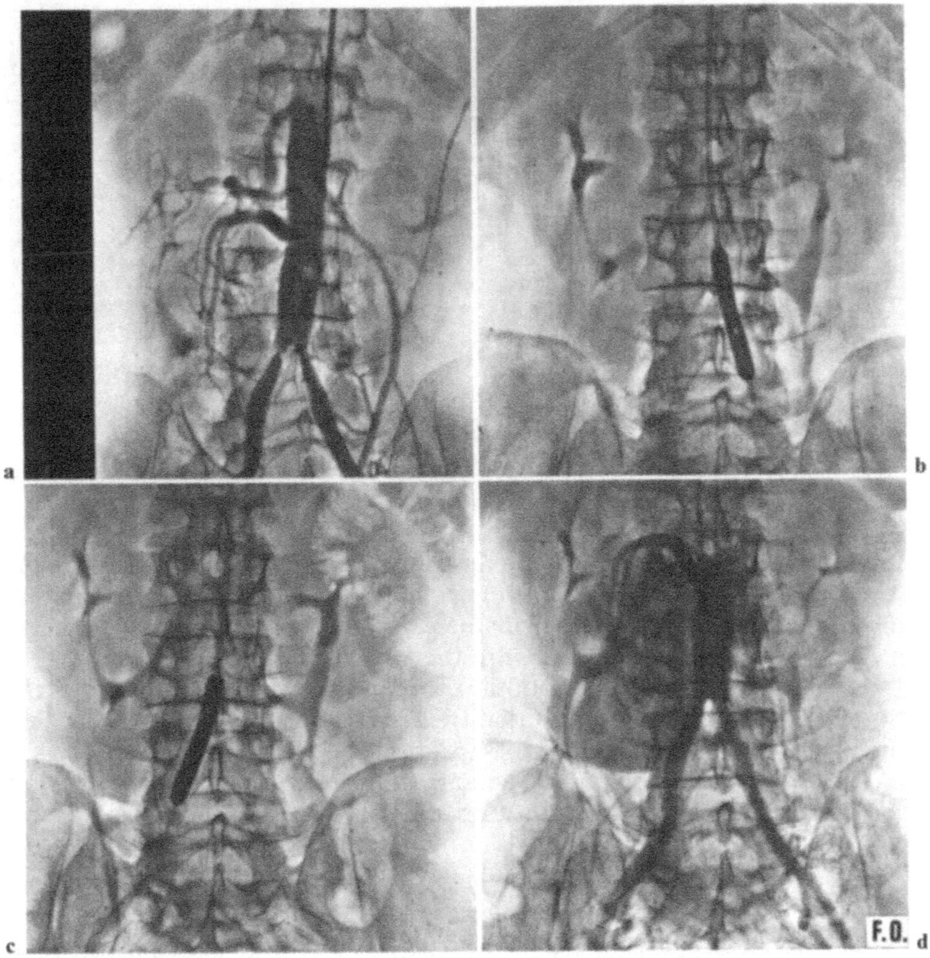

Fig. 8a–d. In a patient with poorly palpable inguinal pulses transaxillary angiography confirmed the clinical suspicion of a stenosis in the central portion of the left and right common iliac artery **a.** After insertion of an 8-mm-balloon into the left **b** and subsequently into the right **c** common iliac artery dilatation resulted in a patent vessel **d**. The Dopplerindex improved from 0.5 to 0.9 on both sides. The walking distance was unlimited

balloon was advanced into the stenosed portion. After inflation of the balloon angiography revealed that the stenosis had been removed. After 3 months the Doppler index was 1, an increase of 0.5.

A 50-year-old male patient had severe bilateral stenosis of the central portion of the common iliac artery (Fig. 8). Dilatation was effected by the Olbert catheter system, the catheter being introduced via the transaxillary route by means of the guide tube technique. Follow-up angiography showed complete elimination of the stenosis. The Doppler index improved bilaterally by 0.4.

Recanalisation of an obstruction of 15 cm length in the middle third of the right superficial femoral artery as well as of an 6 cm long obstruction in the

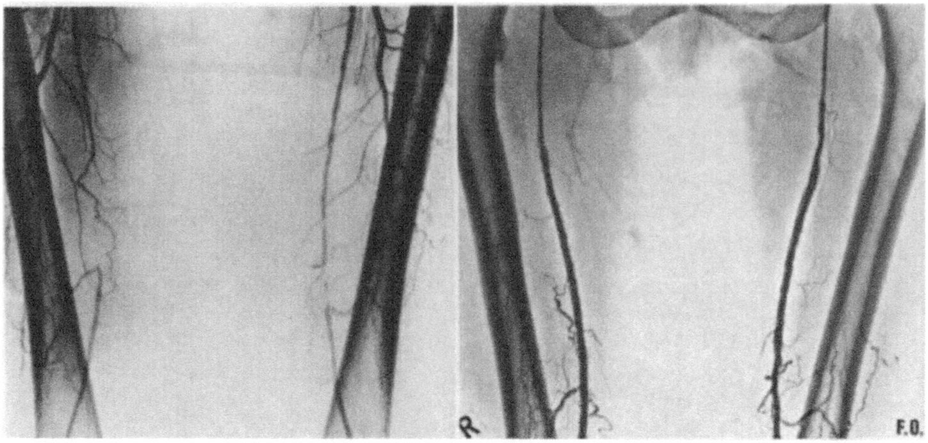

Fig. 9. The 10 cm long occlusion in the right femoral artery and the 6 cm long occlusion in the left femoral artery are recanalized successfully

transition area from the middle to the lower third of the left superficial femoral artery (Fig. 9). Recanalization led to complete restoration of the arterial blood flow. There was an improvement of the Doppler index by 0.4 for the right and by 0.3 for the left superficial femoral artery.

Figure 10 shows a stenosis of the central subclavian artery two fingers from its origin from the arch of the aorta. Blood pressure values differented about 50 mm Hg – on the right arm 120/80 and on the left arm 70/0.

After recanalization, follow-up angiography revealed complete restoration of the arterial blood flow with a pressure of 120/80 on both arms.

Discussion

Use of the Olbert catheter system for the treatment of stenoses and occlusions in the peripheral vessels has considerably reduced the incidence of complications. Haematomas at the site of puncture and reocclusions occur less frequently. On account of its pressure stability the balloon may also be used to dilate fairly hard stenoses, since the lumen of the balloon will not be dilated before or behind the stenosis so that no undue damage will be inflicted on the vascular wall.

Throughout the procedure the catheter system remains "splinted" by a guide wire. Initially, an 0.35 mm Teflon Coated Spring Guide (USCI) is used, which is replaced by an 0.25 mm diameter Cordis guide wire in order to permit intraoperative visualisation of the successful dilatation by injection of a contrast medium. The necessary rinsing of the catheter with heparin is effected by connecting a haemostasis valve (Cordis Cat. No. 501-621) to the dilatation catheter.

Thanks to guide tube systems the catheter may be painlessly exchanged for another one with a different balloon length or width. This greatly simplifies dilatation of the distal abdominal aorta and the pelvic vessels immediately after transaxillary angiography.

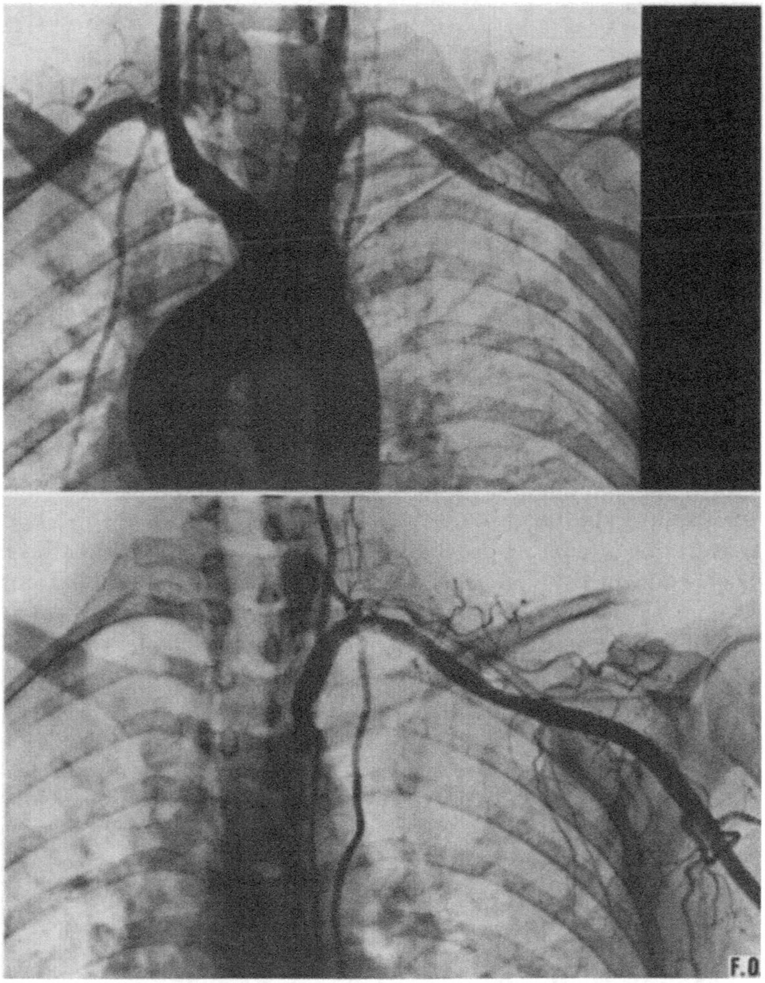

a

b

Fig. 10a, b. Angiography of the aortic arch showed a considerable stenosis of the left subclavian artery 2 fingers width above its origin from the aorta **a**. After dilatation with an 8 mm balloon catheter the vascular lumen was normal and blood pressure values were the same on either side **b**

References

1. Hanecka L, Olbert F (1977) Ballonkatheter. OE Patent, 17 February 1977, Patent No. 348,094
2. Olbert F, Hanecka L (1977) Transluminale Gefäßdilatation mit einem modifizierten Dilatationskatheter. Fortschr Med 95(13): 867–869
3. Olbert F, Hanecka L (1978) Transluminal vascular dilatation with a modified dilatation catheter. In: Zeitler, E. Grüntzig A, Schoop W (eds) Percutaneous vascular recanalization. Springer, Berlin Heidelberg New York, pp 32–38
4. Olbert F, Schidrich W, Schlegl A (to be published) Ein neuer Dilatations-Katheter. Gemeinsame Herbsttagung der Bayerischen und Berliner Röntgengesellschaft 25–27 Sept. 1981, Nürnberg. Wachholz, Nürnberg

III. Percutaneous Transluminal Angioplasty: Mechanism and Morphology

10. The Morphological Concept of Percutaneous Transluminal Angioplasty

H. J. Leu

Introduction

Since the introduction of percutaneous transluminal angioplasty (PTA), the question of the destiny of the obliterating arteriosclerotic material after the perforating or dilating procedure has been widely discussed. Several possibilities have been mentioned, such as compression of the intimal cushions, lysis of intimal appositions, dilatation of the vessel wall including the media, radial rupture of the intima, and loosening of intimal plaques with embolization into the periphery [1–8]. In reality the spectrum of morphological alterations is as complex as the morphological pattern of arteriosclerosis itself. Any of the mentioned possibilities may occur. Only by evaluating the type of arteriosclerotic lesion can we understand the chances of PTA and the possible reasons for failure and for certain complications. In spite of the latter, PTA has gained a definite position within the therapy spectrum of obliterating arterial disease.

Morphological Types of Arteriosclerosis and Alterations Following PTA (Table 1)

Dilating Types of Arteriosclerosis

True Aneurysm

The vascular lumen is dilated. The media is atrophic and decreased in diameter. The smooth musculature is partly replaced by collagen fibers. Thickening and sclerosis of the intima is scarce; apposition of thrombotic material may occur. Cellular organization of the thrombus is minimal and limited to the marginal areas, whereas the majority of the thrombotic material consists of fibrinous homogenized cell-free masses which may even be accessible by therapeutic fibrinolysis at a late date. Parts of these masses may easily embolize into the periphery. This hardly ever gives rise to clinical symptoms. This may be due to spontaneous lysis within the small peripheral blood vessels. When embolism with clinical consequences occurs this is mostly due to popliteal aneurysms (traumatic influence of joint movements?).

Percutaneous Transluminal Angioplasty
(ed. by C. T. Dotter, A. Grüntzig, W. Schoop, E. Zeitler)

Table 1. Chances of dilatation with different types of arteriosclerosis

Type of arteriosclerosis	Chances of dilatation
Dilating types	
True aneurysm	TD not indicated Danger of embolism
Mönckeberg's arteriosclerosis of media	TD only necessary in the case of additional intimal sclerosis
Obliterating types	
Soft cushions (juvenile type)	Well compressible Risk very low
Additional thrombi	May easily be perforated and compressed Danger of embolism
Intimal plaques	Not compressible Intimal ruptures possible, leading to successful dilatation
Intimal fibrinous insudations Intimal hemorrhages	Danger of dissection, perforation, and loosening of plaques
Fatty degeneration of intima	Danger of dissection within the intima
Obliteration by dense connective tissue	Perforation impossible Dilatation impossible Danger of dissection
Inflammatory arterial occlusions	
Thromboangiitis obliterans Takayasu's disease Pathergic granulomatoses Polyarteritis nodosa	Perforation of thrombi not possible because of early organization by dense connective tissue Danger of perforation

TD, transluminal dilatation

Arterial aneurysms are, of course, no indication for PTA. As they are sometimes difficult to recognize angiographically, PTA may be performed erroneously. The fibrinous masses in the aneurysms are easily perforated and compressed but the probability of embolization of thrombotic material into the periphery is very high (Fig. 1a). Two such cases have been observed by us, one ending with amputation above knee level.

Mönckeberg's Arteriosclerosis of the Media

The media is atrophic and calcified. The rigid walls keep the lumen of the artery wide open. Unless there is additional intimal sclerosis, there is no stenosis of the lumen and therefore no indication for PTA.

Obliterating Types of Arteriosclerosis: Alterations Following PTA

Juvenile Arteriosclerosis

The "soft" intimal cushions consist of loose mesenchymal connective tissue which is edematous and contains few and tender collagen fibers. Intimal deposits

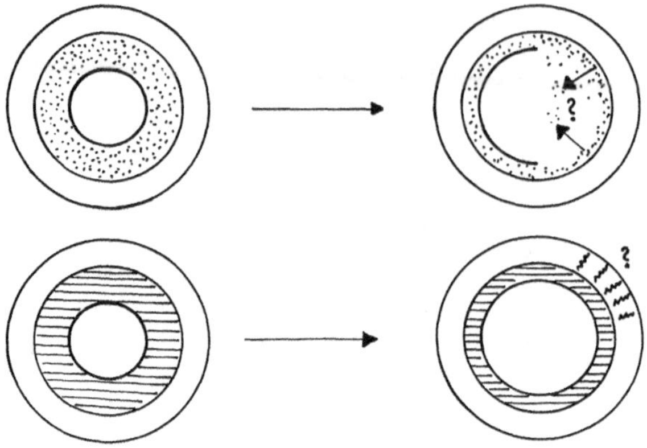

a b

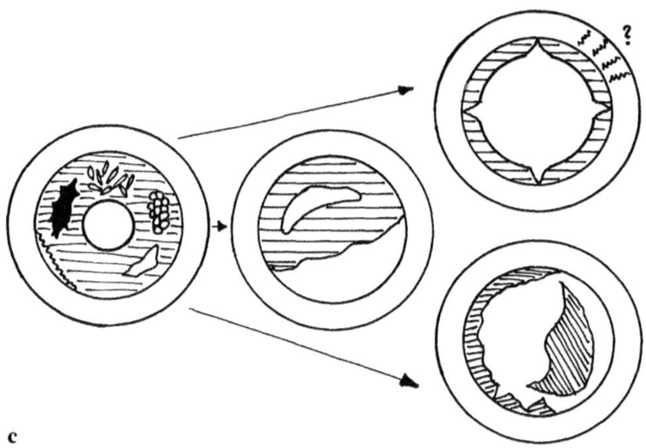

c

Fig. 1a–c. The possible effects of PTA. **a** compression or possibly pulverization of appositional thrombi; **b** compression of soft intimal cushions, possibly lacerations of media; **c** radial intimal ruptures with or without additional lacerations of media or dissection between intima and media or loosening and embolization of intimal plaques

(fat, cholesterin granulomas, calcifications) are usually lacking. This material is ideal for dilatation because it has a soft consistency and can easily be compressed by the balloon catheter. On the other hand, these cushions are well fixed to the arterial wall and the danger of loosening a plaque is minimal. It is unknown why this soft material remains in a compressed state and does not expand again by edematous insudations (Fig. 1b).

Intimal Plaques with Hyalinization and Calcification

The intimal plaques consist of dense collagen fibers including deposits of cholesterin and calcifications. They are hardly compressible. If the pressure of the balloon is high enough, radial ruptures of the intima ending at the internal elastic lamella may occur. This enables the vessel wall to be dilated to a certain degree. The fissures are soon covered by new connective tissue and the surface is smoothed again by this procedure. The lumen may remain more or less permanently dilated (Fig. 1c).

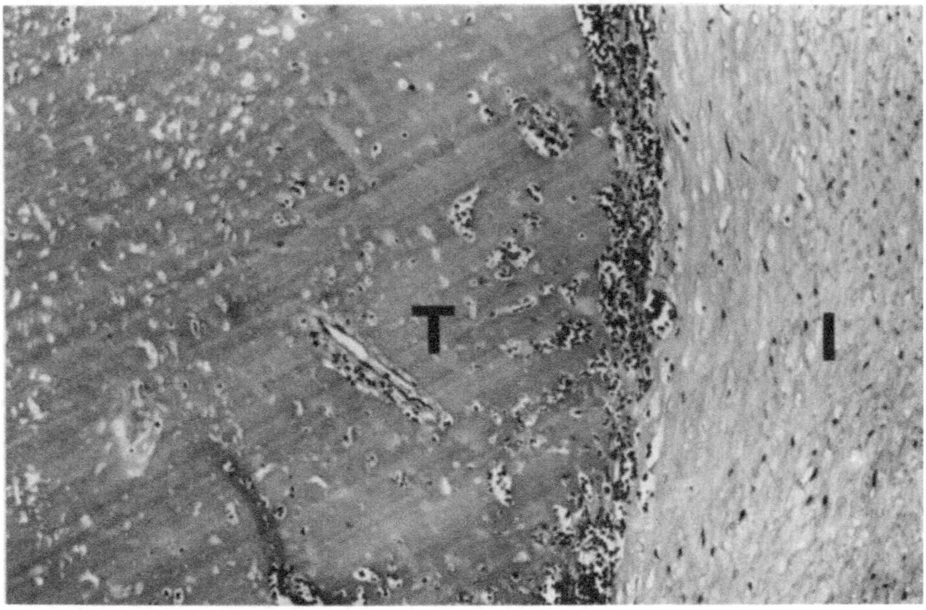

Fig. 2. Occluded artery with homogeneous fibrinous thrombotic masses on sclerotic intima. *T*, thrombus; *I*, intima. HZ 25722/71. F.74/30. Hemalaun-eosin, × 125

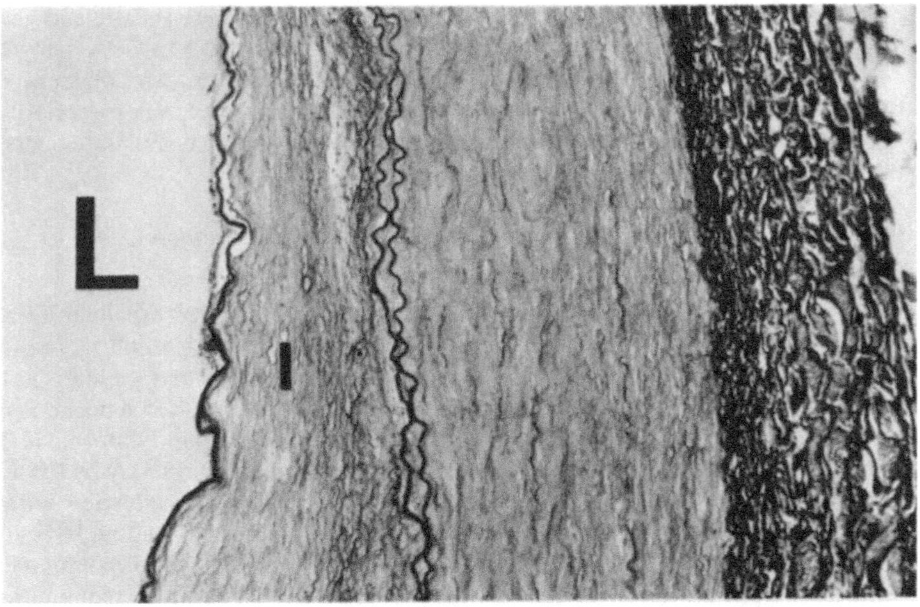

Fig. 3. Five days after PTA. The intima (*I*) is compressed, no overlying thrombotic material is present, the lumen (*L*) is patent. AZ 522/79. F.74/17. Elastin, × 80

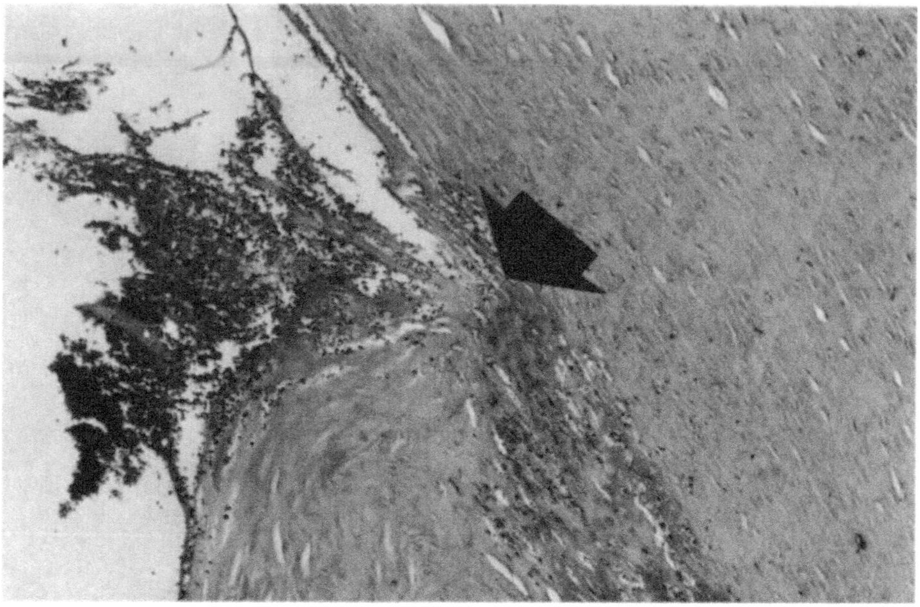

Fig. 4. Ruptured intima (*arrow*) a few days after PTA. The lumen is dilated. HZ 4566/82. F.74/25. Hemalaun-eosin, × 80

Additional Thrombi Covering Intimal Sclerotic Plaques

As long as the thrombotic material remains in a fibrinous state and is not organized and integrated into the vessel wall by connective tissue, perforation and dilatation is easy, but there is always the risk of inducing embolism of such material into the periphery. Small emboli are probably well tolerated and removed by spontaneous lysis. Larger emboli may necessitate surgical intervention (Figs. 1a, 2, and 3).

Intimal Plaques with Fatty Degeneration, Fibrinous Insudation, and Hemorrhages

The intimal proliferations consist of alternating areas of dense collagen fibers, insudations of blood and fibrin, fatty degeneration, cholesterin granulomas, and calcifications (Fig. 4). Additional thrombotic appositions may or may not be present. A compression of such material by the balloon catheter is not or is only partly possible. Spontaneous dissection between intima and internal elastic lamella is occasionally observed. In these cases intimal plaques may be loosened by the catheter and may embolize into the periphery, usually necessitating surgical removal. Areas with fatty degeneration, hemorrhage, and fibrinous insudation are easily penetrated by the catheter. This may lead to wall dissection within the intima. Even perforation of the catheter through the atrophic media and adventitia may occur. Examples of these complications are demonstrated in Figs. 5–7.

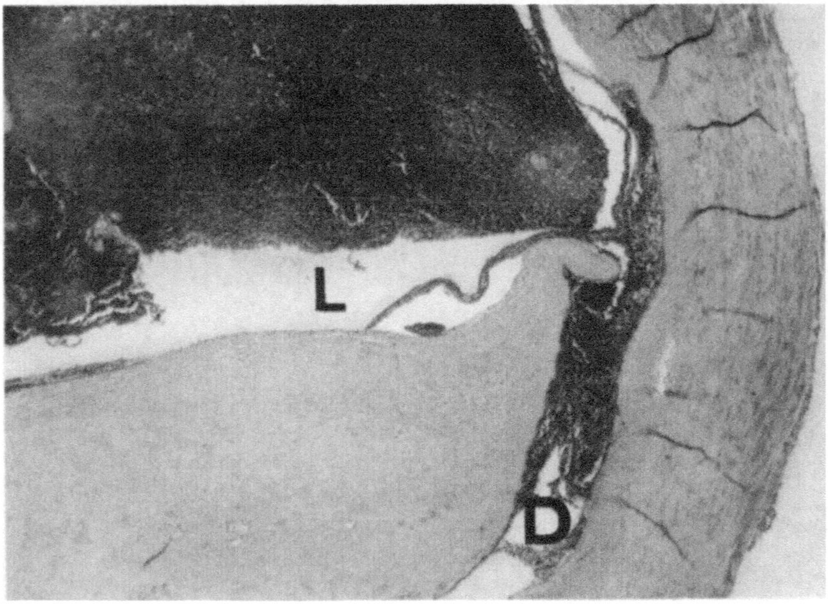

Fig. 5. Spontaneous dissection between intima and media (*D*) 24 h after PTA. *L*, lumen. HZ 9364/80. F.74/23. Hemalaun-eosin, × 30

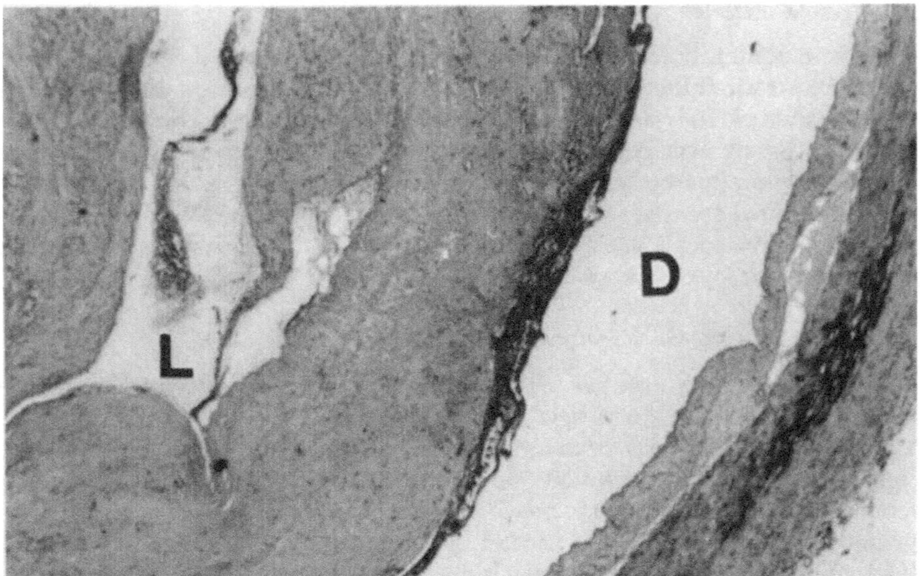

Fig. 6. Dissection by the catheter (*D*). *L*, residual lumen. The dissection lies between intima and media. HZ 13616/81. F.72/35. Hemalaun-eosin, × 30

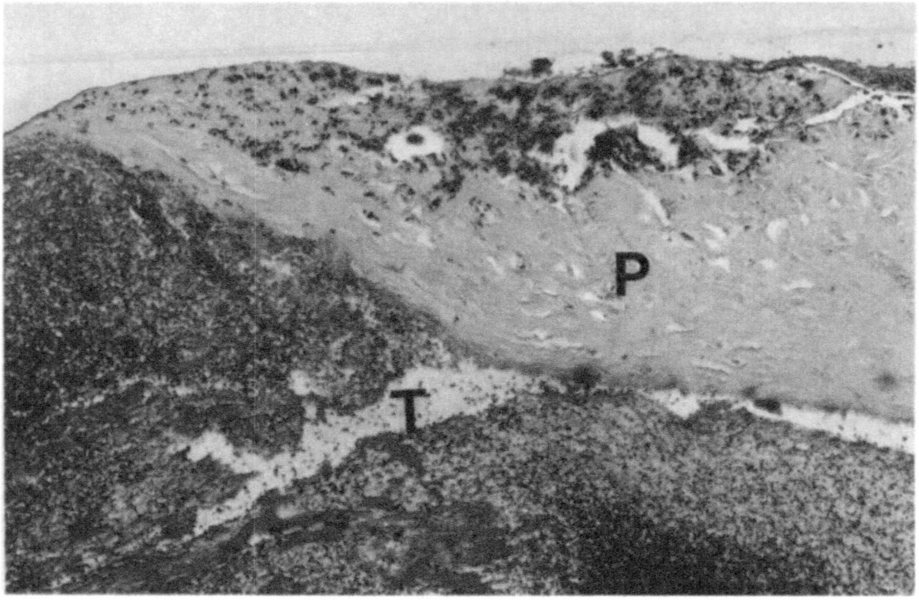

Fig. 7. Intimal plaque which was loosened during PTA and embolized into the periphery. The surgically removed plaque consists of dense collagen tissue (*P*) with apposition of thrombotic material (*T*). HZ 12207/81. F.74/22. Hemalaun-eosin, × 80

Obliterated Arteries

Complete obliteration of the arterial lumen may be due to a central thrombus which allows the catheter to penetrate and which also permits a dilatation of the central area of the vessel lumen. Obliteration by dense connective tissue, however, hardly ever permits perforation and dilatation with lasting succes. If perforation is apparently successful, the catheter usually forms a new lumen through intimal areas of insudation and fatty degeneration. This new channel is usually soon occluded again by thrombus formation. The chances of successful PTA are very low in these cases.

Inflammatory Arterial Diseases

Any inflammatory arterial disease, such as thromboangiitis obliterans, Takayasu's disease, pathergic granulomatoses, and collagen diseases, is complicated by the early formation of occluding thrombi. These thrombi are – unlike thrombi in arteriosclerotic arteries – quickly organized by dense connective tissue containing newly formed vasa vasorum. This dense tissue cannot be penetrated by the catheter. The media and adventitia are edematous and inflamed and may rupture easily. The danger of wall dissection and perforation of the catheter through the vessel wall is high. PTA is therefore not indicated in inflammatory arterial diseases. In later stages of the disease secondary arteriosclerosis develops and cannot be distinguished morphologically from genuine arteriosclerosis. Against these late alterations PTA may be successful with no increased risk of complications.

Combined Types of Arteriosclerosis

All the morphological features of arteriosclerosis which have been described above may occur in combination. Even combinations of dilating and obliterating types of arteriosclerosis and of genuine and secondary arteriosclerosis may be found. Unfortunately, radiology does not permit the distinction of these types. Even aneurysms may not be recognized if the lumen is filled by thrombi with a residual filiform vascular channel which simulates a narrowed lumen within an arteriosclerotic artery. Furthermore, the morphological pattern may vary in different segments of the same artery. This explains why it can never be foreseen what may happen during PTA and why PTA should only be performed with a trained vascular surgeon standing by. In spite of the various pitfalls and possible complications, the number of cases which have to be corrected by reconstructive surgery is astonishingly small.

Contribution to the Discussion on the Effects of PTA

A tube with contractile or elastic walls, such as a healthy artery, does not permit a mechanical dilatation which remains permanent. A tube with rigid walls, such as an arteriosclerotic vessel, reacts to a dilatating force according to physical laws. This means that an increase in the volume can be obtained either by rupture of the walls or by decrease in the thickness of the inner wall layers.

Rupture of the Wall

Ruptures may occur either in the thickened intima or in the fibrotic media. According to physical laws the resulting fissures run in a radial direction. This may actually happen in the intimal fibrotic layer. Crevasses which penetrate the whole intima to the internal elastic lamella produce an increase of the luminal surface. Later on the crevasses are organized by connective tissue but the lumen remains dilated.

It is as yet unknown whether a similar process may occur in the media. Morphological examinations including electron microscopy have not shown evidence of such a process so far, but this does not exclude the possibility of the development of microfissures within the fibrotic medial layer. Whether such traumatic fissures would lead to a permanent increase of the circumference depends on the state of the media musculature. If some of the contractile properties of the smooth muscles were left, the original circumference would probably be reestablished by contraction. If the walls were completely fibrotic a permanent dilatation would seem possible, but might be lost again later by shrinking of the scar tissue.

Compression of the Intima

"Compression" with permanent result can occur in two ways. Compression of appositional thrombotic material and of arteriosclerotic intimal plaques must be distinguished. Thrombotic material overlying the intima consists of homogeneous fibrinous masses with no or very little cellular attachment to the intima. Such material, which regularly occurs in arteriosclerotic vessels, is no longer detectable in arteries successfully treated by PTA. It appears that such material is not flattened against the walls but is pulverized by the compressing force and later swept away by the restored bloodstream. The embolization of these tiny particles usually has no clinical consequences; the fibrinous material is probably dissolved by spontaneous lysis.

A permanent compression of arteriosclerotic intimal plaques is hardly imaginable. However, examination by electron microscope shows that intimal plaques are often far from being compact. They frequently consist of debris of necrotic material, fatty deposits, cholesterin, and fibrin mixed with some collagen fibers and very few and widely scattered fibroblasts. A continuous endothelial lining is usually lacking, the surface being partly uncovered, partly lined by single, unconnected fibroblasts (pseudoendothelial lining). Such a tissue is easily compressible and the fluid components may be squeezed out into the vessel lumen at the proximal and distal end of the balloon. It remains unexplained, however, why such a compressed intimal proliferation does not expand again in a short period. Hypothetical explanations are: (a) that the compression may stimulate fibroblastic activity and that the resulting scar tissue may decrease by shrinking, (b) that microfissures may occur and undergo the same shrinking process, and (c) that parts of the debris might be removed by the reestablished bloodstream. None of these explanations, however, is completely convincing. As long as our knowledge is so limited, we must assume that there is not just one mechanism responsible for the various effects produced by PTA but that several may operate, either alone or in combination.

Summary

The morphological pattern of arteriosclerosis, which varies from case to case and sometimes even from segment to segment of the same artery, determines the outcome of PTA. Soft intimal cushions containing edematous fluid and few and tender collagen fibers as well as old fibrinous thrombotic material may be compressed with permanent success. The possible loosening and embolization of small fibrin particles seems to be well tolerated. This is probably due to spontaneous lysis of small emboli. Even concentric hyaline intimal proliferations may be distended by occurrence of radial ruptures. This permits a certain dilatation of the intimal ring. Intimal plaques in combination with intimal hemorrhage, fibrinous insudation, and spontaneous dissection between intima and media may be loosened by the catheter and carried into the periphery. This complication usually necessitates surgical intervention. Completely obliterated arteries are difficult to penetrate by the catheter if the occlusion consists of dense connective tissue without a residual central channel. In these cases the danger of dissection or perforation of the catheter through the atrophic media is high. Arteries in patients with inflammatory diseases are usually occluded by well-organized thrombi which can hardly be penetrated by the catheter. Perforation through the edematous and inflamed vessel wall may easily occur.

References

1. Baughman KL, Pasternak RC, Fallon JT, Block PC (1978) Coronary transluminal angioplasty in autopsied human hearts. Circulation 58 (2): 11–80
2. Block PC, Myler RK, Stertzer S, Fallon JT (1981) Morphology after transluminal angioplasty in human beings. N Engl J Med 305: 382
3. Castanega-Zunida WR, Formanek A, Tadavarthy M (1980) The mechanism of balloon angioplasty. Radiology 135: 565
4. Freudenberg H, Wefing H, Lichtlen PR (1978) Risks of transluminal coronary angioplasty: a postmortem study. Circulation 58 (2): 11–80
5. Lee G, Ikeda RM, Joye JA, Bogren HG, De Maria AN, Mason DT (1980) Evaluation of transluminal angioplasty of chronic coronary artery stenosis: value and limitations assessed in fresh human cadaver hearts. Circulation 61: 77
6. Leu HJ, Grüntzig A (1978) Histopathologic aspects of transluminal recanalization. In: Zeitler E, Grüntzig A, Schoop W (eds) Percutaneous vascular recanalization. Springer, Berlin Heidelberg New York, pp 39–50
7. Pasternak RC, Baughman KL, Fallon JT, Block PC (1980) Scanning electron microscopy after coronary transluminal angioplasty of normal canine coronary arteries. Am J Cardiol 45: 591
8. Simpson JB, Robert EW, Tillingham ME, Myler R, Harrison DC (1978) Coronary transluminal angioplasty in human cadaver hearts. Circulation 58 (2): 11–80

11. Pathological Basis for Percutaneous Catheter and Balloon Revascularization

D. Sinapius

Five years ago I histologically examined ten occluded segments of the superficial femoral artery, taken during saphenous vein bypass operation after application of percutaneous transluminal angioplasty (PTA) [2]. I have already indicated the dilating effect of PTA, which should become more evident using the balloon catheter. In order to demonstrate this, after application of the balloon catheter we examined ten additional segments of the superficial femoral artery, taken at autopsies on subjects of various ages and with different degrees of atherosclerosis.

We endeavored to answer the following questions:

1. Is any dilating effect apparent in microscopic sections after postmortem balloon catheter application?
2. Are there similar alterations of the vessel wall throughout life which are not to be attributed to the effect of PTA?
3. Are fibrous plaques and atheromas compressible by PTA?
4. Does PTA cause destruction of the vessel wall (mainly of the intima) which might lead to thrombosis in live patients?

In our 1978 publication a bulging effect of PTA, combined with a thinning of the media and forming of clefts between the layers of the intima or between intima and media, was shown [2]. Similarly, in these postmortem cases dilation of the lumen, thinning of the media, and cleavage of fibrous intima or cleavage between intima and media could be seen (Fig. 1). Dilation and cleavage were only missing in fibrous and rigid areas of several stenosed segments (Fig. 2). Atheromatous parts of the plaques were not compressible by PTA (Fig. 3). In this point I agree with Hempel [1], but I cannot confirm the findings of Leu and Grüntzig [3]. Moreover, fibrous plaques also seem not to be compressible.

Thinning of the tunica media is a frequent finding resulting from loss of elasticity. It is apparent in advanced age and also beneath atherosclerotic plaques. It should not be mistaken in histopathological examinations for a stretch effect due to the balloon catheter.

In the cases presented here, no ruptures of the intima were seen which could have produced thrombosis during life. The clefts do not communicate with the lumen (Figs. 1 and 3). Thus these ruptures should not be regarded as an effect of PTA. Only in one case is a deeper tear of intima and media seen, and this was probably caused by application of the balloon catheter (Fig. 4). But this tear does not communicate with the lumen.

Percutaneous Transluminal Angioplasty
(ed. by C. T. Dotter, A. Grüntzig, W. Schoop, E. Zeitler)

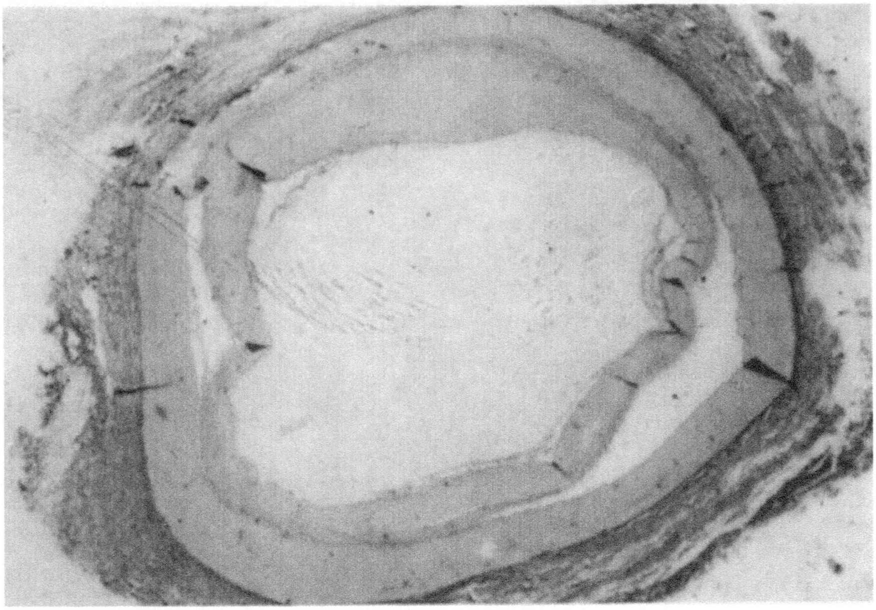

Fig. 1. Postmortem PTA by balloon catheter of the superficial femoral artery: dilation of the lumen, thinning of the media, clefts in the intima. A 76-year-old man. Elastica, × 14

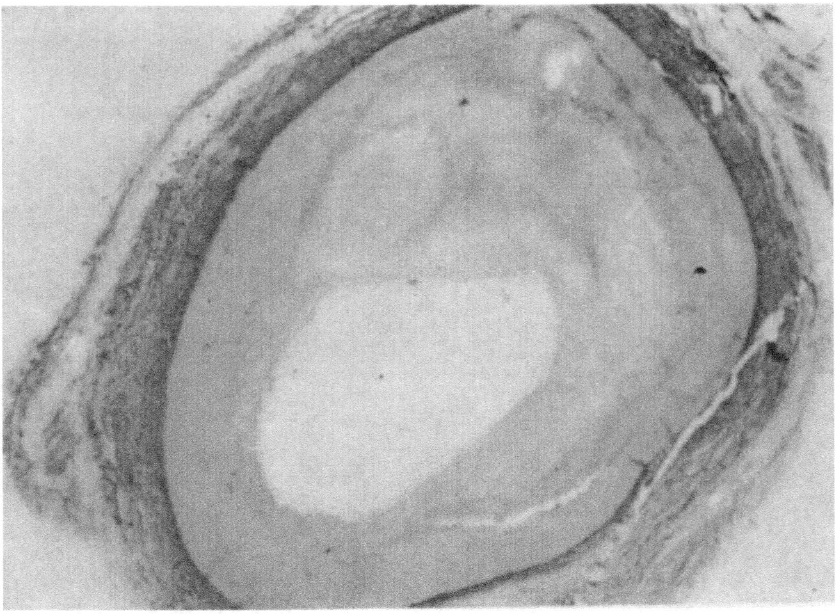

Fig. 2. Postmortem PTA by balloon catheter of another segment of the same artery as Fig. 1, severely stenosed by a fibrous rigid plaque. No dilation of the lumen, no thinning of the media, no clefts in the intima. Elastica, × 14

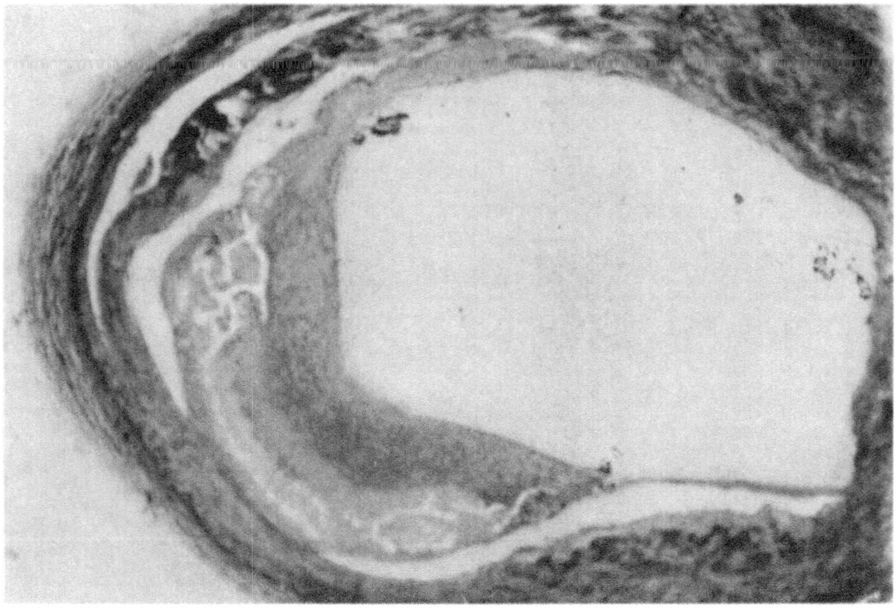

Fig. 3. Postmortem PTA by balloon catheter. Moderate dilation of the lumen of the superficial femoral artery in a segment with moderately stenosing atherosclerosis. Clefts between deep intima and media and in the media not communicating with the lumen. Atheroma in deep intima (*left*) not compressible. A 67-year-old man. Goldner, × 14

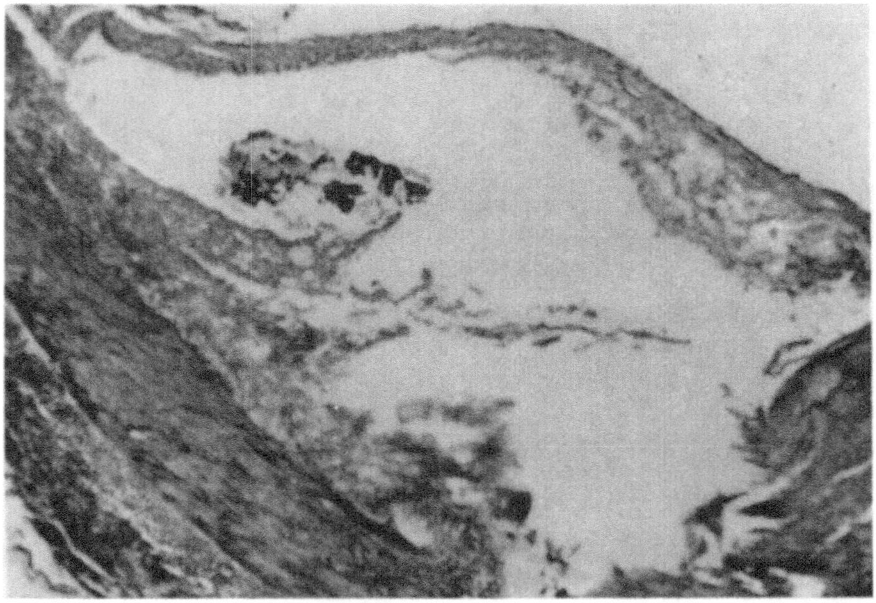

Fig. 4. Postmortem PTA by balloon catheter. Deep tear of the intima and media, possibly caused by the PTA procedure. No communication between the cleft and the lumen. A 72-year-old man. Goldner, × 35

References

1. Hempel KJ (1969) Morphologische Befunde zur Kompressibilität atheromatöser und thrombotischer Intimaveränderungen. In: 2nd Angiologisches Symposion. Aggertalklinik Engelskirchen
2. Jester HG, Sinapius D (1978) Morphologic alterations after percutaneous transluminal recanalization of chronic femoral atherosclerosis. In: Zeitler E, Grüntzig A, Schoop W (eds) Percutaneous vascular recanalization. Springer, Berlin Heidelberg New York, p 51
3. Leu HJ, Grüntzig A (1978) Histopathologic aspects of transluminal recanalization. In: Zeitler E, Grüntzig A, Schoop W (eds) Percutaneous vascular recanalization. Springer, Berlin Heidelberg New York

12. Results of Animal Experiments With Balloon Dilatation

C. L. Zollikofer, W. R. Castaneda-Zuniga, and K. Amplatz

Introduction

We have recently described a new concept, based on animal and human cadaver studies, which suggests that intimal disruption and medial stretching rather than remodeling or compression of atherosclerotic plaques represent the probable mechanism for increase in the diameter of the lumen after percutaneous transluminal angioplasty (PTA) [1, 2]. Similar findings have been reported by other authors, although some of them do not exclude plaque compression and mention the possibility of desquamation of superficial plaque elements [3–6].

Certainly this new concept has established some major progress in understanding the pathophysiological effects of angioplasty, but some major questions remained unanswered. How do the balloon size, the duration and pressure of balloon inflation, and the compliance of the balloon material influence the result of angioplasty? What are the advantages or disadvantages of polyethylene (PE) versus polyvinyl chloride (PVC)? Can the compliance of a normal artery or an atherosclerotic lesion be measured in order to determine the optimal amount of dilatation?

To answer these questions normal and atherosclerotic aortas in rabbits and normal carotid arteries in dogs were studied after angioplasty, using varying sizes of balloon and varying pressure and duration of balloon inflation. PE and PVC balloons from different manufacturers were used. To study the compliance of the arteries and the balloon catheters, pressure-volume curves during inflation of the balloons were recorded.

Experiments and Results

Rabbit Aortas

Aortas of atherosclerotic and normal New Zealand rabbits were dilated. Balloon sizes were approximately 25% and 50% larger than the internal diameters of the aortas and inflation times ranged from 15 to 60 s. The animals were killed within 15–30 min after dilatation. Dilated and control aortic segments were studied histologically and by electron microscopy.

Percutaneous Transluminal Angioplasty
(ed. by C. T. Dotter, A. Grüntzig, W. Schoop, E. Zeitler)

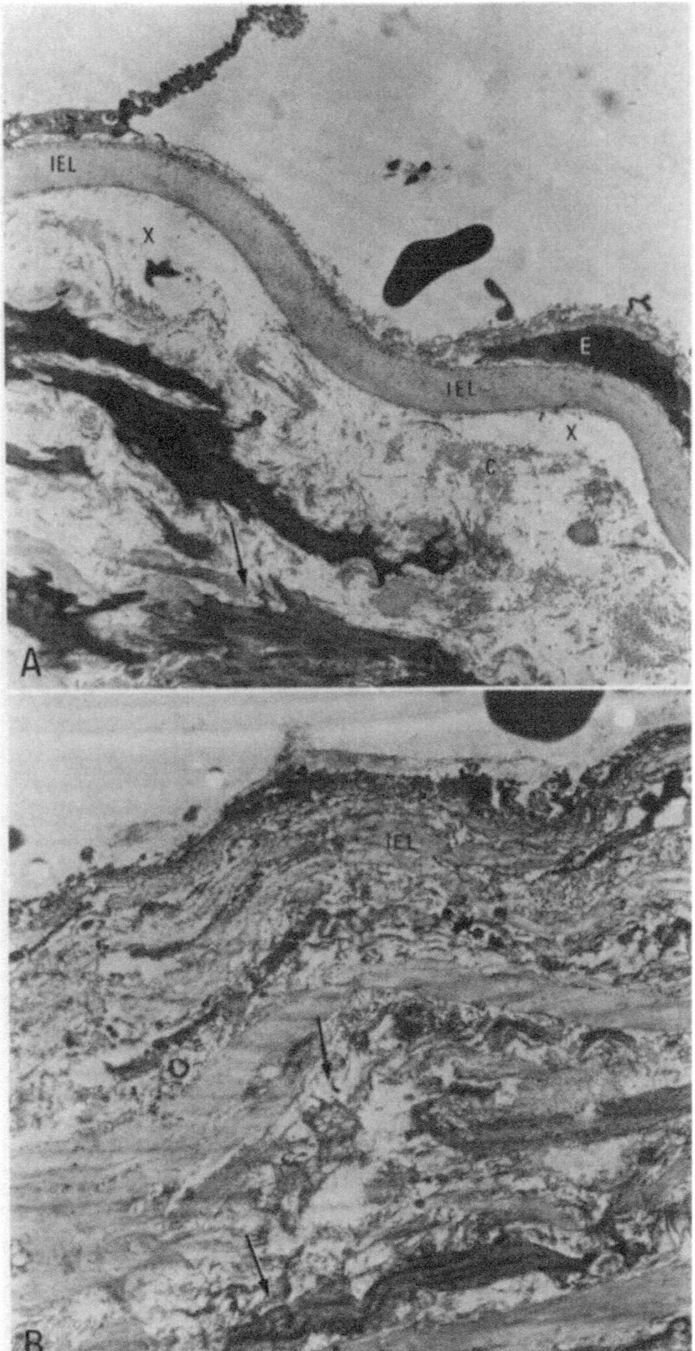

Fig. 1A, B. Transmission electron micrograph (× 5,000 approx.) **A** Normal rabbit aorta, over dilated by 50%, 30 s. Note partial destruction of endothelium (*E*). Internal elastic lamina (*IEL*) is intact. Detachment of collagen fibrils (*C*) from *IEL* with edema (*X*). Degenerating myocyte (*arrow*). **B** Normal rabbit aorta over dilated by 50%, 60 s. Endothelium is completely destroyed. *IEL* is fragmented. Most of the myocytes are degenerating and show hydropic changes (*arrows*). The wall looks compressed, collagen and elastic laminae are arranged in a disorderly manner. There has been progressive damage between 30 and 60 s

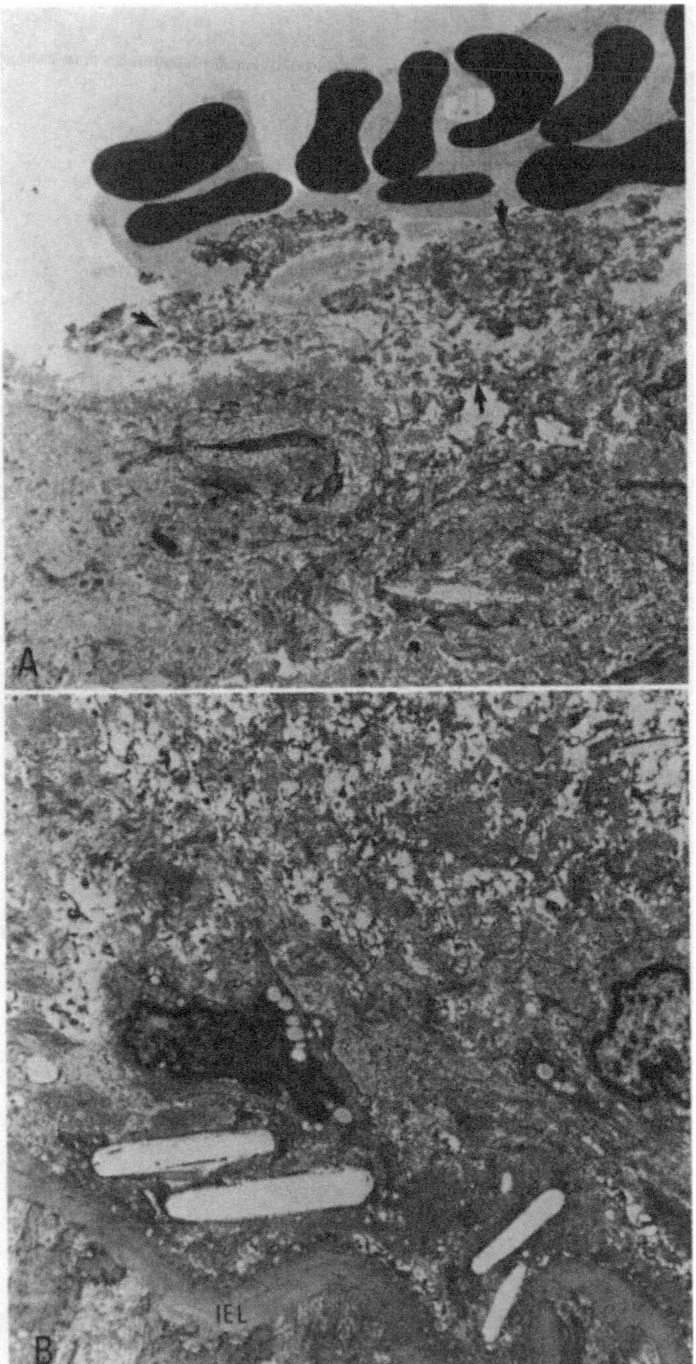

Fig. 2A, B. Transmission electron micrograph (× 5,000 approx.) Atherosclerotic rabbit aorta over dilated by 25%, 30 s. **A** Surface of plaque shows some loosened plaque material partially desquamated (*arrows*). **B** Deeper layers of the plaque adjacent to the internal elastic lamina (*IEL*) show no signs of compression

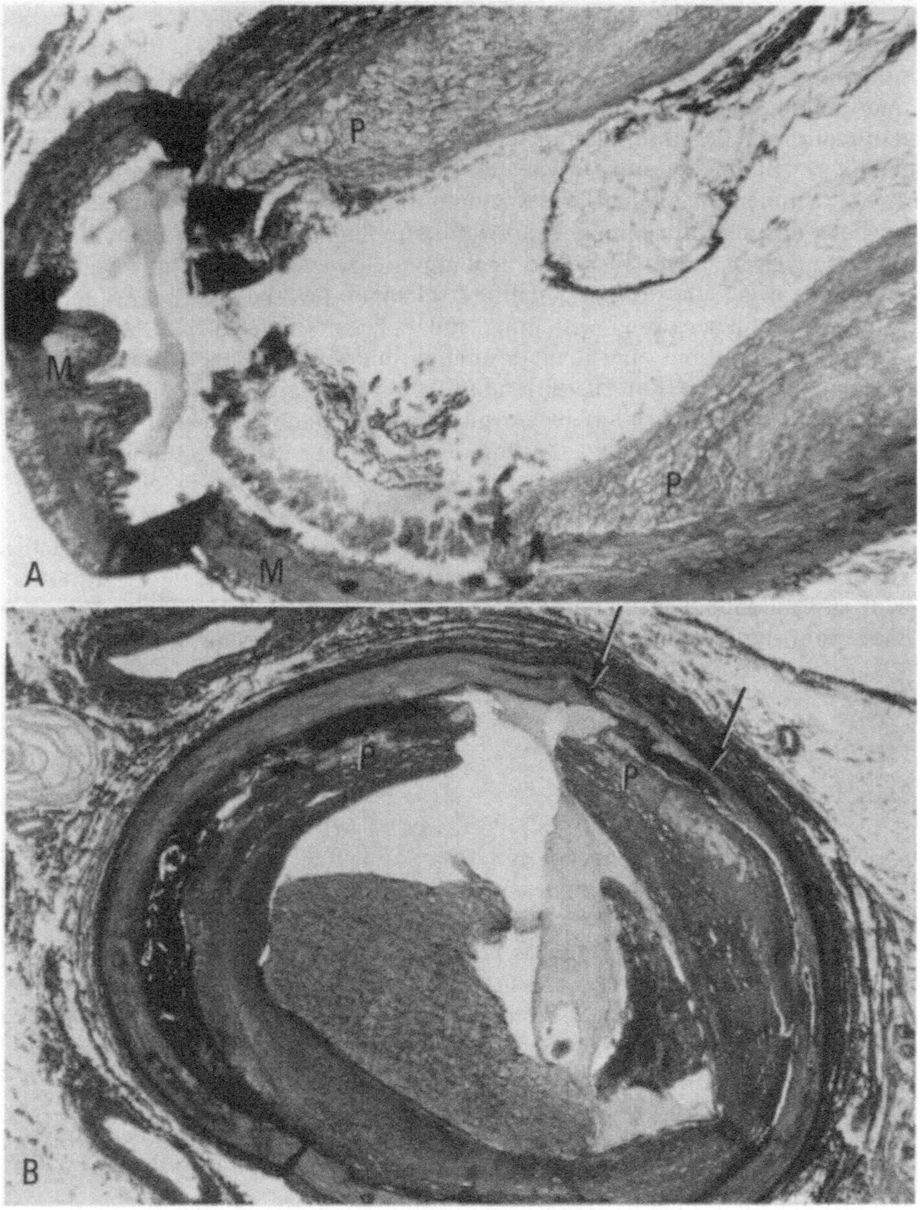

Fig. 3. A Photomicrograph of atherosclerotic rabbit aorta over dilated by 50%, 60 s. Note disruption of plaque (*P*) with partial dehiscence and marked stretching and partial disruption of media (*M*). **B** Photomicrograph of human femoral artery dilated 1 week previously (Courtesy of PD Dr. J. Schneider, Dept. of Pathology, University of Zürich). Note partial dehiscence of plaque (*P*) with rupture. Note tears in media (*arrow*). In *A* And *B* increase of lumen occurred with stretching and tearing of media where plaque is no longer adherent to underlying media

There was definite progression of acute changes with increasing balloon diameter and time in both the normal and atherosclerotic animals. In the nonatherosclerotic animals, changes varied from focal denudation of the endothelium and slight changes in the innermost part of the wall to complete denudation of the endothelium, clot formation, and continuously penetrating damage, with degenerating myocytes, edema, stretched and torn elastic fibers, and detachment of collagen fibers with increasing time and balloon size (Fig. 1). In the atherosclerotic animals there were only slight changes to the media where the latter was protected by overlying plaque. However, if the plaque ruptured or dissected away there were marked changes in the media, which were progressively penetrating with time and balloon size.

Apart from some superficial desquamation on the plaque surface (Fig. 2A), no signs of compression of the plaque (Fig. 2B) were seen. Dilatation of the vessel wall occurred in places were there was no plaque or were the plaque had ruptured or dissected away. As Fig. 3 shows, the postdilatational changes in atherosclerotic rabbit aortas are comparable to the histological changes seen in patients who have successfully undergone dilatation.

Moreover, we found the atherosclerotic wall to be more vulnerable. Changes observed by light microscopy and electron microscopy were more pronounced with shorter and lesser dilatation than was the case with the normal aortas. Also dissection into the media occurred only in the atherosclerotic animals.

Dog Carotid Arteries

Normal canine carotid arteries were dilated by 20%–100% using PE and PVC Grüntzig balloons. The animals were killed and the specimens were studied by light and electron microscopy immediately and at varying intervals of up to 3 months following balloon dilatation. In a second series of dogs, carotid arteries were dilated with increasing pressure of up to 12.5 atm using both PE and PVC balloons of sizes varying between the same and 100% larger than the internal diameter of the carotid arteries. The changes observed by light microscopy and the ultrastructural changes observed by electron microscopy were related to the balloon material and the size and the pressure of the balloons.

In the first part of the study acute, subacute, and chronic changes correlated well with the amount of overstretching (Fig. 4). Healing of the damaged media occurred, with intimal hyperplasia and extensive fibrosis replacing the damaged myocytes. At pressures of 4 atm a progression of histological changes was seen not only with increase in balloon size but also with PE balloons as compared to PVC balloons. As anticipated, the second part of the study also showed increasing damage to the arterial wall with higher inflation pressures. If the balloons were not or were only slightly oversize the histological changes were more severe with PVC balloons than with PE balloons because their higher compliance allowed increase of balloon diameter with rising inflation pressure (Fig. 5).

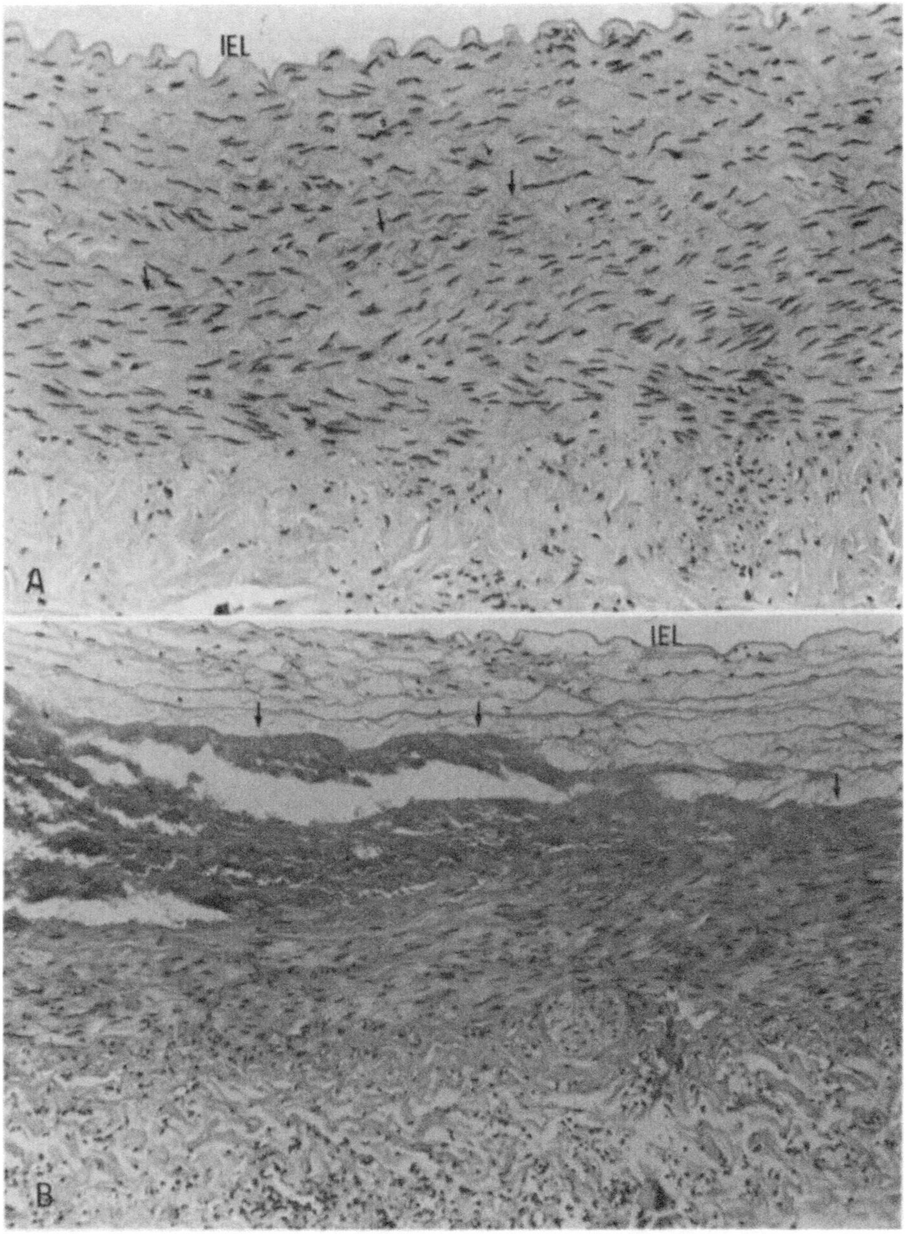

Fig. 4A, B. Photomicrographs of a canine carotid artery 24 h after dilatation show progressive damage with increasing balloon size. **A** 30% overdilatation with PE balloons shows denudation of endothelium. There is some edema in the inner part of the wall. Apart from some corkscrew nuclei the myocytes appear intact. Note normal undulation of elastic fibers (*arrows*). *IEL,* internal elastic lamina. **B** 100% overdilatation with PE balloon shows extensive dissection into the media with hemorrhage (*arrows*). The inner half of the media shows loss of most nuclei of the myocytes and marked stretching of the *IEL* and other elastic laminae

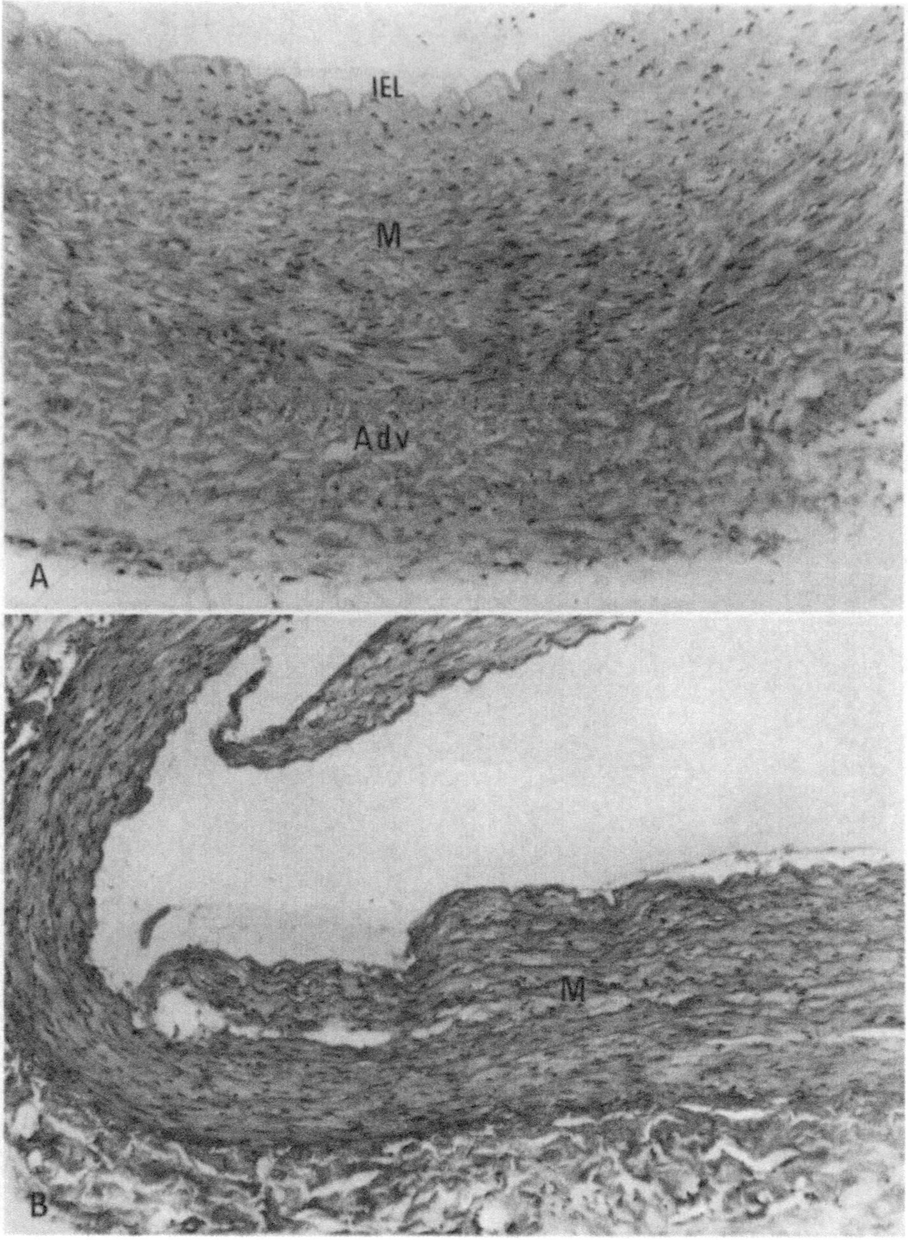

Fig. 5A, B. Photomicrograph of a canine carotid artery 4 mm in diameter 30 h after dilatation. **A** Segment dilated with 4-mm PE balloon. There is denudation of the endothelium with stretching of the internal elastic lamina (*IEL*) and some damage to the inner third of the media (*M*) with edema and loss of some of the nuclei of myocytes. *Adv,* adventitia. **B** Segment dilated with 4-mm PVC balloon. Note extensive damage with dissection and partial disruption of the media (*M*). The entire wall shows extensive changes with numerous corkscrew nuclei

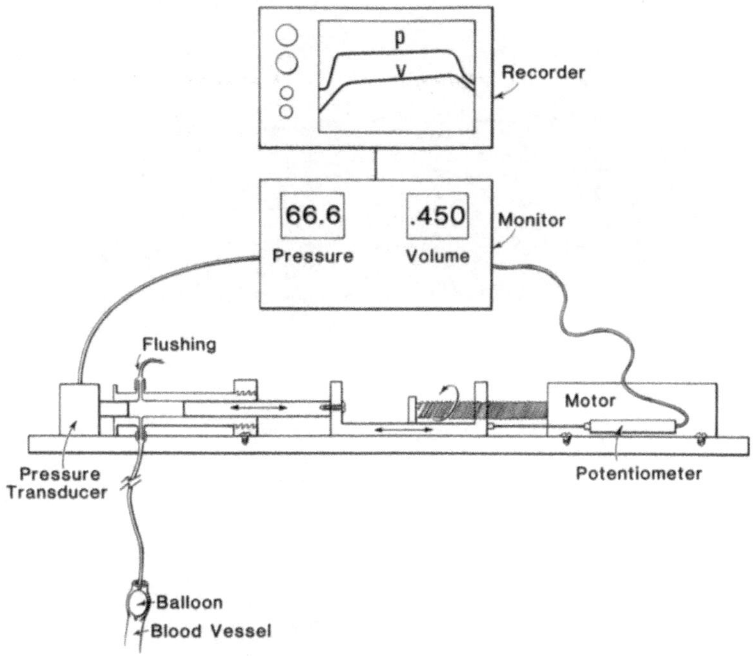

Fig. 6. Apparatus for simultaneous recording of balloon pressure and flow into and out of the balloon (Medi-Tech Inc., Watertown MA 02172). *p*, pressure curve; *v*, volume curve

Compliance Studies

To evaluate further the impact of the balloon compliance on the result cf PTA, PE and PVC balloons were tested in vitro and in vivo. An apparatus which allowed simultaneous and continuous monitoring of balloon pressure and flow into and out of the balloon (Fig. 6) was used. A servomotor pump compensating for volume or pressure changes within the balloon allowed pressure-volume curves to be recorded during arterial dilatation and in vitro tests.

Balloon Compliance

In vitro tests were performed with the balloon in water at 37° C, or in animal and human cadaver arteries. In vivo, normal canine carotid arteries were dilated with balloons of sizes varying between the same and 100% larger than the lumen of the arteries. Pressures varied from 4 to 12.5 atm. Inflation times were three times 1 min.

When testing the balloons in water, fairly characteristic volume-pressure curves were obtained for PE and PVC balloons. As Fig. 7 shows, PE balloons exhibit a much lower compliance than PVC. No spontaneous rupture of the PE balloons occurred at constant pressure of 4.5 atm even after several minutes. There were also differences in compliance among PE and PVC balloons from different manufacturers. Most striking was the difference between the PE

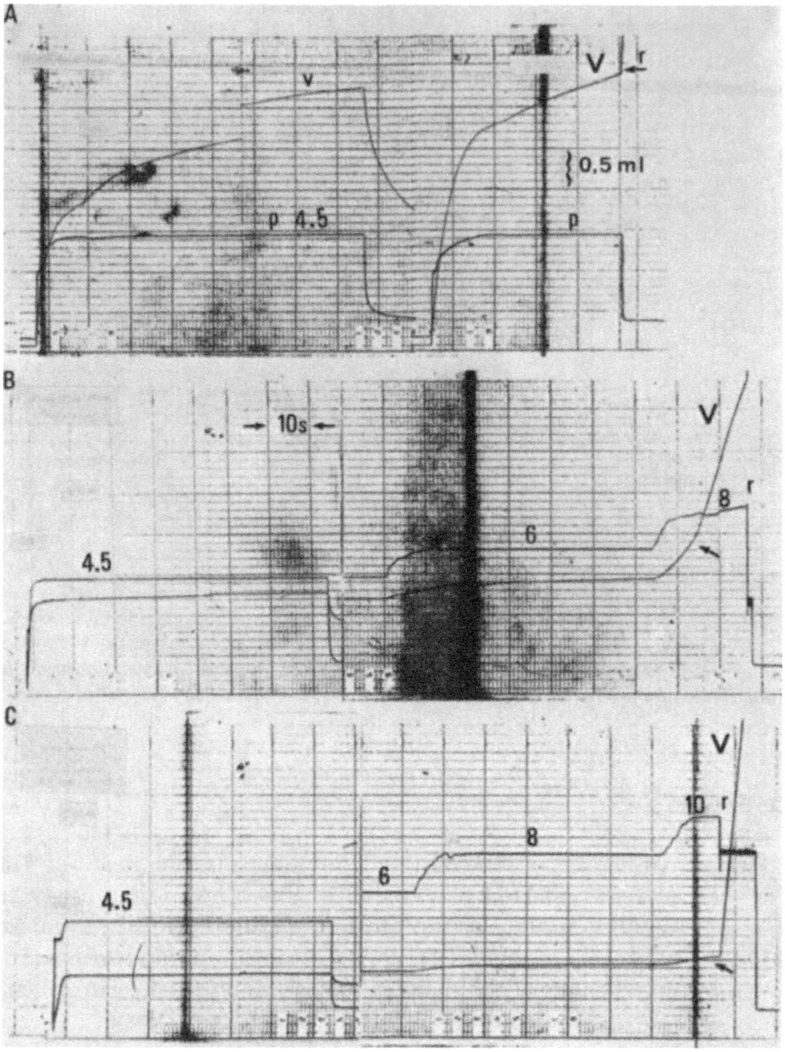

Fig. 7A–C. Pressure-volume tracings to characterize balloon compliance. **A** 6-mm, 2-cm PVC balloon. Note the significant volume increase over 2 min with spontaneous rupture (*r*) of the balloon after 45 s, of the second inflation at 4 1/2 atm. *p*, pressure; *v*, volume curve. **B** 6-mm, 2-cm PE 1 balloon. Much less volume increase over 2 min at 4 1/2 atm than in **A**. Only when pressure is raised from 6 to 8 atm there is significant volume increase (*arrow*), with rupture after 20 s (*r*). **C** 6-mm, 2-cm PE 2 balloon. Volume increase over 2 min at 4 1/2 atm is almost zero. Even when pressure is increased from 6 to 10 atm, volume increase (*arrow*) is limited until rupture of the balloon (*r*)

materials 1 and 2 if the pressure of inflation was raised from normal working pressure of 4.5 to near bursting pressure. Figure 7 shows considerable stretching of the PE material 1 with increasing pressure. In other words, the compliance or the "banana effect" at high pressure was much less with the PE material 2 than with PE 1.

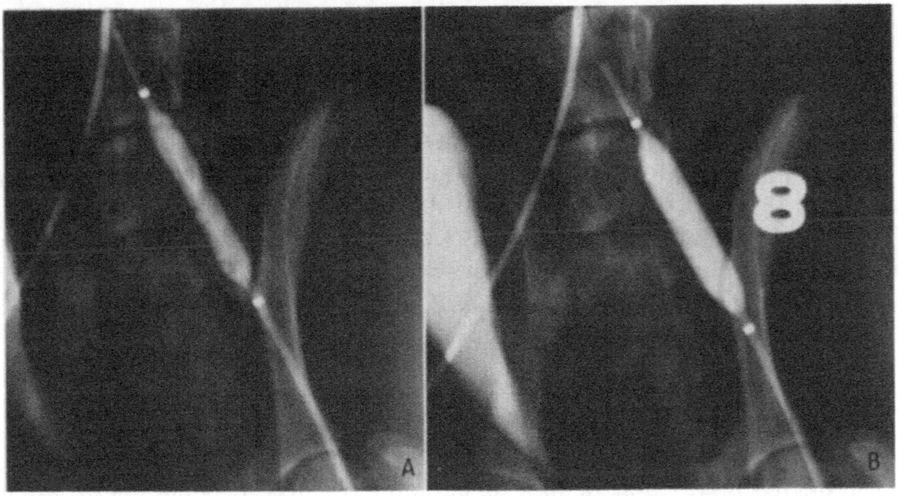

Fig. 8A, B. Dilatation of canine iliac artery with 8-mm PE Balloon. **A** At 4 1/2 atm actual diameter of balloon is only 6.6 mm. **B** Only after artery has ruptured at 10 atm the balloon does gain its supposed diameter of 8 mm

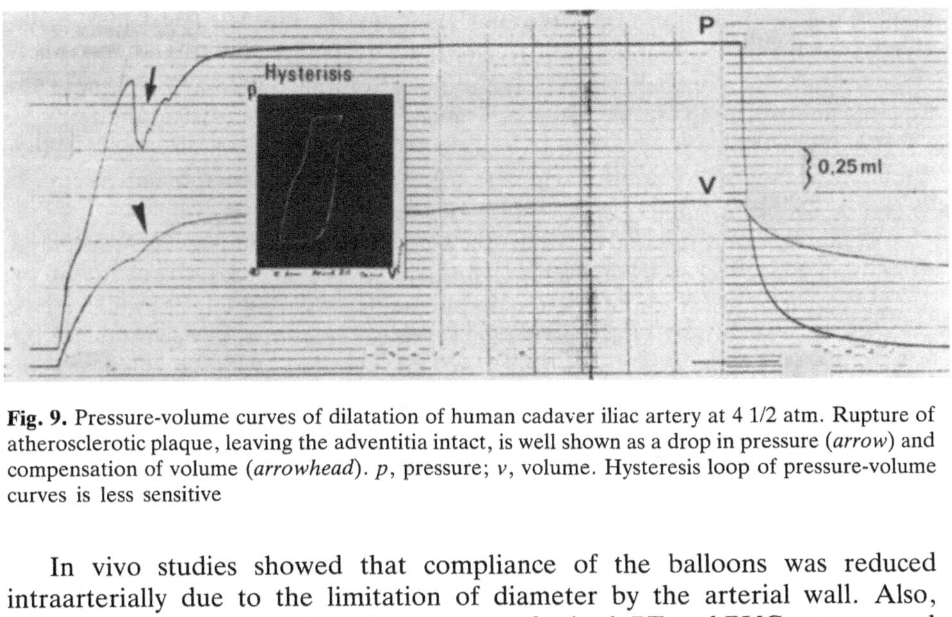

Fig. 9. Pressure-volume curves of dilatation of human cadaver iliac artery at 4 1/2 atm. Rupture of atherosclerotic plaque, leaving the adventitia intact, is well shown as a drop in pressure (*arrow*) and compensation of volume (*arrowhead*). *p*, pressure; *v*, volume. Hysteresis loop of pressure-volume curves is less sensitive

In vivo studies showed that compliance of the balloons was reduced intraarterially due to the limitation of diameter by the arterial wall. Also, bursting pressures were about 2 atm greater for both PE and PVC as compared to the balloons tested outside the arteries. Furthermore, 50%–100% oversized balloons did not reach their supposed diameter at normal working pressures in healthy arteries or hard lesions (Fig. 8).

Arterial Compliance

To optimize results in PTA the compliance of a vascular lesion ought to be known. By using a noncompliant system with recording of pressure-volume curves we hoped to show the arterial compliance. When dilating normal canine arteries the so-called creep or compliance of the slowly stretching arterial wall could not be detected. Increasing volume of the balloon with multiple dilatations of an artery was too inconsistent and could not be differentiated from the balloon's own compliance. However, a sudden tearing of the media or breaking of an atherosclerotic plaque in cadaver arteries as well as disruptions of artificial stenoses in in vitro studies are well documented on pressure-volume curves (Fig. 9). The pressure curves proved to be more sensitive than the volume curves. The plotting of volume against pressure curves with inflation and deflation of the balloon – "hysteresis loop" – was of no benefit (Fig. 9).

Discussion and Conclusions

The degree of vascular damage is definitely related to balloon size, inflation pressure, and duration of inflation in normal as well as in atherosclerotic arteries. The most important mechanisms which increase the arterial lumen in PTA seem to be: (a) rupture and splitting of the atherosclerotic plaque or dehiscence of the plaque from the underlying media; and (b) stretching of the arterial wall with damage to the myocytes and stretching and possibly tearing of elastic fibers in areas where there is minimal intimal thickening or where the plaque has ruptured or has dissected away from the underlying media.

Desquamation of superficial plaque elements was shown by electron microscopy but it is doubtful whether this amounts to a significant degree of increase in lumen unless major parts of the plaque are loosened.

Again no compression of atherosclerotic plaques could be demonstrated. Although the atherosclerotic animal model may be criticized because of the difference in composition of the human plaque, our own findings as well as those of others [3–5] show that the histological changes seen in atherosclerotic rabbits and human arteries after angioplasty are comparable. Whether and how the healing process and formation of scar tissue in the damaged atherosclerotic artery differ from those in the normal canine and rabbit arteries cannot be answered at this time. Long-term studies using the atherosclerotic animal model will be necessary to explain why scarring and thrombus formation do not reduce lumen size after angioplasty.

Because of their considerably lower compliance PE balloons seem to be preferable to PVC balloons. Damage to the arterial wall is better controlled, especially with the PE material 2, because the diameter and shape of the balloon are much better retained and change only little with increasing inflation pressure. Therefore, higher pressure can be applied, which may be necessary in hard or fibrotic lesions. Also the dilating force is better concentrated on the actual lesions. Expansion of the balloon distal and proximal to a localized lesion which may cause damage to an uninvolved segment is minimal (Fig. 10).

Although it was not possible to differentiate the creep of the arterial wall from the balloon's own compliance in normal arteries, a sudden change in the mechanical properties of the arterial wall was well documented on pressure-vol-

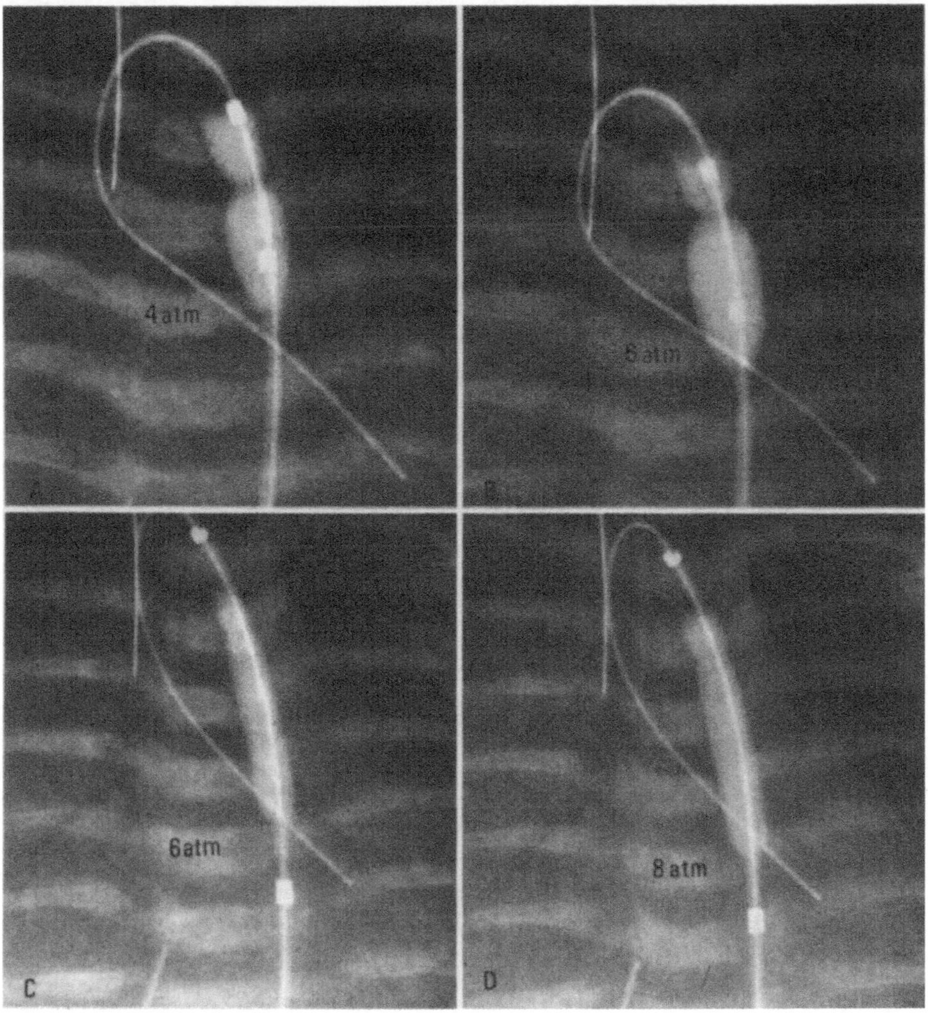

Fig. 10A–D. **A** and **B** show extensive ballooning of PVC balloon in localized aortic lesion. **C** and **D** PE 2 balloon retains shape well even with pressures up to 8 atm. There is almost no waist seen at area of lesion

ume curves during balloon inflation. Using a noncompliant syringe system for continuous pressure recording during balloon inflation, it was possible to demonstrate a sudden yield of the vessel wall or disruption of an atherosclerotic plaque. We think this may be important for optimization of results in PTA. Such a system made available for clinical use may help to determine at which point dilatation of a stenosis should be terminated.

Summary

Observations made in the atherosclerotic animal model are analogous to the findings in human atherosclerotic vessels after percutaneous transluminal angioplasty (PTA). Histological changes after PTA are definitely related to balloon size, pressure, and duration of balloon inflation, as well as to the balloon material. The two most important mechanisms which are responsible for the increase in the arterial lumen after PTA seem to be: (a) rupture and splitting and dehiscence of the atherosclerotic plaque from the underlying media, and (b) stretching of the arterial wall at places where the media is freed from the encasing effect of the thickened intima.

Because of their lower compliance polyethylene (PE) Grüntzig balloons are more effective and safer than polyvinyl chloride (PVC) balloons. This is especially true in hard and localized lesions where high inflation pressure may be neccessary. The use of a noncompliant syringe system with continuous recording of the balloon pressure during inflation may be helpful in determining when to terminate the dilatation of a stenosis and so optimizing results in PTA.

References

1. Castaneda-Zuniga WR, Formanek A, Tadavarthy M et al. (1980) The mechanism of balloon angioplasty. Radiology 135: 565–571
2. Castaneda-Zuniga WR, Amplatz K, Laerum F et al. (1981) Mechanics of angioplasty: an experimental approach. Radiographics 1: 1–14
3. Block PC, Baughman KL, Pasternak RC et al. (1980) Transluminal angioplasty: correlation of morphologic and angiographic findings in an experimental model. Circulation 61: 778–785
4. Block PC, Fallon JT, Elmer D (1980) Experimental angioplasty: lessons from the laboratory. AJR 135: 907–912
5. Hoffmann MA, Fallon JT, Greenfield AJ et al. (1981) Arterial pathology after percutaneous transluminal angioplasty. AJR 137: 147–149
6. Saffitz JE, Totty WG, McClennan BL et al. (1981) Percutaneous transluminal angioplasty. Radiology 141: 651–654

13. Radiological Pattern at and After Angioplasty

F.-J. Roth, G. Cappius, and E. Fingerhut

The idea of an angioplasty is to increase the insufficient blood flow in occlusive arterial disease. In performing angioplasty, one must deal with injury at the puncture site and in the treated segment of the artery caused by the introduction and dilatation of the treating balloon catheter.

In this chapter only the injury of the vessel wall caused by the dilating force of the balloon catheter will be discussed. The extent of the damage to the vessel wall depends on the forces of the dilating balloon and the mechanism of angioplasty itself. The mechanisms of angioplasty are:

1. A compression of the atheromatous material causing the vascular obstruction [6, 7].
2. The overstretching of the vessel wall [5].

In our experience, these two mechanisms may occur alone or together. The overstretching is the more frequent and important one. For the purposes of analysis, one may distinguish between the postangioplasty arteriogram taken immediately after the Dotter procedure and the follow-up arteriogram.

The Postangioplasty Arteriogram

The injury caused by means of the dilating balloon depends on the size of the diameter of the balloon compared to the diameter of the vessel and on the dilating force. If the postangioplasty arteriogram demonstrates a patent artery with a smooth wall, it may be assumed that there is no severe injury of the vascular wall.

Often a residual stenosis (Table 1) is demonstrated arteriographically. When we evaluated 334 consecutive angiograms from our clinical series of 2,257 angioplasties performed in the last 5 years, we observed a residual stenosis in 66%; the lumen was normal in size in the remaining 34%. The degree of the stenosis was calculated by the method described in 1972 by Alter et al. [1]. In the postangioplasty arteriogram one often sees irregularity of the wall of the artery (Table 1), probably caused by compression of the core substance. This occured in 70% of our patients; a smooth vessel wall was observed in only 8%.

In many instances the postangioplasty arteriogram reveals a separate margin of the contrast column (Fig. 1). This represents a splitting of the intima. It is caused by a partial overstretching of the vascular wall. The ruptured intima heals

Percutaneous Transluminal Angioplasty
(ed. by C. T. Dotter, A. Grüntzig, W. Schoop, E. Zeitler)

Table 1. Radiographic pattern of 334 consecutive postangioplasty arteriograms

	n	Wall irregularity	Smooth wall	Separate margin of contrast column	Intramural cleft	Overstretching	Residual stenosis (%)		
							∅	≤ 50	> 50
Iliac artery stenosis	109	66 (60%)	14	50 (46%)	7	2	29	74	6
Groin artery stenosis	26	18 (69%)	2	15 (58%)	1		6	20	
Femoropopliteal artery stenosis	75	61 (81%)	5	44 (59%)	1	3	28	46	1
Femoropopliteal artery occlusion	124	92 (74%)	7	60 (48%)	6	4	49	71	4
Total	334	237 (70%)	28 (8%)	169 (51%)	15 (4.5%)	9 (2.7%)	112 (34%)	211 (63%)	11 (3%)

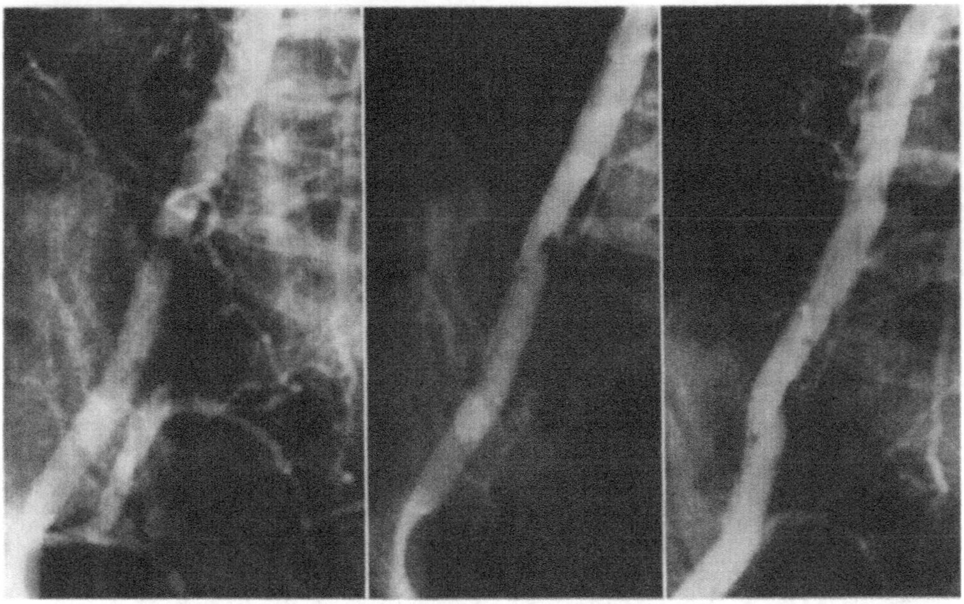

a b c

Fig. 1. a Stenosis of external iliac artery. **b** Postangioplasty arterogram: slight residual stenosis, separate margin of contrast column (intimal split). **c** Control arteriogram 6 months after angioplasty: disappearance of the intimal split and the residual stenosis

and enlargement of the lumen is observed in the control arteriogram (Fig. 2). This process takes 1–2 weeks, as demonstrated in 1980 by Block et al. [2] in experimental angioplasty in rabbits. We sometimes observed this phenomenon in our patients, too; the intimal split occurred in 51%.

If the localized injury to the vascular wall is more severe, the split may extend through the intima into the media (Fig. 3), and rarely into the adventitia. Usually, overstretching does not involve the entire vascular wall. Angiographically, the intramural cleft (Fig. 3) corresponds with the damage to the vascular wall [2, 3, 10, 11]. This injury tends not to be reversible. A control arteriogram may reveal localized ectasia in the dilated arterial segment (Fig. 3). Such damage is found arteriographically in 4.5%.

Overstretching (Fig. 4) is seldom observed. It is defined as a focal ectasia of the entire vascular wall with tearing of the elastic fibers following angioplasty, without evidence of splitting of the intima and media in the postangioplasty arteriogram.

If the guide wire and consequently the balloon catheter slide subintimally, a neolumen will be produced (Fig. 5). The postangioplasty arteriogram may reveal a double-barreled lumen. This was observed in our material only once in 2,257 angioplasties. This injury is believed to be a dissection. Dissection is a rare complication of angioplasty. Usually these patients need surgery, not because of severe deterioration caused by angioplasty but because the catheter treatment failed to improve the condition.

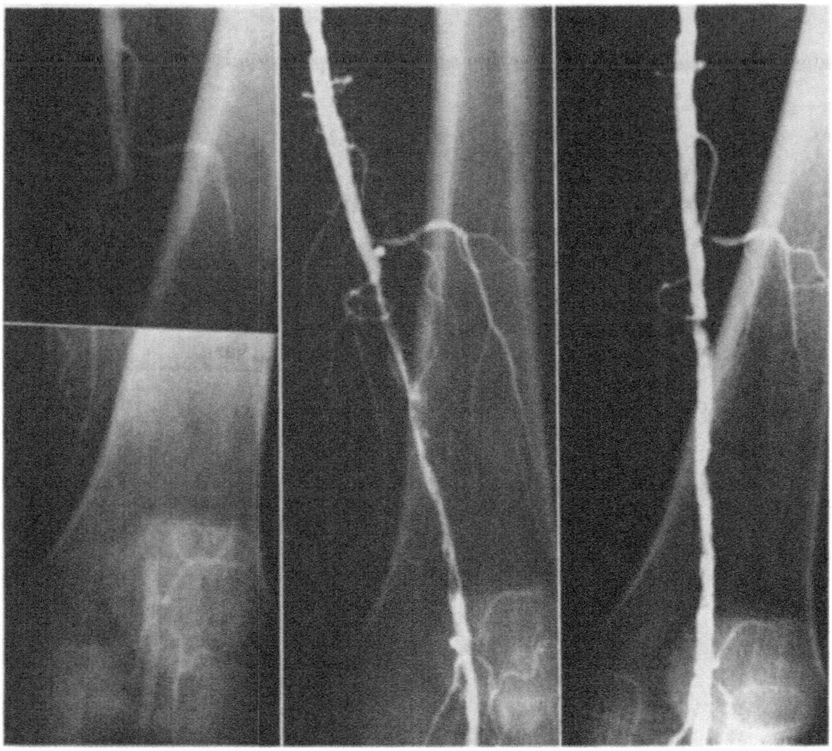

a b c

Fig. 2. **a** Occlusion of the superficial femoral artery. **b** Postangioplasty arteriogram: significant residual stenosis, separate margin of contrast column. **c** Control arteriogram 1 year after angioplasty: enlargement of lumen, stenosis in the area of the former occlusion because of recurrence

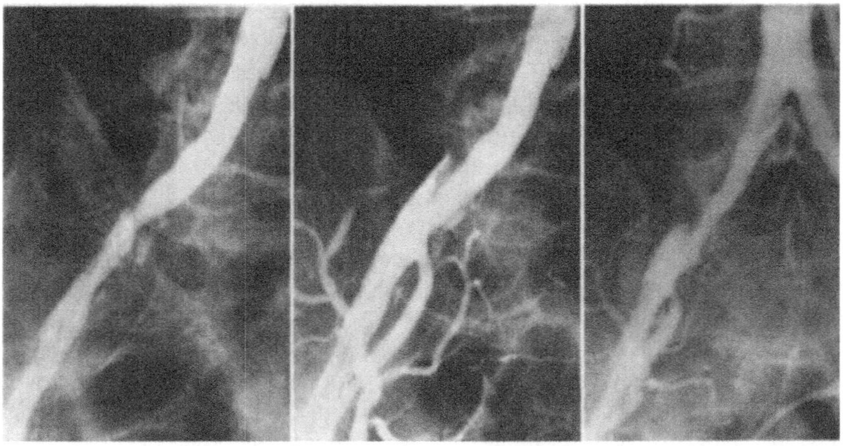

a b c

Fig. 3. **a** Stenosis of the external iliac artery. **b** Postangioplasty arteriogram: intramural cleft (medial split). **c** Control arteriogram 27 months after angioplasty: localized ectasia in the area of the former stenosis

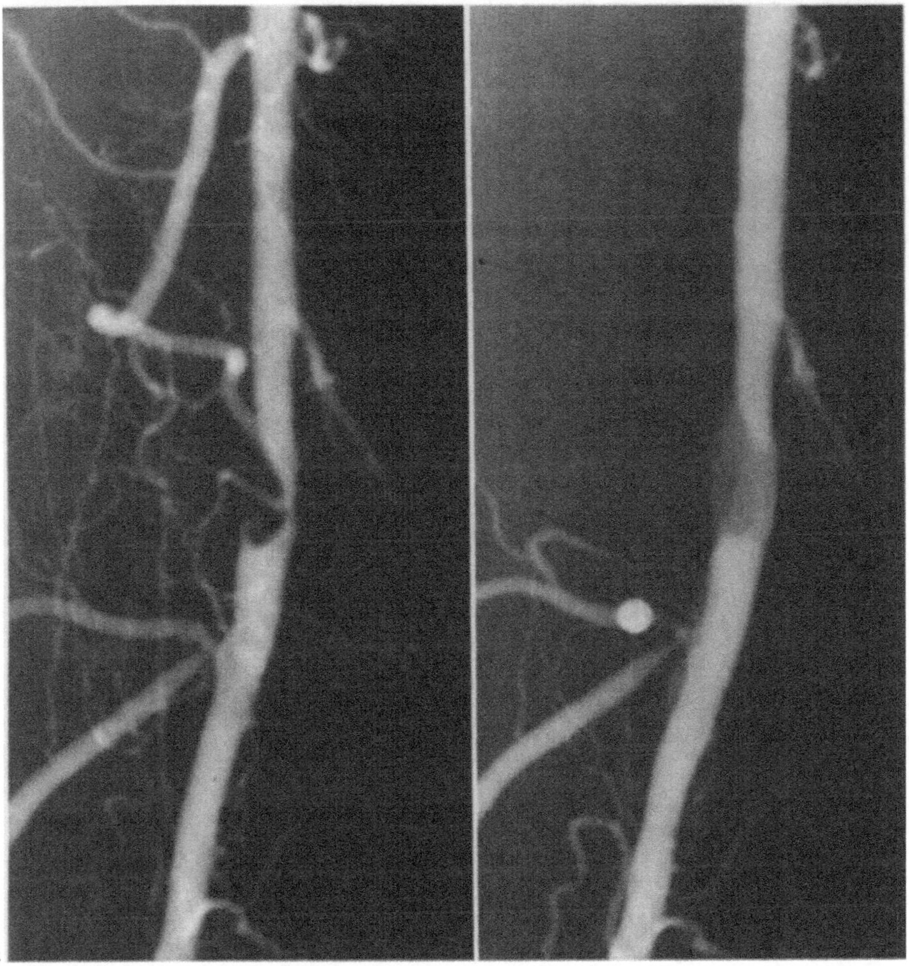

Fig. 4. a Stenosis of the superficial femoral artery. **b** Postangioplasty arteriogram: focal overstretching of the vascular wall

In 3 out of 2,257 cases a false aneurysm was found, caused by a perforation by the guide wire or by a rupture of the intima and media extending through the adventitia. We observed two aneurysms after angioplasty and one as an unexpected finding when an arteriogram was repeated because of acceleration of the atherosclerotic disease on the contralateral side (Fig. 6).

Rarely, spasm of the treated artery occurs following angioplasty (Fig. 7). In the case of successful angioplasty the collateral vessels will be reduced in size or disappear.

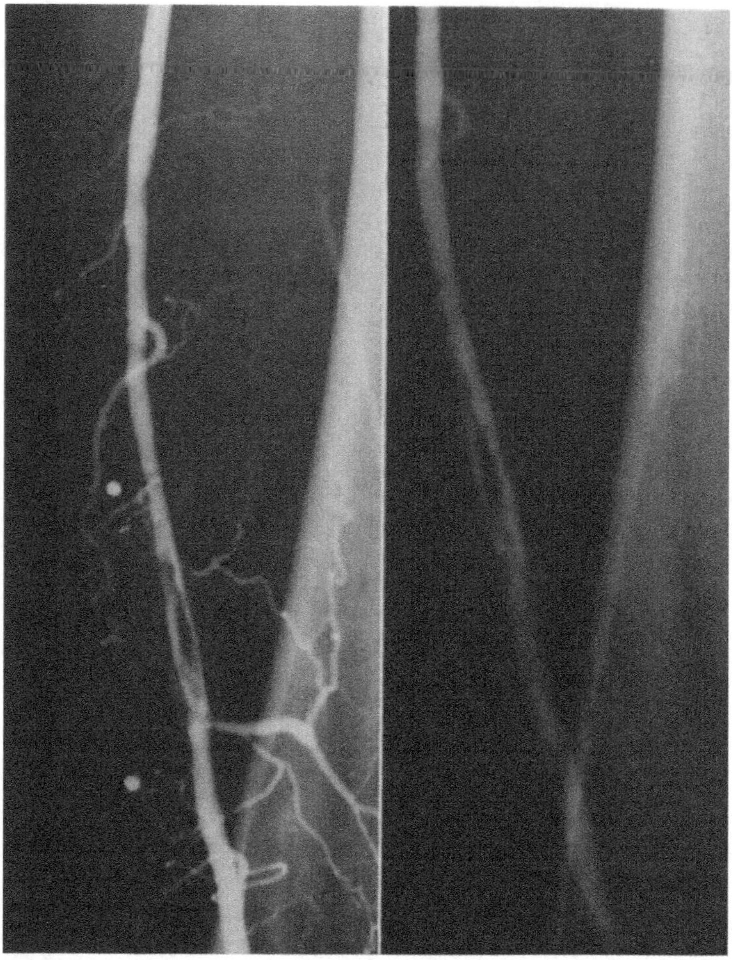

a b

Fig. 5. a Arteriogram immediately after angioplasty of an occlusion of the superficial femoral artery: dissection producing a double-barreled lumen. **b** Control arteriogram 10 days after angioplasty: no change, patent superficial femoral artery with double-barreled lumen (neolumen)

The postangioplasty arteriogram may reveal one or more of the following patterns:

- Residual stenosis
- Irregularity of contrast column
- Separated margin of contrast column
- Overstretching (local ectasia)
- Spasm
- Intraluminal clot formation
- Disappearance of collateral vessels
- Neolumen (dissection)
- Aneurysm (perforation)
- Intramural cleft.

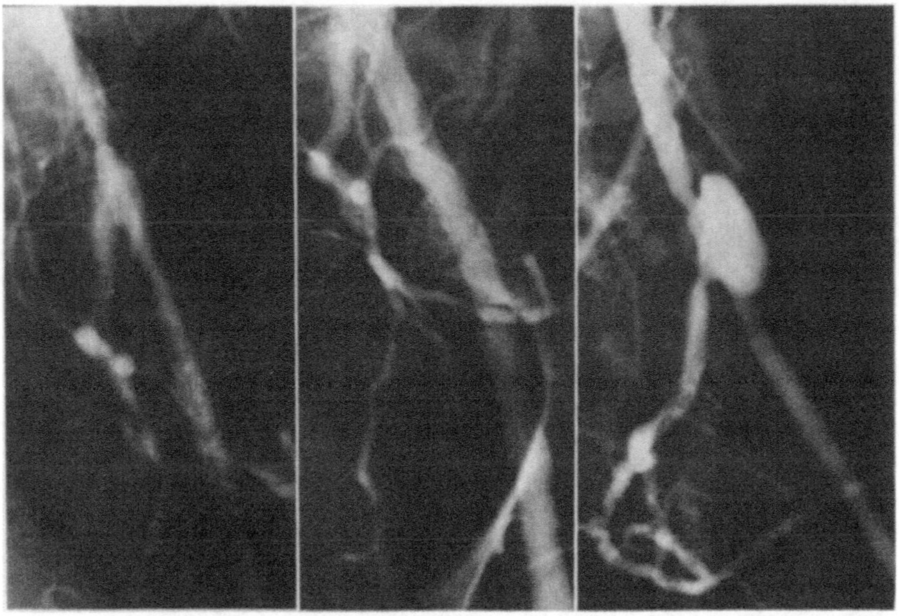

a b c

Fig. 6. a Stenosis of common iliac artery. **b** Postangioplasty arteriogram: patent common iliac artery. **c** Control arteriogram 1 year after angioplasty: false aneurysm in the area of the former stenosis

The Follow-up Arteriogram

The follow-up arteriogram is performed days, weeks, or years following angioplasty because of recurrence or acceleration of the atherosclerotic disease. One finds that the irregularities in the contrast column are smoothed (Fig. 1c). The separate margin of the contrast column disappears within 2–4 weeks (Fig. 1). Often an increase in luminal size (Fig. 2) is observed. These changes are caused by healing of the injury of the intima and media; there is also a retraction of the intimal flap raised by the dilating forces of the balloon catheter [2].

In cases of recurrence, an unusually long stenosis (Fig. 8) is often found in the formerly occluded arterial segment. In a few cases we observed a local ectasia in the dilated arterial portion, especially if the postangioplasty arteriogram revealed an intramural cleft (Fig. 3).

Discussion

In performing angioplasty one must expect a controlled focal injury of the intima and media. Desquamation of endothelium, a rupture of atherosclerotic plaques, and localized splitting of the intima and media [2–5, 10–12] are the changes to

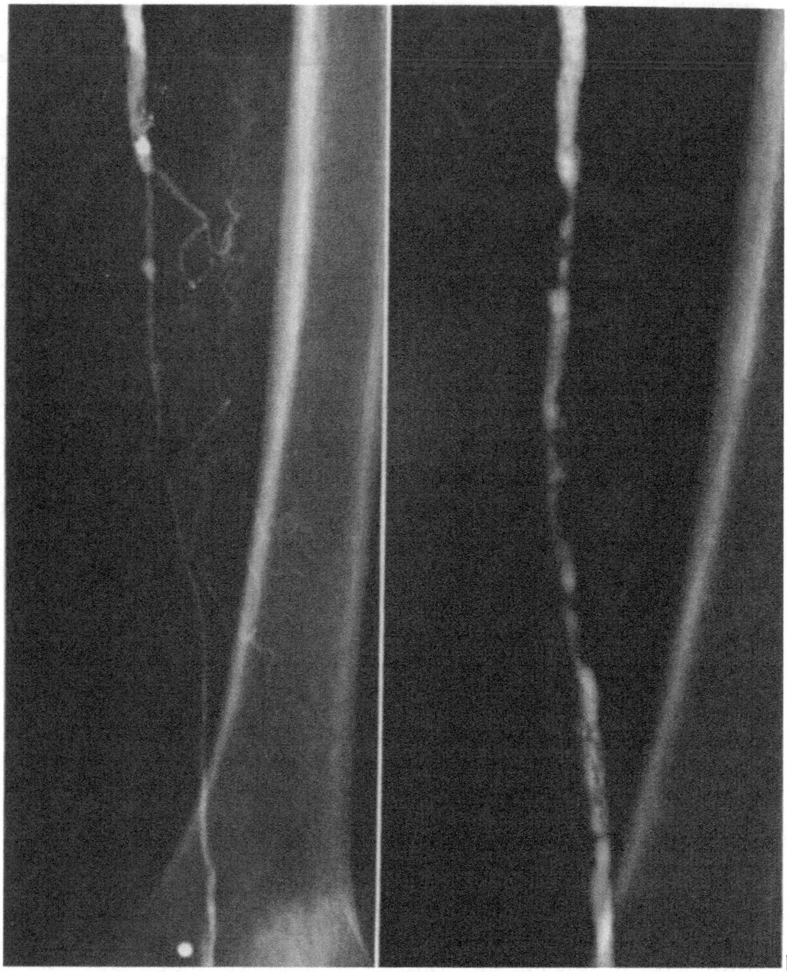

a b

Fig. 7. a Postangioplasty arteriogram following recanalization of a superficial femoral artery with a long occlusion: poor primary results with a long residual stenosis. **b** Control arteriogram 7 days after angioplasty: enlargement of lumen

Fig. 8. a Occlusion of superficial femoral artery. **b** Postangioplasty arteriogram: separate margin of contrast column. **c** Arteriogram because of recurrence 7 months later: long stenosis in the area of the former occlusion. **d** Postangioplasty arteriogram after repeated angioplasty: separate margin of contrast column, patent superficial femoral artery

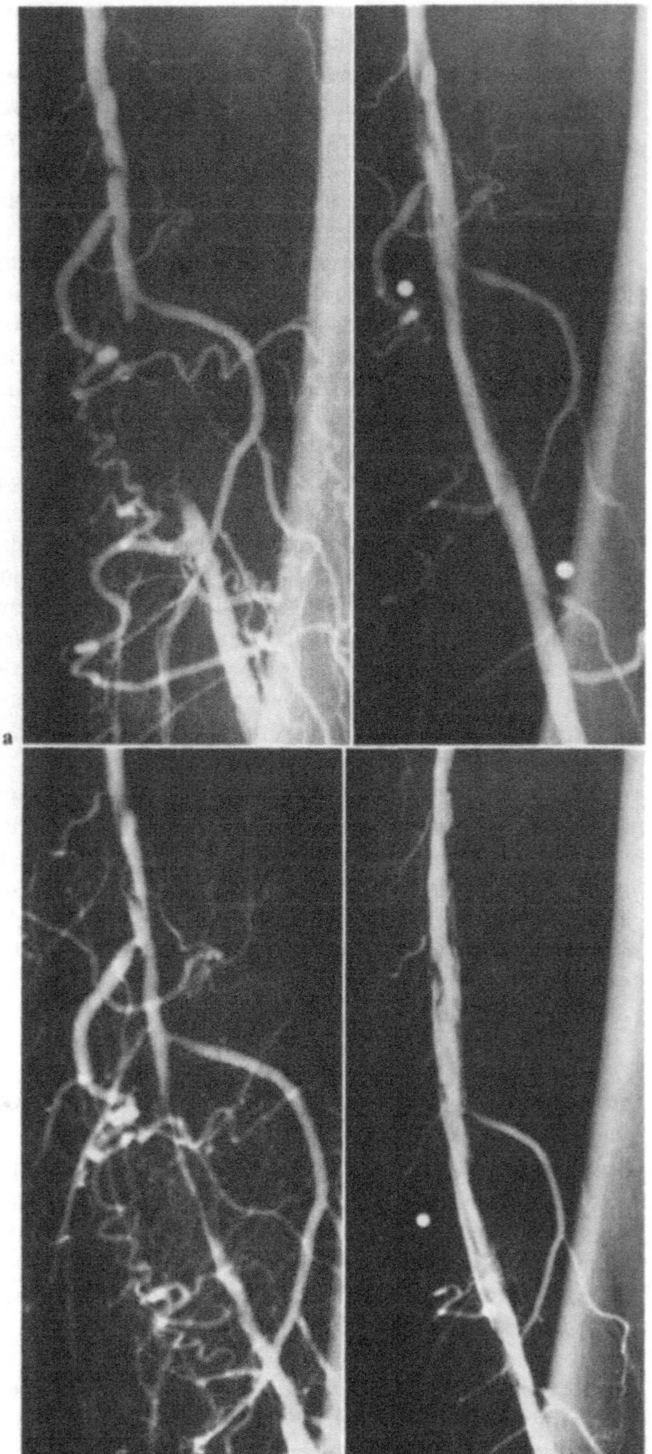

Fig. 8a–d

be found. The first two alterations mentioned are hardly visible in the postangioplasty arteriogram.

Splitting of the intima may be demonstrated angiographically as a separate margin of the contrast column [2]. The postangioplasty arteriogram demonstrated this injury in 51% of our patients. In our experience this damage to the arterial wall is reversible (Fig. 1). On the other hand, medial splits occurred in only 4.5% of our 334 patients. This damage to the vascular wall is not completely reversible (Fig. 3) and the control arteriogram may reveal a focal ectasia.

In the control arteriogram a moderate enlargement of the luminal size (Figs. 1, 2, and 7) is often observed. This change is caused by the healing of the damaged intima and media as well as the ruptured atherosclerotic plaques [2]. The damage to the intima and media should not be thought of as a dissection. Only if the guide wire and the catheter slide subintimally and a double-barreled lumen (Fig. 5) is produced should these changes be called a dissection.

In 66% of our evaluated material a residual stenosis was evident in the postangioplasty arteriogram. In only 3% (Table 1) was the degree of the stenosis over 50%. In most instances the residual stenosis was clinically without hemodynamic effect. In our experience the slight residual stenosis does not tend to cause recurrence. On the other hand, a significant residual stenosis may produce recurrence. Often the slight residual stenosis disappears in the follow-up because of healing of the injured vascular wall [2–4, 8].

In cases of recurrence an unusually long stenosis is sometimes observed in the previously treated arterial segment (Fig. 8). These stenoses are believed to be a response of the intima and media to the localized injury due to the dilating balloon catheter.

In performing angioplasty one should be aware that one is causing controlled focal damage to the intima and media, and may be to the adventitia. The severity of the injury depends on the diameter and force of the dilating balloon. In order to prevent damage to the vascular wall an appropriate balloon diameter has to be chosen. It is recommended that a balloon diameter 1 mm smaller than the arterial diameter demonstrated by the arteriogram be used. In any case, the balloon diameter should not exceed the vessel diameter.

Summary

A series of 334 postangioplasty arteriograms is evaluated. Residual stenosis, mostly without hemodynamic effect, are observed in 66%. In 70% irregularity of the vascular wall is observed, and in 51% a separate margin to the contrast column (intimal split) can be seen. Occasionally (in 4.5%), splitting of the media (intramural celft), spasm, dissection, or overstretching are found in the postangioplasty arteriogram.

The control arteriogram taken days, weeks, or months after angioplasty reveals a smoothing of the vascular wall and an increase in luminal size produced by healing of the focal vessel wall injury. In cases of recurrence, an unusually long stenosis sometimes occurs in the area of the former occlusion. These changes are probably the response of the intima and media to the focal injury from the dilating forces of the balloon. It is emphasized that in order to avoid severe injury to the vascular wall the balloon catheter should not be larger than the diameter of the artery.

References

1. Alter M, Kieffer S, Resch J, Ansari K (1972) Cerebral infarction: clinical and angiographic correlations. Neurology 22: 590–601
2. Block PC, Fallon JT, Elmer D (1980) Experimental angioplasty: lessons from the laboratory. AJR 135: 907–912
3. Block PC, Baughman KL, Pasternak RC, Fallon JT (1980) Transluminal angioplasty: correlation of morphologic and angiographic findings in an experimental model. Circulation 61: 778–785
4. Block PC, Myler RK, Stertzer S, Fallon JT (1981) Medical intelligence: morphology after transluminal angioplasty in human beings. N Engl J Med 305: 382–385
5. Castaneda-Zuniga WR, Formanek A, Tadavarthy M, Vlodaves Z, Edwards JE, Zollikover C, Amplatz K (1980) The mechanism of balloon angioplasty. Radiology 135: 565–571
6. Dotter CT (1978) Transluminal angioplasty – pathologic basis. In: Percutaneous vascular recanalization. Springer, Berlin Heidelberg New York, pp 3–12
7. Dotter CT, Judkins MP (1964) Transluminal treatment of arteriosclerotic obstruction: description of a new technic and a preliminary report of its application. Circulation 30: 654–670
8. Fallon JT (1980) Pathology of arterial lesions amenable to percutaneous transluminal angioplasty. AJR 135: 913–916
9. Grüntzig A, Hoppff H (1974) Perkutane Rekanalisation chronischer arterieller Verschlüsse mit einem neuen Dilatationskatheter. Modifikation der Dotter-Technik. Dtsch Med Wochenschr 99: 2502–2509
10. Höhn P, Wagner R, Zeitler E (1975) Histologische Befunde nach der Katheterbehandlung arterieller Obliterationen nach Dotter und ihre Bedeutung. Herz/Kreisl 7: 13–23
11. Leu HJ, Grüntzig A (1978) Histophatologic aspects of transluminal recanalization. In: Percutaneous vascular recanalization. Springer, Berlin Heidelberg New York, pp 39–50
12. Pasternak RC, Baughman KL, Fallon JT, Block PC (1980) Scanning electron microscopy after coronary transluminal angioplasty of normal canine coronary arteries. Am J Cardiol 45: 591–598
13. Porstmann W (1973) Ein neuer Korsett-Ballonkatheter zur transluminalen Rekanalisation nach Dotter unter besonderer Berücksichtigung von Obliterationen an den Beckenarterien. Radiol Diagn (Berl) 14: 239–244
14. Simpson JB, Robert EW, Billingham ME, Myler RK, Harrison DC (1978) Coronary transluminal angioplasty in human cadaver hearts. Circulation [Suppl 2] 58: 11–80
15. Zeitler E, Grüntzig A, Schoop W (eds) (1978) Percutaneous vascular recanalization: technique, application, clinical results. Springer, Berlin Heidelberg New York
16. Zeitler E, Schoop W, Zahnow W (1971) The treatment of occlusive arterial disease by transluminal catheter angioplasty. Radiology 99: 19–26

IV. Medical Treatment

14. Percutaneous Transluminal Angioplasty: Adjunct Drug Therapy

E.-I. Richter and E. Zeitler

Accessory drug treatment before, during, and after percutaneous transluminal angioplasty (PTA) has the following goals:

1. To avoid platelet aggregation leading to early rethrombosis
2. To avoid acute thrombosis during the procedure when flow is minimized by the dilating catheter
3. To avoid mechanically induced spasm
4. To maintain peripheral perfusion during the catheter dilatation and the subsequent manual compression of the arterial puncture site after catheter removal.

Mechanical alterations of the intimal layer of arteries during PTA, as well as vascular wall damage at the puncture site from catheter introduction, require a check on the coagulation system. At the recanalization site all medications that prevent platelet aggregation and formation of a fibrin network in the artery and the catheter are of value in avoiding rethrombosis and embolization. However, anything hindering thrombus development presents an increased risk of bleeding from the site of arterial access, with the associated complications of hematoma or pseudoaneurysm formation. After a clean intrainguinal puncture, the risk of bleeding after treatment is minimized by manual compression and a pressure bandage for 2 days. Unless a hematoma develops, any medical measures within the scope of PTA should be designed to preclude clot formation at the site of the mechanically caused intimal lesion.

Coagulability must be decreased during treatment, since the intraarterial catheter reduces the velocity of the blood, and laminar flow may become turbulent. Above all, the inner and outer surface of the catheter within the vessel is a site of increased thrombogenesis, which varies depending on the catheter material. It is important to prevent blood entering the catheter.

Various forms of adjunct drug therapy have been used so far:

1. Heparin treatment after effective PTA [7, 10, 11, 22, 26–28]
2. Dextran infusion after effective PTA [2, 4, 9, 25]
3. Aggregation inhibitors after effective PTA: acetylsalicylic acid (ASA) 0.5 g three times daily [11, 27, 28] or Anturane (a sulfinpyrazone derivative which is a salicylate antidote and potentiates the action of coumarin derivatives 200 mg four times daily [7, 8]
4. Heparin administered intraarterially after the puncture but before dilatation: 5,000 IU [5, 6, 12, 17, 29]; 10,000 IU [1, 2, 11, 26–28]

Percutaneous Transluminal Angioplasty
(ed. by C. T. Dotter, A. Grüntzig, W. Schoop, E. Zeitler)

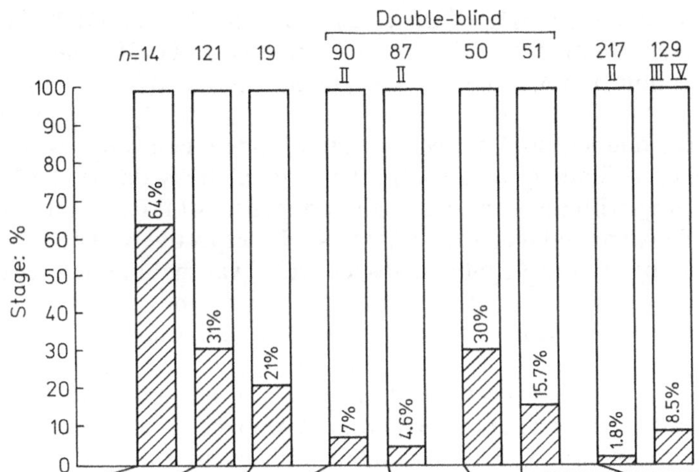

Drugs	Without	Heparin 5000 IU i.a +25000 IU 2-7 days		ASA +Heparin +Heparin pump Infusion 2 days	ASA +Heparin i.a. 5000 IU Φ	ASA	Asasantin	Asasantin+ Heparin 5000 IU
Cathether	Dotter	Dotter	Dotter	Dotter or single Teflon	Dotter	Ödman gray (70) Grüntzig (31)		Single Teflon+ Grüntzig
Within	10	7	10	10		14		14 days
Author	Zeitler	Wierny	Zeitler	Zeitler et al.		Hess et al.		Zeitler et al.
Year	1969	1973	1973	1973		1978		1981

Fig. 1. Rate of rethrombosis after successful PTA of leg arteries with the additional use of various drugs. *ASA*, acetylsalicylic acid; *Asasantin,* 330 acetylsalicylic acid + 75 mg dipyridamole

5. Platelet aggregation inhibitor (ASA) plus heparin administered intravenously after PTA [11, 27, 28]
6. Pre- and posttreatment with aggregation inhibitor only [28]: ASA, 0.5 g three times daily 2 days before and 10–14 days after PTA; or dipyridamole plus ASA, two or three times one tablet for 1 day before and for 1 day after PTA [11, 23, 24, 28]
7. Pretreatment with aggregation inhibitor ASA 0.5 g three times daily for 2 days, plus posttreatment with aggregation inhibitor ASA 0.5 g three times daily for 10–14 days, plus heparin infusion until effective coumarin levels are established after successful PTA [15, 16, 27]
8. Sufficient anticoagulation with coumarin before and after PTA [11, 25]
9. Fibrinolysis with streptokinase or urokinase during or after PTA [13, 18, 20, 21]

Quite similar results were obtained by using the various forms of additional drug therapy (Fig. 1). Of the patients treated with heparin alone after PTA (initial 5,000 IU plus pump infusion of 1,000–1,500 IU/h for 2 days), 20% had rethrombosis within 10 days. An initial dose of 10,000 IU heparin following arterial puncture but before PTA, with subsequent heparin treatment, resulted in rethrombosis in 31% of 121 cases [26] within 7 days. Of 30 patients given the combined treatment with heparin (initially 5,000 IU plus 1,500 IU/h) and aggregation inhibitor (ASA 0.5 g three times daily), 10% suffered rethrombosis.

In a double-blind study [14, 28] with premedication with an aggregation inhibitor in both groups (ASA 0.5 g three times daily), and with treatment continuing with the same ASA dose after successful PTA, the rethrombosis rate at 10 days was reduced to 7.0% and 4.6% respectively. The difference between the groups (90 and 87 patients respectively) was that the first received additional heparin according to the schedule previously shown.

The combined treatment with heparin and Acetosal (ASA) was found to increase the risk of posttreatment bleeding at the puncture site. Of the 90 patients given the combined treatment, 11 had posttraumatic bleeding; this occurred in only six in the ASA group. Grüntzig initially treated his patients with heparin and van Andel his patients with coumarin until a sufficient anticoagulation effect was obtained (thrombo test to a level of about 10%), but both later revised their regimens. Van Andel had to give blood transfusions to four patients because of copious posttreatment bleeding.

A double-blind study [14] carried out with different catheters demonstrated that the number of rethromboses within 2 weeks was significantly less with ASA (330 mg) combined with dipyridamole (75 mg) three times daily than with ASA (330 mg) alone three times daily 2 days before to 2 weeks after PTA.

Taking into consideration the various forms of accessory drug treatment and the frequency of rethrombosis within the first 2 weeks after succesful PTA (Fig. 1), the positive effects of oral medication with aggregation inhibitors become evident. However, it is yet to be determined whether an additional intraarterial application of heparin during catheter treatment is meaningful. Comparison of the rethrombosis rates in two double-blind studies [14, 28] shows that intraarterial application of heparin reduces the rethrombosis rate. Fibrinogen uptake studies have shown not only that an intimal lesion is produced at the site of the therapeutic dilatation, but also that fibrinogen is deposited [3, 27].

After antegrade catheter angiography in one leg, uniform fibrinogen accumulation, proportional to leg diameter and without a discerniable peak, was established by means of the fibrinogen uptake test. Only at the puncture site, with its local thrombosis, was an increased fibrinogen accumulation of 5%–10% demonstrable (Fig. 2). In contrast, increased fibrinogen deposition was demonstrable, even without hemodynamically effective stenosis (Fig. 3), at the site of the catheter dilatation.

The technique for the fibrinogen uptake test was as follows. Immediately after effective PTA the patients received 100 μCi ^{125}I-fibrinogen intravenously. During the following 7 days the activity was measured at 14 positions in each extremity. Single values were expressed as percentages of activity, with background measured over the precordium. The results are demonstrated as an activity profile (Figs. 2–4). The left side of the graph represents the puncture site at the groin. Anatomic reference points from thigh to foot are shown from left to right.

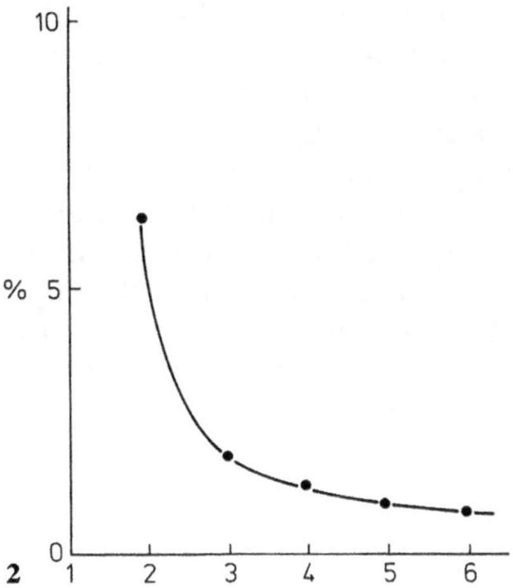

2

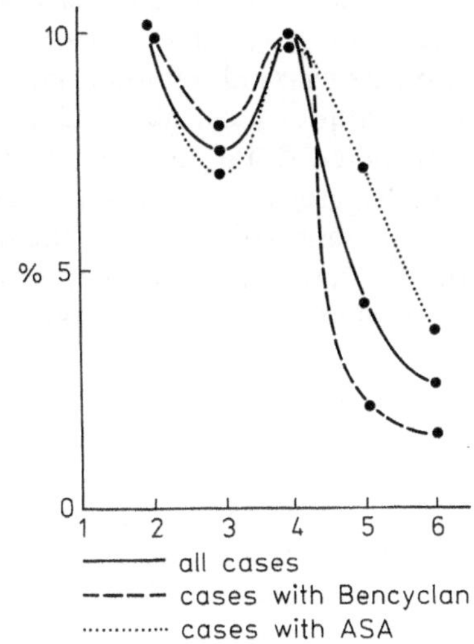

3

Fig. 2. Fibrogen uptake test following antegrade catheter angiography of the leg

Fig. 3. Fibrogen uptake test after PTA with administration of acetylsalicylic acid (*ASA*) or Bencylan

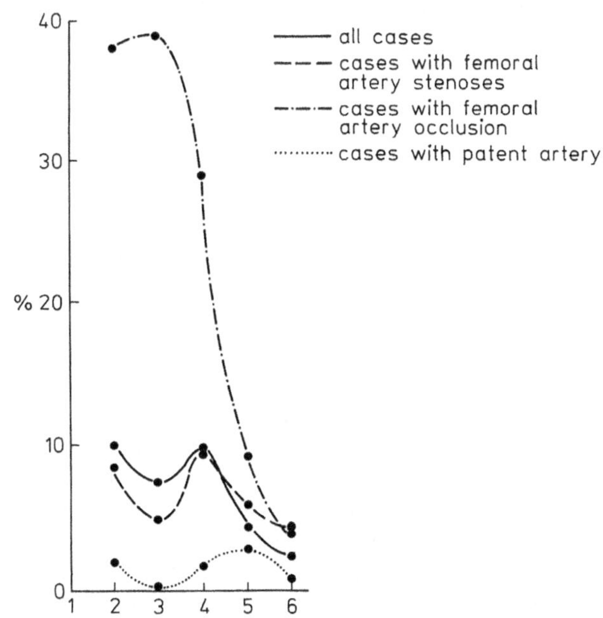

Fig. 4. Results of fibrinogen uptake test after PTA of occluded distal femoral artery

Examination of 80 patients after angiography served as the basis for this evaluation (Fig. 2). Increased activity was noted in hematomas at the puncture site in the groin. In orthograde angiography of legs performed with catheters in subjects who did not undergo PTA, a uniform decrease in activity from thigh to foot without local accumulation was ascertained. After effective PTA of the obstructed distal superficial femoral artery and additional medical treatment with aggregation inhibitors alone, the fibrinogen uptake test showed an accumulation of activity in the area of the dilated arterial obstruction in the thigh in 23 patients after successful dilatation (Fig. 3). This proves that after angioplasty increased deposition of fibrinogen occurred at the site of the mechanical dilatation.

The mean values of the fibrinogen uptake test performed after hemodynamic and angiographic studies clearly demonstrate minor fibrinogen deposition occurring at the site of residual stenosis; a high concentration of labeled fibrinogen appears only at rethrombosis (Fig. 4).

These results, along with the fact that thrombotic deposition may also occur on the catheter surface and between guide wire and catheter, confirm the necessity for additional treatment with drugs in order to avoid early relapses. With such a regimen, even dilatations leaving residual stenoses may have a good prognosis.

Dipyridamole is said to potentiate the effect of prostacyclin on the blood platelets [19]. Both in a double-blind study by Hess and in our own patient series with continuous drug administration, a reduced thrombosis rate was found within the first 2 weeks if the dose of ASA was reduced from 500 mg three times daily to 330 mg, with the addition of 75 mg dipyridamole three times daily.

As the result of all these studies, we consider the following form of adjuvant drug treatment to be optimal at present:

1. Pretreatment over 1–2 days with the aggregation inhibitor ASA (330 or 500 mg), alone or in combination with dipyridamole (75 mg) three times daily
2. Injection of 5,000 IU heparin intraarterially after entering the correct artery with the catheter and before passage of the obstruction
3. Posttreatment over 2–6 days with aggregation inhibitors (ASA, ASA + dipyridamole, etc.)
4. Initiation of coumarin treatment on the 1st or 2nd day after effective PTA, depending on the individual risk of bleeding. The aggregation inhibitor therapy can be stopped when effective coumarin levels are reached
5. If coumarin treatment is contraindicated, the treatment with aggregation inhibitors (e.g., Acetosal, ASA, ASA + dipyridamole) is continued over a long-term period to prevent natural progression of the disease

Particularly in those cases when guide wire or catheter must be advanced into the popliteal artery, arterial spasm must be avoided. Although the avoidance of mechanical traumatization of the intima is a key factor in preventing spasm, high-grade spasm in the popliteal artery can still be prevented by injecting 3 ml lidocaine 1% intraarterially while the catheter lies in the artery and prevents quick peripheral dispersion of the drug.

With mere slow blood flow, the anesthetic can exert a time-limited influence on the intima. The greatest efficacy is again obtained when lidocaine is applied while the catheter lies within the arterial obstruction and further slows the blood flow distally. However, the effect is minor when injection occurs before the catheter has passed the arterial obstruction. A randomized study disclosed that 3 ml lidocaine 1% injected intraarterially immediately after the catheter had passed the obstructing lesion significantly reduced the angiographically demonstrable frequency and intensity of arterial spasm in the popliteal artery. A recommended alternative is the addition of lidocaine 1% to the contrast medium.

During catheter treatment, peripheral perfusion is reduced for a variable period. In this interval the coagulability of the blood must be reduced by concomitant drug therapy and distal circulation enhanced by the use of vasodilators. This applies not only for the time of catheter manipulation, but also for the time of groin puncture site compression when it is necessary to maintain good perfusion. For this reason several authors recommend the intraarterial administration of vasodilators. Tolazoline, adenosine triphosphate, and similar substances are in use. We very slowly inject into the artery a combination of adenosine triphosphoric acid and a adenosine diphosphate (Laevadosin) in a dose of 2 ml dissolved in 10 ml of physiological saline solution. Evidence of the therapeutic efficacy of vasodilators has not yet been made available by a controlled study.

Adjunct medical therapy before, during, and after PTA is of great importance in ensuring the success of the mechanical treatment. The avoidance of early rethrombosis by platelets or agglutinative thrombus is of major import. The best prophylaxis against early rethrombosis after successful PTA is quick release of the arterial blood flow and the reduction of the thrombocyte tendency to aggregation by drug therapy. Immediately after catheter removal, the patient himself can augment circulation by active foot movement.

References

1. Andresen I, Gjioudal T (1967) Transluminal Behandlung av arteriosclerosis obliterans. Tidsskr Nor Laegeforen 47: 1057
2. Berglund G, Bodvall B, Eldh J, Yolên S (1969) Nytt behandlings alternativ vid arteriell insufficiens i benen. Lakartidningen 66: 129
3. Blana W (1976) Der Fibrinogen-Uptake-Test bei Patienten mit arterieller Verschlußkrankheit nach Angiographie unter besonderer Berücksichtigung der Dotter-Behandlung. Dissertation, Universität of Mainz
4. Brahme F, Swedenborg J, Tibell B (1969) Evaluation of transluminal recanalization of the femoral artery. Acta Chir Scand 135: 679
5. Dembski JC, Zeitler E (1978) Selective arterial clot lysis with angiography catheter. In: Zeitler E, Grüntzig A, Schoop W (eds) Percutaneous vascular recanalization. Springer, Berlin Heidelberg New York, pp 157–159
6. Dotter CT (1978) Transluminal angioplasty – pathologic Basis. In: Zeitler E, Grüntzig A, Schoop W (eds) Percutaneous Vascular Recanalization. Springer, Berlin Heidelberg New York, pp 3–12
7. Dotter CT, Roesch J, Judkins P (1968) Transluminal dilatation of atherosclerotic stenosis. Surg Gynecol Obstet 127: 794

8. Dotter CT, Rösch J, Anderson JM, Antonovic R, Robinson M (1974) Transluminal iliac artery dilatation. Nonsurgical catheter treatment of atheromatous narrowing. JAMA 230: 117
9. Dotter CT, Rösch I, Seaman AJ (1974) Selective clot lysis with low-dose streptokinase. Radiology 111: 31–37
10. Dow JD, Hardwick C (1966) Transluminal arterial recanalization. Lancet I: 73
11. Grüntzig A (1977) Die perkutane transluminale Rekanalisation chronischer Arterienverschlüsse mit einer neuen Dilatationstechnik. Witzstrock, Baden-Baden
12. Grüntzig A, Senning A, Siegenthaler W (1979) Nonoperative dilatation of coronary artery stenoses: percutaneous transluminal coronary angioplasty (PTCA). N Engl J Med 301: 61–68
13. Hess H (1982) Systemische und selektive Streptokinase-Therapie bei arteriellen Verschlüssen. Internist (Berlin) 23: 405–409
14. Hess H, Müller-Faßbender H, Ingrisch H, Mietaschk A (1978) Verhütung von Wiederverschlüssen nach Rekanalisation obliterierter Arterien mit der Kathetermethode. Dtsch Med Wochenschr 103: 1994–1997
15. Horvath L (1980) Percutaneous transluminal angioplasty. Importance of anticoagulant and fibrinolytic drugs. AJR 135: 951–954
16. Horváth L, Varró J (1978) Complications of the transluminal angioplasty excluding the puncture site complications. In: Zeitler E, Grüntzig A, Schoop W (eds) Percutaneous transluminal recanalization. Springer, Berlin Heidelberg New York, pp 126–139
17. Martin M, Zeitler E (1978) Percutaneous transluminal recanalization (PTR) and fibrinolysis: fibrinolytic treatment of femoral reocclusions subsequent to PTR procedures. In: Zeitler E, Grüntzig A, Schoop W (eds) Percutaneous vascular recanalization. Springer, Berlin Heibelberg New York, pp 152–156
18. Martin M, Schoop W, Zeitler E (1970) Thrombolyse bei chronischer Arteriopathie. Angiologie: 8. Huber, Bern
19. Mills DCB, Smith JB (1971) The influence on platelet aggregation of drugs that affect the accumulation of adenosine 3′:5′-cyclic monophosphate in platelets. Biochem J 121: 185
20. Müller-Fassbender H, Hess H (1975) Spätlysebehandlung chronischer arterieller Verschlüsse. Ein Weg zur Verbesserung der Ergebnisse. Münch Med Wochenschr 117/37: 1461–1462
21. Müller-Fassbender H, Hess H (1978) Percutaneous transluminal recanalization combined with fibrinolysis. In: Zeitler E, Grüntzig A, Schoop W (eds) Percutaneous transluminal recanalization. Springer, Berlin Heidelberg New York, pp 148–151
22. Palayew MJ, Sedlezky J, Sigman HH (1969) Occlusive peripheral arteriosclerosis: treatment by percutaneous transluminal recanalization – "Dotter procedure". Can Med Assoc J 101: 66
23. Schwarten DE, Yune HY, Klatte EC, Grim CE, Weinberger MH (1980) Clinical experience with percutaneous transluminal angioplasty (PTA) of stenotic renal arteries. Radiology 135: 601–604
24. Staiger J, Mathias K, Friederich M, Heiss HW, Konrad S, Spillner G (1980) Perkutane Katheterrekanalisation (Dotter-Technik) bei peripherer arterieller Verschlußkrankheit – Einfluß von Thrombozytenaggregationshemmern auf die Rezidivhäufigkeit nach einem Jahr. Herz/Kreisl 12/9: 383–386
25. van Andel GJ (1976) Percutaneous transluminal angioplasty. Excerpta Medica, Amsterdam
26. Wierny L, Plass R, Porstmann W (1974) Long-term results in 100 consecutive patients treated by transluminal angioplasty. Radiology 112: 543–548
27. Zeitler E (1978) Drug treatment before and after percutaneous transluminal recanalization (PTR). In: Zeitler E, Grüntzig A, Schoop W (eds) Percutaneous transluminal recanalization. Springer, Berlin Heidelberg New York, pp 73–77
28. Zeitler E, Reichold J, Schoop W, Loew D (1973) Einfluß von Acetylsalicylsäure auf das Frühergebnis nach perkutaner Rekanalisation arterieller Obliterationen nach Dotter. Dtsch Med Wochenschr 98: 1235–1288
29. Zeitler E, Grüntzig A, Schoop W (1973) Percutaneous vascular recanalization. Springer, Berlin Heidelberg New York

15. Platelet Activation at the Time of Percutaneous Transluminal Angioplasty

W. Blättler, N. Foullon, G. Cappius, and F.-J. Roth

There is good reason to assume that the procedure of percutaneous transluminal angioplasty (PTA) may activate platelets as well as the coagulation system. Such an activation is presumably triggered by blood contact with catheters and guide wires, but it may also occur at the site of angioplasty. Thus it is likely that this process may have a bearing on the immediate outcome of the operation. The incidence of early reocclusion of dilated stenoses and occlusions may therefore largely depend on the primary prevention of the deposition of platelets and fibrin.

In an attempt to elucidate the role of platelets during and immediately after PTA, we determined the levels of platelet-derived proteins in plasma during and up to 4 h after the procedure. Betathromboglobulin (BTG) and platelet factor 4 (PF4) were the two proteins studied.

Patients and Methods

We studied 13 patients with peripheral vascular occlusive disease (four women, nine men; mean age 63 years, range 52–79). All patients had complete obliteration of the femoral or popliteal artery (length of the obstruction 1.5–10 cm). Ten patients were in stage II, two in stage III, and one in stage IV. PTA was performed using Teflon-coated guide wires, Teflon catheters, and polyvinyl chloride balloon catheters. The contrast materials were either sodium ioxaglate/meglumine ioxaglate or iopamidole. The patients had no intravenous line and were not given a premediaction. Their usual oral therapy was maintained except for aspirin and dipyridamole, which were stopped 4 days before PTA the latest.

Heparin was given intraarterially to some patients after penetration of the occlusion. A bolus of 5,000 units was given to four and one of 2,500 units to another four patients. The other patients received heparin only with the saline used for catheter rinsing (400–1,000 units).

Blood was obtained at the following intervals: before start of the procedure, after introduction of the probing catheter, after penetration of the occlusion, after balloon dilatation, and after the manual compression of the puncture site was accomplished. Further samples were secured 1, 2, and 4 h after the end of the procedure. Blood was taken by separate venipunctures from forearm veins

Percutaneous Transluminal Angioplasty
(ed. by C. T. Dotter, A. Grüntzig, W. Schoop, E. Zeitler)

using butterfly sets and a two-syringe technique. Blood was added to precooled anticoagulant (tubes from the BTG kit) and incubated at 4° C for 30–60 min. It was then centrifuged at 5,000 *g* at 4° C for 20–30 min; 1.5 ml of the supernatant was aspirated below the surface and centrifuged for 2 min at 12,000 *g* in an Eppendorf centrifuge. The decanted plasmas were stored at −20° C until assay. BTG was quantitated using the kit of Amersham, PF4 using the kit of Abbott.

Results

The preinfusion values were 38 ± 22 ng/ml (SD; range 18–95) for BTG and 9.0 ± 6.4 ng/ml (SD; range 1.6–21.9) for PF4. Five out of 13 patients had values above 30 and 10 ng/ml respectively, which are our upper limits of normal.

A dramatic increase in both platelet proteins was observed after dilatation of the occlusion in all but one of the patients not given a bolus of heparin before that (Fig. 1). The mean peak values were 81 and 49 ng/ml respectively. The mean increase as compared to the preinfusion value was 48 ng/ml (range 14–123) for BTG and 67 ng/ml (range 4–144) for PF4. One and two hours after the end of PTA PF4 values had returned to preinfusion levels, while BTG remained elevated.

When a bolus of heparin was given (Fig. 2), a mean BTG increase of 5.8 ng/ml (range −11 to 37) was observed. The PF4 increase was 75 ng/ml (range 34–100). By 1 h after PTA, BTG values were below preinfusion and PF4 values had returned to that level. At 2 and 4 h BTG values were slightly elevated, while PF4 levels remained on the baseline.

A comparison of the peak BTG value with the total dose of heparin administered (Fig. 3) established a dose-response relationship. The BTG rise was prevented in all patients receiving 5,000 units or more, while it occurred in all but one of the patients receiving 1,000 units or less.

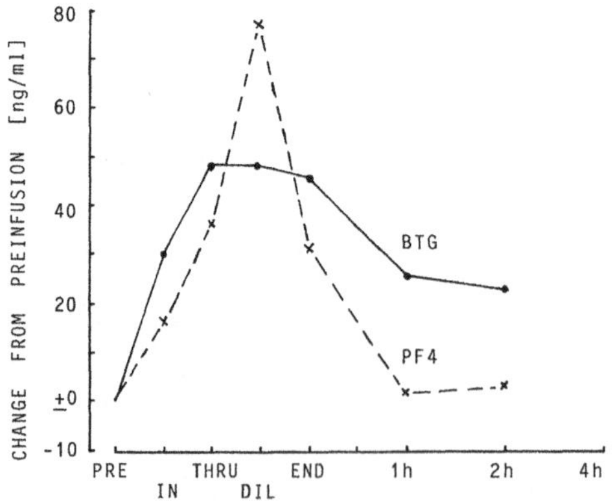

Fig. 1. The changes in BTG and PF4 from preinfusion values (ng/ml) are given for different steps during PTA and for various time intervals thereafter. The data are the means of values in five patients who received no bolus of heparin. *PRE,* before start of the procedure; *IN,* after introduction of the catheter; *THRU,* after penetration of the occlusion; *DIL,* after balloon dilatation; *END,* after manual compression of puncture site

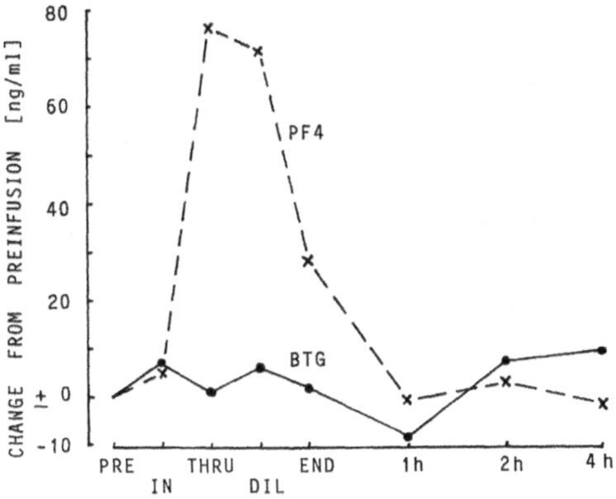

Fig. 2. The changes in BTG and PF4 during and after PTA are plotted as in Fig. 1. The data are the means of values in eight patients who received a bolus of heparin (2,500 or 5,000 units). *PRE,* before start of the procedure; *IN,* after introduction of the catheter; *THRU,* after penetration of the occlusion; *DIL,* after balloon dilatation; *END,* after manual compression of puncture site

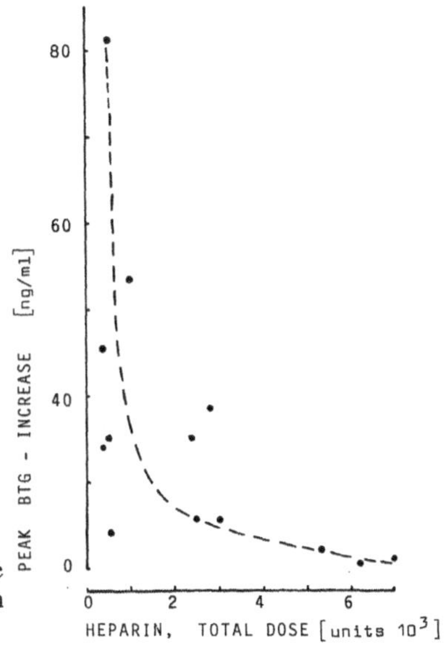

Fig. 3. The peak BTG increase over preinfusion value (ng/ml) is plotted against the total dose of heparin administered during PTA

Discussion

Our study establishes that an activation of platelets occurs at the time of PTA. Two phases may be discerned: one during and another one after PTA. During PTA, and exessive rise in levels of BTG and PF4 is often encountered. Heparin prevents the BTG increase in an almost dose-related manner. This phenomenon points to the generation of thrombin as the cause of the platelet activation. The rise of PF4 observed upon heparin injection is due to desorption of the peptide from the endothelial surface – a well-known effect of heparin.

After PTA, a striking discrepancy between BTG and PF4 values was found in about half the patients, whether heparin had been administered or not (Fig. 4). A plot comparing the corresponding BTG and PF4 data discloses that the preinfusion values fit a straight line, reflecting the fact that both values are

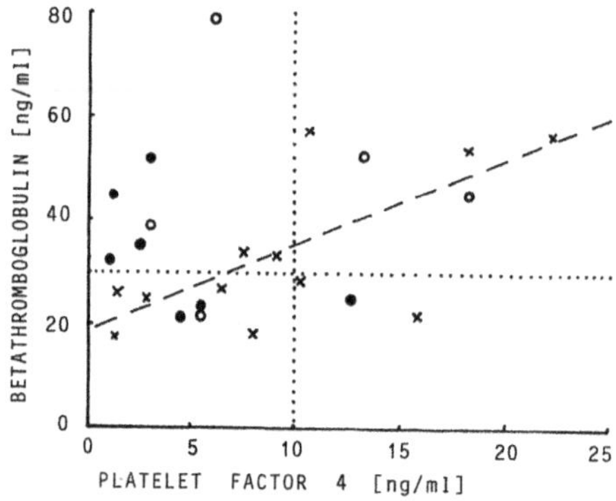

Fig. 4. A plot of absolute values (ng/ml) of BTG vs. PF4. The *dotted lines* represent our upper limits of normal for each protein. × denotes preinfusion data; ●,○ denote values from the last specimen obtained from each patient, ● referring to patients who received a bolus of heparin and ○ referring to those who did not

elevated to the same extent – if at all. The data points obtained from the last sample in each case either fitted the very same line or lay completely apart from it. These patients had clearly elevated BTG but perfectly normal PF4 levels. This platelet protein pattern is known to occur typically in localized deep venous thrombosis.

Thus we tentatively conclude that two distinct phases of platelet activation occur:

1. During PTA, a tremendous platelet stimulation happens, presumably as a consequence of thrombin formation. This activation can be prevented by heparin at a bolus dose of 5,000 units.
2. After PTA, a pattern of platelet protein elevation reflecting local thrombosis is observed in about half the patients. The clinical bearing of this second phase of platelet activation, particularly its relation to early reocclusion, remains to be elucidated. So far, the data favor drugs with antithrombin activity as possible tools for the prevention of early reocclusion.

16. Results With Additional Use of SP 54 in Percutaneous Transluminal Angioplasty

L. Horváth, K. Fendler, and I. Illés

The idea of using sulfated polyanions – such as SP 54 (Benechemie, Munich) – was prompted by several factors. First of all, it is well-known that intravascular thrombi may be dissolved by natural human fibrinolytic activity. The stimulation of this process has been widely used for a long time in the form of low-dose subcutaneous heparin therapy in major surgery. But in this case the use of heparin serves other purposes too. Depending on their molecular compounds heparin and heparin-like drugs may stimulate fibrinolytic activity [1]. When this was investigated it was found that even old clots can be dissolved if they are not organized [2, 3]. So what would happen during and following percutaneous transluminal angioplasty (PTA) if we purposefully stimulated the fibrinolytic enzyme system? SP 54 as a sulfated polyanion has seemed a suitable substance to use in combination with PTA. Among members of the sulfated polyanion group, the capacity to activate the fibrinolytic system increases with the degree of depolymerization. Being a compound with a very low molecular weight, SP 54 shows the optimum effects; it develops no more than traces of anticoagulant activity, thus achieving adequate therapeutic mobilization and reactivation of the physiological enzyme system with negligible effects on blood coagulation [4]. And it does not involve hypocoagulemia with the dangerous tendency to hemorrhage. The optimum single dose of SP 54 is 1–2 mg/kg. A peak in the fibrinolytic action develops after 30–60 min following intravenous administration of SP 54. With intramuscular injection the peak of fibrinolytic activation occurs 1–2 h later, decreases in the next 4–6 h and is still measurable even after 24 h. An increase in the fibrinolytic activity of about 300% can be achieved using this drug. Its other effects (lipolysis, reduction of blood viscosity, antisludging effect, antiaggregation effect, etc.) are favorable in atherosclerotic diseases.

Sp 54 is indicated in acute thrombotic and embolic conditions, including deep venous thrombosis, pulmonary embolism, postoperative thrombosis and its prevention, coronary occlusion and fresh infarction, and thrombosis of the portal and mesenteric venous system, as well as in thrombotic complications of cardiovascular surgical interventions. With respect to chronic diseases, it is indicated in atherosclerotic and diabetic arteriopathies of any vessel and of any stage, in hyperlipemia, in fatty liver, and in fat embolism. Contraindications are thrombocytopenic bleeding and hemorrhagic diathesis. Some caution is necessary in panmyelopathy, allergic history, and hypersensitivity.

The protocol of medication for PTA at our institute is as follows:

1. Premedication: salicylic acid 0.5–1.0 g three times daily for 3 days;

Percutaneous Transluminal Angioplasty
(ed. by C. T. Dotter, A. Grüntzig, W. Schoop, E. Zeitler)

2. Intraoperatively: heparin 2,500–5,000 units in saline solution; SP 54 50 mg i.a. when the lesion is passed; Rheomacrodex 50–100 ml i.a. in small doses;
3. Postoperatively: SP 54 100 mg s.c. or i.v. twice daily; Rheomacrodex 250–500 ml i.v. daily. Both of these are continued during hospitalization (3–5 days);
4. As outpatient: SP 54 50–100 mg orally twice daily; nicotinic acid 100 mg or more orally three times daily; vitamin E 100 mg/day orally; dicumarol (for the high-risk group). All these are given long-term (years).

We have used SP 54 in PTA in 116 patients, 86 of whom were included in a randomized study. The patients also treated with anticoagulants or any other drug active on the coagulation or fibrinolytic system were not included.

However, anticoagulants and SP 54 were included in the medication in the so-called high-risk group (smokers, immobiles, diabetics). In some cases the dose of SP 54 was increased (remaining clots, etc.) and they were included in the study.

The cumulative patency rate after 3 years is 83% in the SP 54 group and 63% in the control group treated with dicumarol (Table 1). It must be emphasized that our cases are not specially selected in respect of the possible results. Of course, the anatomical contraindications, smoking habit, and some other factors are respected. But in candidates for amputation we always try our best not to lose a limb, even in smokers. This group of patients does not influence our statistics favorably. The cumulative reocclusion rate in the first 24 h is 3%, in the 1st week 6%, in the 1st year 11%, and in the 2nd year 15%. The corresponding figures for the control group are 9%, 14%, 22%, and 30%. We saw reasonable thrombolysis in 11 patients, the result being thrombolysis in 11 patients, the result being evaluated either by angiography or blood flow measurements (pulse volume recording, etc.). Occasional dissolution not essentially influencing the blood supply could have been undetected in both groups.

Old clots can be resolved in the venous system too [7]. It has also been proved that stimulation of the endogenous fibrinolytic enzyme system can be employed to remove clots, thrombotic depositions, and emboli. Following PTA, the fibrinolytic substances face the thrombus on a larger surface, and this may be the reason for increased effectiveness [5, 6]. It has been found that

Table 1. Frequency of reocclusion after PTA (cumulative)

	Reoccl. within 1 day	Reoccl. within 1 week	Reoccl. within 1 year	Reoccl. within 2 years	Reoccl. within 3 years	Thrombo-lysis
Dicumarol (86 cases)	8 (9%)	12 (14%)	19 (22%)	26 (30%)	32 (37%)	
SP 54 (86 cases)	3 (4%)	5 (6%)	9 (11%)	13 (15%)	15 (17%)	11
χ^2-test	$p < 0.05$	$p < 0.05$	$p < 0.05$	$p < 0.05$	$p < 0.05$	

$p < 0.05$ (significant)

hemodynamic studies show an increasing flow rate through the recanalized arterial segment during subsequent weeks. Such an increase may be experienced following PTA in combination with SP 54, but in a higher degree and over a much longer period of time.

Fibrinolytic therapy is incorporated into the technique of transluminal angioplasty in our institute, as anticoagulation has sometimes been. Polyanions are less risky to use than anticoagulants: we have had no major complication so far. The follow-up is simpler and there is no need to check blood prothrombin time weekly. This medication reduces the risk and may improve the results of PTA in a group of patients who would otherwise have a poor prognosis.

References

1. Halse T, Philipp K, Ruf F (1950) Tierexperimentelle Untersuchung über intravasale Thrombolyse mit Heparin und Thrombocid. Langenbecks Arch Chir 263: 459
2. Gottlob R, Blümel G (1969) Experimentelle Grundlagen der Lysierbarkeit alter Gerinnsel. In: Müller-Wieland K (ed) Fibrinolyse-Therapie. Schattauer, Stuttgart
3. Lübcke P, Weber J, Bartscher U (1979) Lysierbarkeit und Frischhaltephänomen von akuten und älteren Phlebothrombosen unter Streptokinase-Einfluß. Herz Kreisl 11: 126
4. Weyer H, Muth HW (1973) Zur Therapie mit dem sulfatierten Polyanion SP 54. Med Welt 24: 800
5. Horváth L (1980) Percutaneous transluminal angioplasty: importance of anticoagulant and fibrinolytic drugs. Am J Roentgenol 135: 951
6. Horváth L, Fiegler M (1982) Treatment of a subclvian stenosis with perorally given fibrinolytic drug and by percutaneous transluminal angioplasty (in Hungarian). Orv Hetil 123: 1051
7. Luebke P, Weber J (1980) Delayed fibrinolysis of venous thrombi in pelvic veins and vena cava. In: May R, Weber J (eds) Pelvic and abdominal veins: progress in diagnostics and therapy. International Congress Series No. 550. Excerpta Medica, Amsterdam, p 345

17. Nafazatrom: A New Antithrombotic Compound

F. Seuter

Introduction

Nafazatrom (BAY G 6575), 3-methyl-1-[2-(2-naphthyloxy)-ethyl]-2-pyrazolin-5-one, is under development as an antithrombotic drug with a novel mode of action [1]. Its antithrombotic activity was demonstrated in experimentally induced thrombosis, especially in models based on the following freezing technique. The blood vessels of rats, rabbits, and guinea pigs were exposed and dissected free from the surrounding tissue. The jugular vein and the carotid artery of rats or guinea pigs and the femoral arteries of rabbits were used in most of the experiments. The vessels were frozen at −12° C to −15° C over a length of approximately 1 cm in a metal groove for 2–5 min and simultaneously compressed by a weight of 200 g (rat, guinea pig) or 500 g (rabbit). In addition, arteries were clamped with a small silver clip (diameter 0.15–0.20 mm) distally to the lesion. The experimental device is described elsewhere [2].

At the end of the experiments, the animals were heparinized and the thrombi were removed under anesthesia from the injured vessel segment. The thrombi were assessed either by the wet weight determined on an analytical balance immediately after removal or by the hemoglobin content determined with a hemoglobin test kit. To study the prevention of thrombosis the test compounds were administered a few minutes before anesthesia. The thrombi were removed from the vessels 4 h after the thrombogenic stimuli. To determine the thrombolytic activity test compounds were administered at 20–48 h after the thrombogenic stimuli, i.e., at a time when the thrombus had already been formed. The drug effects were determined by comparing the size of thrombi in treated and in control animals.

Results and Discussion

Prevention of Thrombosis

The effects of BAY G 6575 on thrombi in the jugular vein of rats 4 h after freezing are shown in Table 1. The minimal effective dose was 0.3 mg/kg orally. At this dose, the thrombus formation was inhibited by 48%. An increase in the dose up to 10 mg/kg did not lead to a greater effect. As previously reported, at

Percutaneous Transluminal Angioplasty
(ed. by C. T. Dotter, A. Grüntzig, W. Schoop, E. Zeitler)

Table 1. Prevention by BAY G 6575 of freezing-induced venous thrombosis in rat

Treatment	Dose (mg/kg orally)	No. in group	Hemoglobin content (µg) of the thrombus
Control		89	192 ± 13
BAY G 6575	0.1	18	145 ± 27 (−25%, NS)
BAY G 6575	0.3	17	100 ± 21 (−48%, $p < 0.01$)
BAY G 6575	1.0	24	106 ± 23 (−45%, $p < 0.01$)
BAY G 6575	10.0	24	105 ± 13 (−45%, $p < 0.01$)

NS, $p > 0.05$

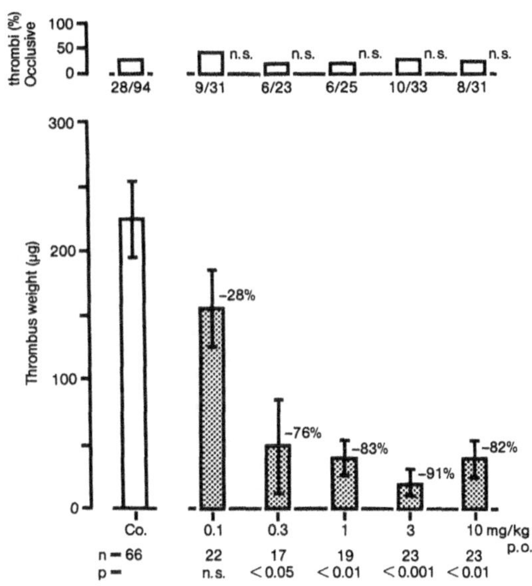

Fig. 1. Prevention of freezing-induced arterial thrombosis in the carotid artery of the rat by BAY G 6575. Thrombus growth time: 4 h. *Co*, control; *n*, no. of animals

least 10 mg acetylsalicylic acid per kilogram orally or 1 mg heparin per kilogram subcutaneously were necessary to induce comparable effects on the size of venous thrombi [3, 4].

The pronounced antithrombotic effects of BAY G 6575 in the carotid artery of the rat are shown in Fig. 1. The weight of arterial nonocclusive thrombi was reduced by 76% after pretreatment with BAY G 6575 at 0.3 mg/kg orally and higher doses.

In the carotid artery, BAY G 6575 reduced not only the size of the thrombi as has been shown for veins, but also completely inhibited thrombus formation in about 60% of the animals (Fig. 2). The incidence of occlusive thrombi was not affected by the drug at any dose used (Fig. 1).

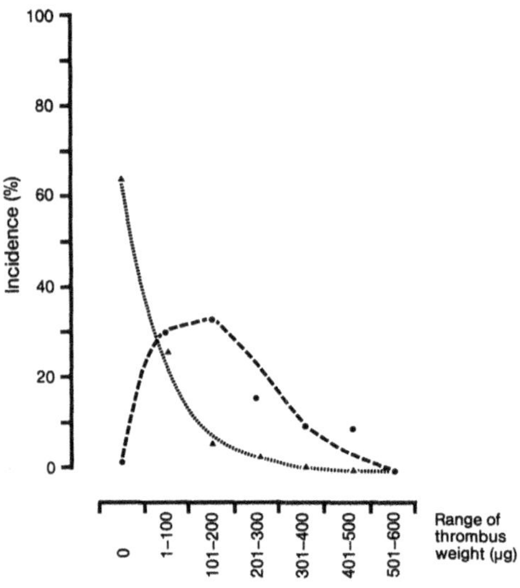

Fig. 2. Effect of pretreatment with BAY G 6575 on thrombus weight in the carotid artery of the rat. Each point represents pooled data obtained with BAY G 6575 at 10.0, 3.0, 1.0, and 0.3 mg/kg orally. ●——● control; ▲···▲ BAY G 6575

Table 2. Prevention of freezing-induced thrombosis in the carotid artery of rats by BAY G 6575 when given by the intravenous route of administration

Dose (mg/kg i. v.)	*n*	Mean thrombus weight (μg) ± SEM	Inhibition (%)	*p*	Occlusive thrombi/total
Control	7	247 ± 64			3/10
1.0	6	36 ± 35	85	< 0.05	4/10
0.3	6	29 ± 24	88	< 0.05	4/10
0.1	6	33 ± 33	87	< 0.05	4/10
0.03	6	63 ± 40	74	< 0.05	3/9
Control	8	172 ± 31			0/8
0.01	6	81 ± 29	53	> 0.05	2/8

Like BAY G 6575, acetylsalicylic acid also prevented freezing-induced thrombosis in the rat [1, 5]. To achieve comparable effects, (about 60% inhibition of mean thrombus weight), tenfold higher doses of ASA were required. Heparin was effective at 1–3 mg/kg s.c. [1].

The antithrombotic activity of BAY G 6575 in the rat carotid artery was also seen when the animals were pretreated with the drug by a parenteral route. The minimally effective intravenous dose (Table 2) was approximately one-tenth of the minimally effective oral dose.

As demonstrated in Fig. 3, BAY G 6575 reduced the arterial thrombus weight in the femoral arteries of rabbits in a dose-related manner. The minimal dose which produced the statistically significant effect was 1 mg/kg orally. As in rats, the incidence of occlusive thrombi was not reduced by the drug.

The activity of BAY G 6575 in preventing thrombosis induced by freezing in the jugular veins of guinea pigs was compared with that of acetylsalicylic acid

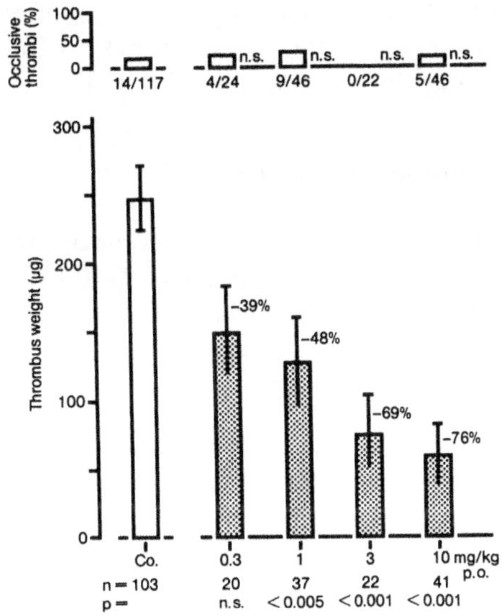

Fig. 3. Effect of pretreatment with BAY G 6575 on freezing-induced thrombosis in the femoral arteries of rabbits. Thrombus growth time: 4 h. *Co*, control; *n*, no. of animals

Table 3. Prevention of freezing-induced thrombosis by BAY G 6575 and acetylsalicylic acid (ASA) in jugular veins of guinea pigs

Compound and dose (mg/kg orally)	Experiment no.	Non occlusive thrombi			
		Inhibition (%) (significance of difference from control)	Occurence (%)		
			No thrombi	Thrombi < 100 µg	Occlusive thrombi (%)
BAY G 6575					
10	1	61 ($p < 0.05$)	42	67	0
10	2	87 ($p < 0.001$)	42	83	0
1	3	69 ($p < 0.05$)	50	80	9
ASA					
10	1	75 ($p < 0.01$)	45	82	8
10	2	77 ($p < 0.001$)	50	60	0
1	3	49 ($p > 0.05$)	22	56	10
Control					
5 ml/kg	1		0	9	0
tragacanth	2		0	18	8
	3		0	10	9

(Table 3). Statistically significant effects were obtained with BAY G 6575 at 1 or 10 mg/kg orally. Acetylsalicylic acid had significant antithrombotic effect at 10 mg/kg but not at 1 mg/kg orally.

Thrombolytic Activity

If administered after induction of thrombosis, BAY G 6575 reduced the weights of thrombi in the jugular veins of rats (Table 4). BAY G 6575 at single oral doses of 0.1 mg/kg at 24 and 26 h after the vessel damage significantly reduced the hemoglobin content of thrombi. There was a further reduction in the hemoglobin content of thrombus with the increase in dose to 2 × 1.0 mg/kg orally (Table 4).

In similar experiments performed on the carotid artery of the rat, BAY G 6575 at 2 × 0.3 mg/kg orally, at 20 and 22 h after induction of the thrombosis, inhibited the weight of the experimentally induced thrombi by 91% (Table 5). Under similar experimental conditions both acetylsalicylic acid and heparin were previously reported to be ineffective [1].

Table 4. Thrombolytic activity of BAY G 6575 on freezing-induced thrombosis in the jugular vein of rats

Treatment	Dose (mg/kg orally)	No. of animals	Hemoglobin content of the thrombus (μg) Mean ± SEM
Control		71	195 ± 16
BAY G 6575	2 × 0.1	24	126 ± 18 (−35%, $p < 0.05$)
	2 × 1.0	18	82 ± 8 (−57%, $p < 0.001$)
	2 × 10	18	82 ± 10 (−58%, $p < 0.001$)
	2 × 100	18	66 ± 7 (−66%, $p < 0.001$)

The drug was given at 24 h after induction of thrombosis and again 2 h later. Thrombus growth time: 28 h

Table 5. Thrombolytic activity of BAY G 6575 on freezing-induced thrombosis in the carotid arteries of rats

Treatment	Dose (mg/kg orally)	No. of animals	Thrombus weight (μg) Mean ± SEM	Incidence of occlusive thrombi	Change in thrombus weight
Control		13	263 ± 41	5/18	
BAY G 6575	2 × 0.1	9	157 ± 76	1/10	− 40%, $p > 0.05$
	2 × 0.3	6	24 ± 23	3/9	− 91%, $p < 0.01$
	2 × 1.0	8	22 ± 25	2/10	− 83%, $p < 0.01$
	2 × 3.0	7	13 ± 9	3/10	− 95%, $p < 0.01$
ASA	2 × 10.0	6	173 + 27	2/8	− 18%, $p > 0.05$
Control		6	212 + 48	3/9	
Heparin	2 × 3.0 s.c.	6	189 ± 48	2/8	− 11%, $p > 0.05$

ASA, acetylsalicylic acid

Table 6. Effects on blood coagulation and fibrinolysis

Test	Concentration (μg/ml)	Dose (mg/kg orally)	Effect
Platelet aggregation[a] (Born technique)	30–100		None (max. 13%)
Partial thromboplastin time	200		None
Thrombin time	300		None
Thromboplastin time (Quick)	300		None
Reptilase time	200		None
Thromboelastogram (coagulation, fibrinolysis)	250		None
Factor XIII activity	3000		None
Euglobulin lysis time (rat)		30	None
Thromboxane generation (rabbit aortic strip)	30		None
Clot retraction (ADP-induced, rat)		100	None

ADP, adenosine triphosphate
[a] Induced by collagen, ADP, ristocetin, etc.

Studies on the Mechanism of Action

Using the tests in Table 6, BAY G 6575 had no significant effect on blood coagulation, fibrinolysis, or other hematological parameters such as hematocrit, hemoglobin, blood sedimentation rate, fibrinogen, and platelet concentration.

An increase in prostacyclin availability due to BAY G 6575 was first studied by Vermylen et al. [6]. Their findings supported the hypothesis that the antithrombotic properties of BAY G 6575 were a consequence of PGI_2 stimulation. Similar results were obtained by MacIntyre and Salzman [7], using rat aortic rings from animals pretreated with BAY G 6575, as well as by Carreras et al. [8], using vascular tissue from diabetic rats.

The basic mechanism, which includes enhancement of PGI_2 availability, may center on the action of BAY G 6575 as a reducing cosubstrate for the hydroperoxide transformation [9], but this warrants further investigation.

General Pharmacology and Toxicity

BAY G 6575 is extremely well tolerated by mice, rats, and rabbits (LD_{50} $> 10{,}000$ mg/kg orally), and in addition to its low toxicity is practically devoid of relevant cardiovascular, autonomic, metabolic, analgesic, and antiinflammatory effects.

Summary and Conclusions

The activity of BAY G 6575 (Nafazatrom; 3-methyl-1-[2-(2-naphthyloxy)-ethyl]-2-pyrazolin-5-one) was evaluated in various models of experimental thrombosis, mainly those of traumatically induced damage of vessel segments. After oral or parenteral pretreatment of rats, rabbits, and guinea pigs with BAY G 6575, the thrombus formation was significantly reduced in the arteries as well as in the veins. The minimally effective doses were 0.3–1.0 mg/kg orally and 0.03–0.1 mg/kg i.v. BAY G 6575 was more potent than acetylsalicylic acid. The incidence of occlusive thrombi was not influenced by the drug.

Of particular interest was the effect of BAY G 6575 on already formed thrombi. The platelet aggregation inhibitor acetylsalicylic acid and the anticoagulant heparin were – as expected – ineffective as thrombolytics under similar experimental conditions. BAY G 6575 in two single doses of 1.0 mg/kg orally significantly reduced the weight of formed thrombi in the arteries as well as in the veins.

The mechanism of the antithrombotic and/or thrombolytic effects of BAY G 6575 is not yet precisely established. The drug did not show any effects on blood coagulation. It did not possess a direct platelet aggregation inhibitory activity, and had no in vitro fibrinolytic effect. The antiaggregatory activity of the vessel wall may be explained by increased availability of prostacyclin, which may be responsible for the antithrombotic activity of the compound.

On the basis of available pharmacologic and toxicological data, the evaluation of BAY G 6575 in the therapy of thromboembolic disorders appears very promising.

References

1. Seuter F, Busse WD, Meng K, Hoffmeister F, Möller E, Horstmann H (1979) The antithrombotic activity of BAY G 6575. Arzneimittelforsch/Drug Res 29 (1): 54–59
2. Schmidt R (1975) Eine neue Methode zur Erzeugung von Thromben durch Unterkühlung der Gefäßwand und ihre Anwendung zur Prüfung von Acetylsalicylsäure und Heparin. Inaugural-Dissertation, Gießen
3. Meng K (1975) Tierexperimetnelle Untersuchungen zur antithrombotischen Wirkung von Acetylsalicylsäure. Ther Ber 47: 69–79
4. Meng K (1976) Tierexperimentelle Thrombose und Behandlung mit Acetylsalicylsäure. Med Welt 27: 1359–1362
5. Meng K, Seuter F (1977) Effect of acetylsalicylic acid on experimentally induced arterial thrombosis in rats. Naunyn-Schmiederberg's Arch Pharmacol 301: 115–119
6. Vermylen J, Chamone DAF, Verstraete M (1979) Stimulation of prostacyclin release from vessel wall by BAY G 6575, an antithrombotic compound. Lancet 1: 518–520
7. MacIntyre DE, Salzman EW (1981) Effects of BAY G 6575 on platelets and on vascular PGI_2 production. Thromb Haemost 46: 19
8. Carreras LO, Chamone DAF, Klerckx P, Vermylen J (1980) Decreased vascular prostacyclin (PGI_2) in diabetic rats. Stimulation of PGI_2 release in normal and diabetic rats by the antithrombotic compound BAY G 6575. Thromb Res 19: 663–670
9. Eling TE, Honn KV, Busse WD, Seuter F, Marnett LJ (1982) Stimulation of PGI_2 biosynthesis by Nafazatrom (BAY G 6575). In: Powles T J et al. (eds.) Prostaglandins and Cancer. New York, Alan Liss Inc., pp. 783–787

V. Primary Results: Leg Arteries

18. Femoropopliteal Arteries

E. Zeitler, E.-I. Richter, and W. Seyferth

Obstructions of the femoral and popliteal arteries present the most frequent indications for percutaneous transluminal angioplasty (PTA). One must also say that occlusions of the superficial femoral artery at its origin, that is at the bifurcation of the common femoral artery, present no primary indication for the percutaneous technique. Proximal femoral occlusions and complete occlusions of the superficial femoral artery are primary indications for a femoropopliteal or a femorotibial bypass.

Special problems arise in antegrade puncture of the femoral artery in the groin. Such punctures can be quite difficult in obese patients, and it is therefore advantageous to hyperextend the hips by placing a cushion beneath the buttocks [23]. In 1%–2% of cases primary puncture of the deep femoral artery occurs, or the needle tip lies in the deep femoral artery and must be guided back into the common femoral artery under fluoroscopic control.

Under fluoroscopic control it is possible, in the overwhelming number of cases, to advance the guide wire successfully into the superficial femoral artery, either directly after the primary puncture, or after a second puncture with observation of the course of the superficial femoral artery after contrast material injection. Before definitive dilatation can proceed, repeat angiography is necessary to delineate the individual obstructive lesions, which are then marked with towel clamps (Figs. 1 and 2).

Independently of the use of polyethylene or Teflon catheters [3, 18–21], one of the most considerable aspects of PTA lies in the safe intraluminal passage of the obstruction. Image intensifier fluoroscopy is essential for such a safe passage. Digital subtraction angiography (DSA) [2, 10, 11, 17], with its reduced requirements for contrast agents, can help monitor the advancement of guide wire and catheter as well as the extent of the dilatation. In cases of occlusion the "explosion method" [7] can sometimes be helpful.

To ensure the intraluminal passage of the obstructive lesion, we employ a Teflon catheter with proximal side holes (Figs. 3 and 4) by which we can follow the progress of the guide wire and catheter by intermittent contrast material injection. Such an arrangement, using a Y-adaptor, also helps avoid entering collateral vessels.

When both the guide wire and initial catheter lie safely intraluminally beyond the obstruction (Fig. 4), an appropriate balloon catheter [5, 6, 13] is chosen for the dilatation, depending upon the size and extent of the obstructing lesion.

Percutaneous Transluminal Angioplasty
(ed. by C. T. Dotter, A. Grüntzig, W. Schoop, E. Zeitler)

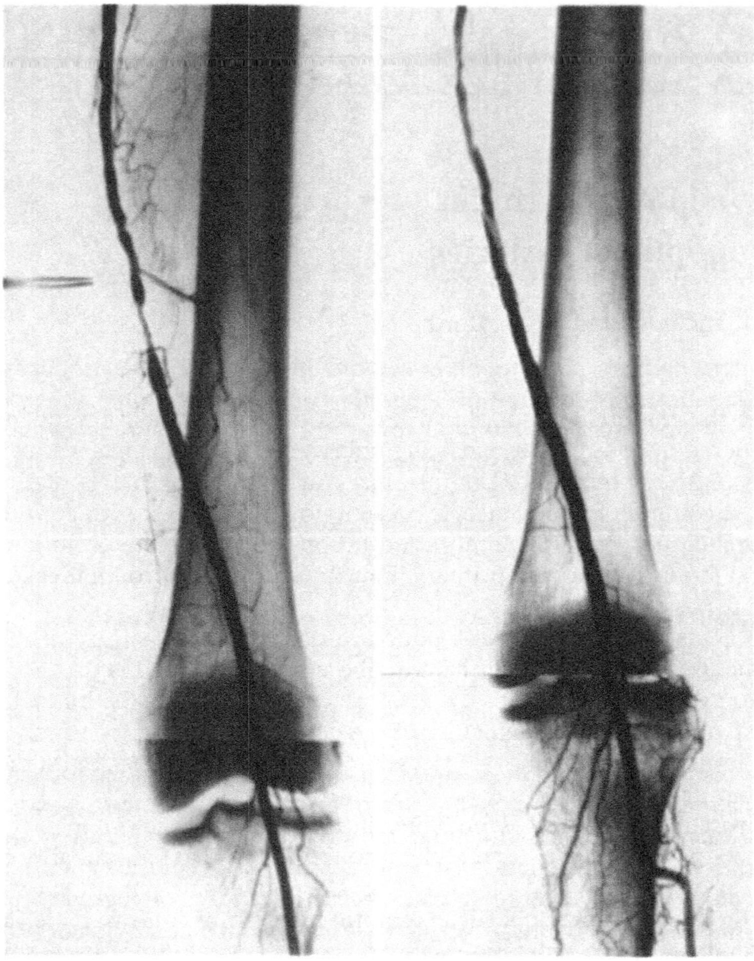
a b

Fig. 1a, b. A 69-year-old man with a pain-free walking distance of 150 m (pace 110 steps/min). **a** Arteriogram prior to treatment showing a high-grade stenosis of the superficial femoral artery. **b** Control angiogram after dilatation. No residual stenosis can be seen. However, one can recognize an intimal flap at the level of the original stenosis

The guide wire remains beyond the obstruction while the Teflon catheter is exchanged for the balloon catheter. Dilatation is performed under manometric control. It is possible to distend the balloon by hand with a 2- to 5-ml syringe, or to use a pressure control pump in the manner of Grüntzig. A 20-ml syringe is recommended for the deflation of the balloon (1; see also Chap. 8 in this volume).

The results of femoropopliteal PTA depend upon:

1. The location of the obstruction [4, 20]
2. The extent of the obstruction [15]
3. The clinical stage (claudication, rest pain, gangrene) [4, 15, 16]
4. The peripheral outflow in the lower leg [16]
5. Concomitant medical therapy [22].

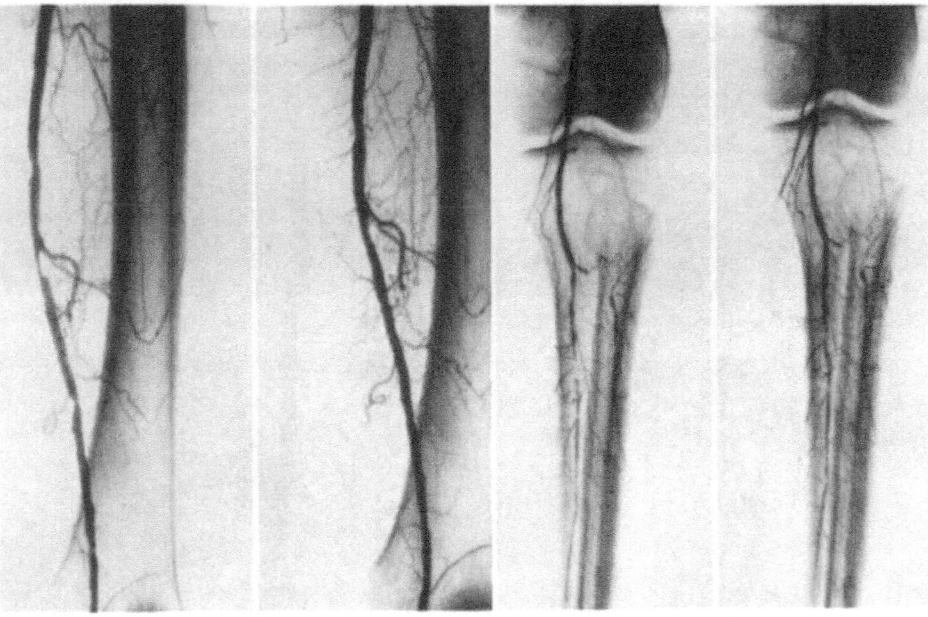

a b c d

Fig. 2a–d. A 63-year-old man with stage IV arterial occlusive disease (Fontaine's classification). Risk factors: cigarette smoking, diabetes mellitus. **a** multiple stenoses of the superficial femoral artery prior to treatment; **b** follow-up angiogram after successful treatment with a Grüntzig balloon dilatation catheter; **c** multiple obstructive lesions in all lower leg arteries; **d** unchanged arteriographic findings in the lower leg. The patient quickly developed gangrenous demarcation, and healing was prompt after the amputation of two toes. At 6 months the pain-free walking distance was 200 m. There is no recurrent gangrene and no rest pain

The primary success rate and 3-year patency rate of our own series in Nuremberg between 1976 and 1982, controlled by means of the life table method, are presented in Figs. 5 and 6. During this period, all patients were treated with aggregation inhibitors (acetylsalicylic acid 330 mg + dipyridamole 75 mg three times daily) before and after PTA. A change in the clinical state was considered to be a positive outcome, objective indications being improvement of the Doppler quotient by more than 0.2 and improvement of the walking distance and of the pulse status, as well as of the result of DSA. DSA was performed in more than 150 patients.

Distal femoropopliteal stenoses are approached by ipsilateral orthograde arterial puncture in the groin. Single stenoses (Fig. 1) can almost always be passed and can generally be well dilated. Multiple stenoses (Fig. 2) can occasionally lead to intimal elevation and partial subintimal dissection resulting from multiple intimal cracks caused by the dilating balloon at various levels. These present the occasion for rare early recurrences (see Chap. 21 in this volume).

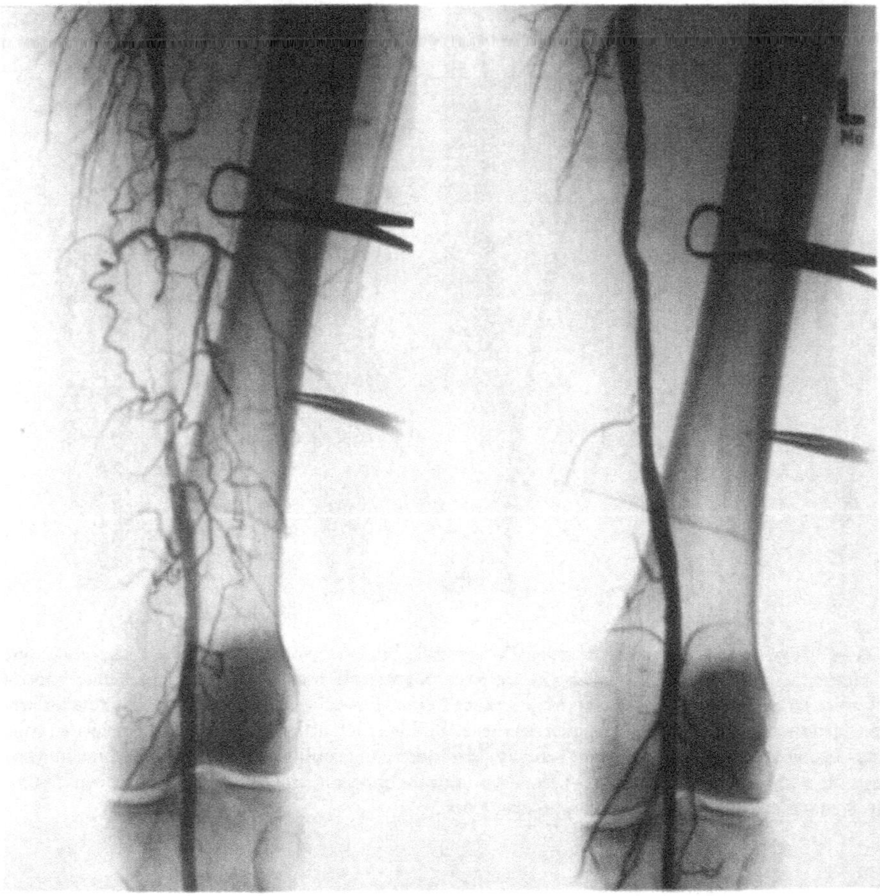

a b

Fig. 3a, b. A 64-year-old woman. Risk factors: diabetes mellitus, hyperlipemia, smoking. Pain-free walking distance was 100 m (at a pace of 110 steps/min). Systolic blood pressure as determined by Doppler technique at the ankle was 60 mm Hg. Arm blood pressure was 150 mm HG, making the Doppler quotient 0.4. **a** Arteriogram prior to PTA with marking of the length of the occlusion and of the proximal stenosis. **b** Arteriogram after successful dilatation. The Doppler quotient at discharge 2 days after the procedure was 0.96. Pain-free walking for more than 5 min (pace 90 steps/min)

Fig. 4a –d. A 43-year-old patient with a femoral occlusion approximately 10 cm in length. Pain-free walking distance was 120 m (at 90 steps/min). Systolic blood pressure at the ankle as measured by Doppler technique was 65 mm Hg, brachial blood pressure 130 mm Hg, Doppler quotient 0.5. The various wall irregularities demonstrate different forms of intimal wall lesions. **a** Arteriogram prior to therapy. **b** Passage of the obstruction with the guide wire and Teflon catheter. **c** Film confirming the location of the balloon catheter in the region of the obstruction. **d** Follow-up angiogram after dilatation. One can detect the effects of overdistension, inhomogeneous contrast density, and a stenosis distal to the lower marking clamp

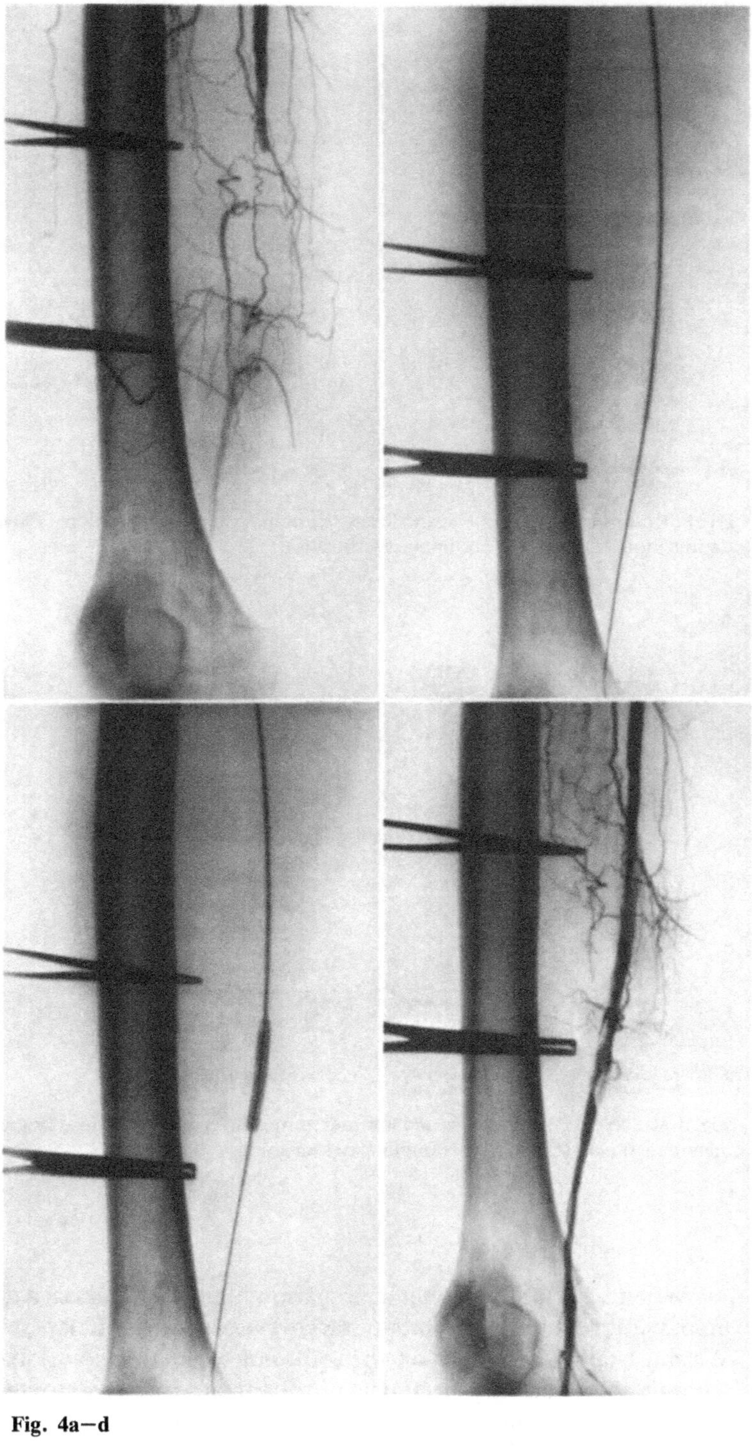

a b c d

Fig. 4a–d

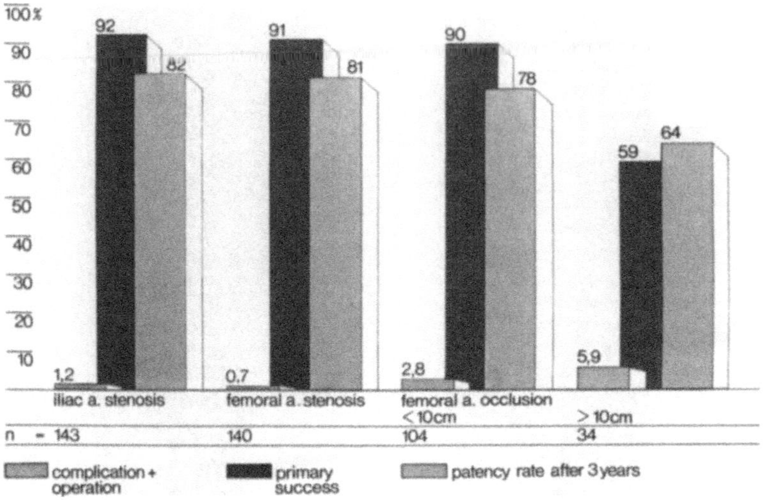

Fig. 5. Results of PTA in pelvic and lower extremity arterial obstructions. Patients with intermittent claudication of stage II (Fontaine classification)

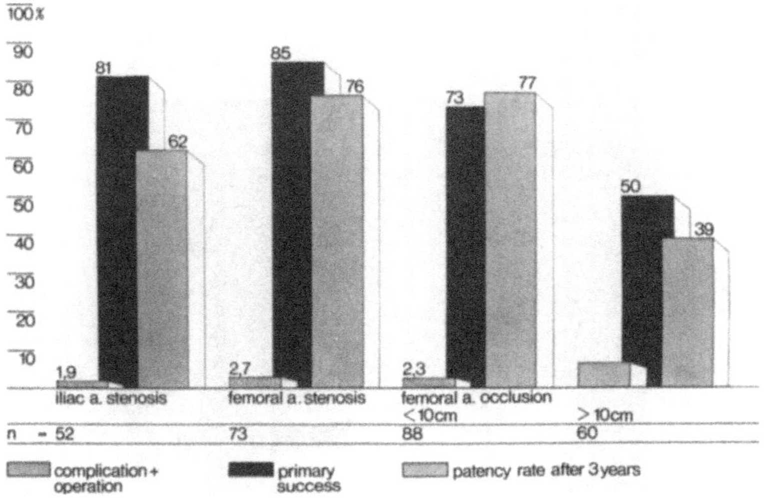

Fig. 6. Results of PTA in pelvic and lower extremity arterial obstructions. Patients with rest pain and gangrene stages III and IV (Fontaine classification)

When additional platelet aggregation inhibitors and intraarterial heparin are employed, rethrombosis is only rarely observed (see Chap. 14 in this volume). We must nevertheless be on the look-out for patients who have been referred without the necessary premedication. In these cases intravenous injection of Aspisol 15–30 min before the dilatation takes the place of the customary premedication with acetylsalicylic acid.

Distal femoral occlusions up to 3 cm in length can usually be recanalized and subsequently dilated to an appropriate luminal size with a balloon catheter. Femoropopliteal occlusions with a length of 4–10 cm can be recanalized in seven out of ten cases (Fig. 3). The long-term follow-up study using the coaxial Dotter dilating set [15, 16] (see also Chap. 21 in this volume) has shown a 10-year-patency rate significantly different from that of occlusions shorter than 3 cm.

Due to their poor initial success and low patency rate, occlusions longer than 10 cm are primary indications for surgery [24]. However, in those patients who present a greater operative risk, whether because of advanced age or because of cardiac, pulmonary, or other systemic medical condition, one may attempt transluminal therapy without elevated risk. These cases predominantly involve patients with rest pain or gangrene (Fig. 5). If recanalization is successful, an adequate lumen may result from use of a single Teflon catheter (Fig. 4) in combination with a Grüntzig, Olbert, or other balloon catheter. Control angiography after PTA often gives information on the further prognosis. For these patients follow-up with Doppler ultrasound technique or intravenous DSA is especially recommended for recognition of early progression or rethrombosis.

Obstructions or occlusions in the region of the distal popliteal artery and proximal trifurcation vessels (Fig. 7) present special technical problems. We employ 3 ml 1% lidocaine intraarterially as a precaution against arterial spasm. Under fluoroscopic control the guide wire and a Teflon catheter with proximal side holes are advanced distal to the obstruction. At this level it is better to use a straight rather than a curved guide wire.

In the arteries of the calf it may suffice simply to pass the obliteration with the Teflon catheter. In the distal popliteal artery better results are achieved by balloon catheter dilatation after the stenosis has been safely passed. A balloon of appropriate luminal diameter (3–5 mm) is recommended [20, 22, 23].

In contrast to the case with the above described lesions, it is advantageous to use a contralateral retrograde technique [14] to approach lesions in the common and deep femoral arteries or in the proximal superficial femoral artery (Fig. 8). This applies especially if a scar exists in the groin on the side of the lesion or if the stenosis occurs at an operative site, such as after bypass. A disadvantage of the contralateral approach is the possible lever effect of the catheter, where the aortic bifurcation serves as a fulcrum. An attempt should nonetheless be made, especially with regard to an obstruction in the groin or in a venous bypass graft.

Today, the vast majority of groups use a balloon catheter for the definitive dilatations of lesions in the femoropopliteal region, independent of the catheter system employed for angiography and the primary passage of the lesion. For the results of a cooperative study by 12 centers on all femoropopliteal obstructions see Chap. 34 in this volume.

If we separate the results of femoral stenoses and occlusions, we see a lower success rate in patients with occlusions. These results do not differentiate the length of the occlusion and the various additional drug therapeutic regimens employed. The results of the Zurich group, who have so far limited PTA mostly

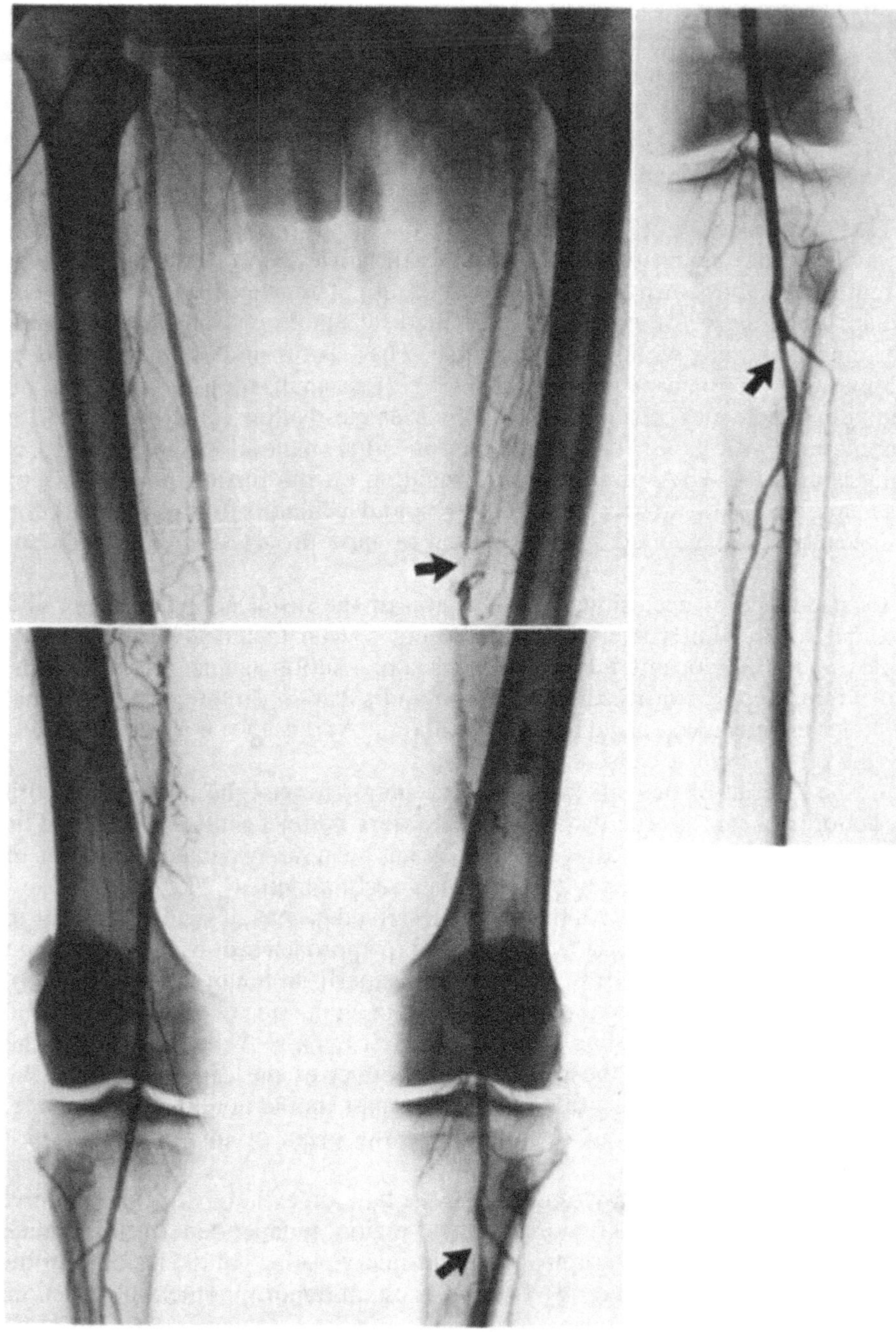

Fig. 7a–c. A 67-year-old man with stage IIb arterial occlusive disease. Pain-free walking distance was 100 m (at 110 steps/min). The left Doppler quotient was 0.4. **a, b** angiogram before PTA: **a** a 2-cm long occlusion of the superficial femoral artery in the aductor canal; **b** stenosis of the tibiofibular trunk; **c** results of dilatation of the tibiofibular trunk with a Teflon catheter of 7 Charrière following recanalization of the femoral artery

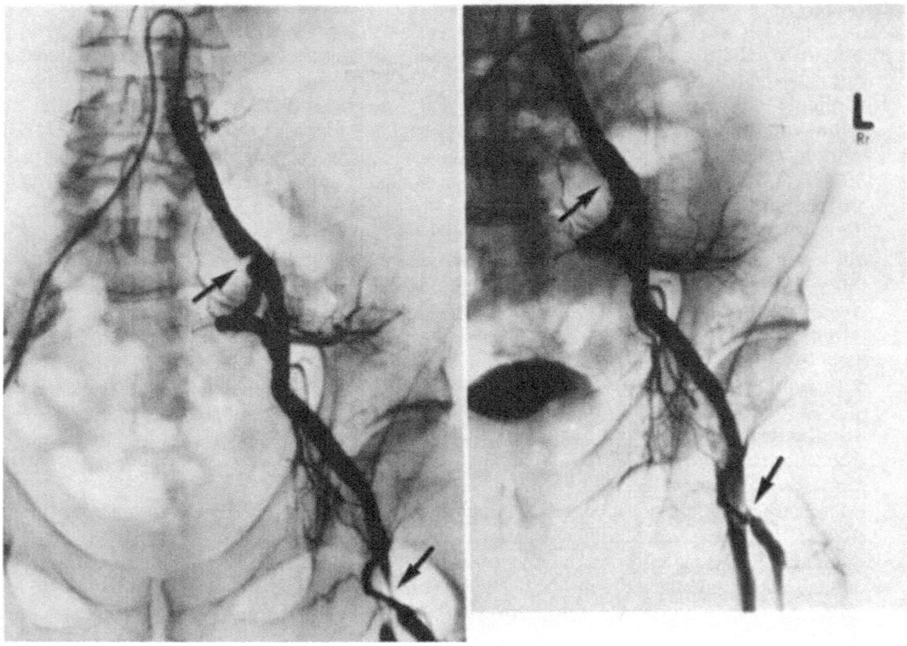

a b

Fig. 8a, b. A 63-year-old man with intermittent claudication; walking distance was less than 50 m (at a pace of 110 steps/min. Doppler quotient 0.25. **a** Left common iliac stenosis and a filiform stenosis of the superficial femoral artery immediately beyond the origin of the deep femoral artery. **b** Angiogram after dilatation: eradication of the common iliac stenosis; dilatation of the proximal femoral segment, with inhomogeneous contrast filling indicating intima fragmentation. Doppler quotient rose to 0.61. Rest pain disappeared. The patient can now walk for 5 min (at a pace of 110 steps/min) without pain

to femoropopliteal occlusions shorter than 3 cm and use follow-up treatment with warfarin, show that it is possible to demonstrate that stricter criteria in selection of patients for PTA and use of anticoagulation give an optimum of success.

There has not yet been a randomized study in patients receiving aggregation inhibitors or warfarin, or a randomized study comparing results of bypass surgery and PTA in patients with femoropopliteal occlusions longer than 3 cm. Nonetheless, today it is possible to say that PTA is the treatment of first choice in all patients with iliac artery stenoses, single and multiple femoropopliteal stenoses, or femoropopliteal occlusions shorter than 3 cm if an experienced angiographer performs the procedure.

For lesions in locations other than those in the lower extremities mentioned above, adequate follow-up studies have not yet been carried out; it is to be hoped that such studies will be undertaken in the near future.

References

1. Abele JE (1980) Balloon catheter and transluminal dilatation: technical considerations. AJR 135: 901–906
2. Crummy AB, Strother CM, Lieberman RP, Stieghorst MF, et al. (1981) Digital video subtraction angiography for evaluation of peripheral vascular disease. Radiology 141: 33
3. Dotter CT, Judkins MP (1964) Transluminal treatment of arteriosclerotic obstruction: description of a new technique and a preliminary report of its application. Circulation 30: 654–670
4. Grüntzig A (1977) Die perkutane transluminale Rekanalisation chronischer Arterienverschlüsse mit einer neuen Dilatationstechnik. Witzstrock, Baden-Baden
5. Grüntzig A, Hopff H (1976) Perkutane Rekanalisation chronischer arterieller Verschlüsse mit einem neuen Dilatationskatheter (Dotter-Prinzip). ROEFO 124: 80
6. Grüntzig A, Kumpe DA (1979) Technique of percutaneous angioplasty with the Grüntzig balloon catheter. AJR 132: 547–552
7. Horváth L, Illés I, Varró J (1978) Complications of the transluminal angioplasty excluding the puncture site complications. In: Zeitler E, Grüntzig A, Schoop W (eds) Percutaneous transluminal recanalization. Springer, Berlin Heidelberg New York, pp 126–139
8. Katzen BT, Chang J (1979) Percutaneous transluminal angioplasty with the Grüntzig balloon catheter. Radiology 130: 623–626
9. Mathias K, Spillner G, Staiger J, Ahmadi A, Werner JP (1979) Perkutane transluminale Revaskularisation von Unterschenkelarterien. Chirurg 50: 158–163
10. Meaney TF, Weinstein MA, Buonocore E, et al. (1980) Digital subtraction angiography of the human cardiovascular system. AJR 135/6: 1153–1160
11. Mistretta CA, Crummy AB, Strother CM (1981) Digital angiography: a perspective. Radiology 139: 273–276
12. Motarjeme A, Keifer JW, Zuska AJ (1981) Percutaneous transluminal angioplasty as a complement to surgery. Radiology 141: 341–346
13. Olbert F, Hanecka L (1978) Transluminal vascular dilatation with a modified dilatation catheter. In: Zeitler E, Grüntzig A, Schoop W (eds) Percutaneous vascular recanalization. Springer, Berlin Heidelberg New York, pp 32–38
14. Roth F-J (1979) Die Dilatation von Stenosen der A. femoralis communis nach der Dotter Technik von der Gegenseite aus. Jahrestagung Dtsche. Ges. f. Angiologie, Heidelberg 1978. Witzstrock, Baden-Baden
15. Schmidtke I, Zeitler E, Schoop W (1975) Langzeitergebnisse der perkutanen Katheterbehandlung (Dotter-Technik) bei femoropoplitealen Arterienverschlüssen im Stadium II. VASA 4: 210
16. Schmidtke I, Zeitler E, Schoop W (1978) Spätergebnisse (5–8 Jahre) der perkutanen Katheterbehandlung (Dotter-Technik) bei femoro-poplitealen Arterienverschlüssen. VASA 7: 4–14
17. Seyferth W, Dilbat G, Marhoff P, Zeitler E (1982) Digitale Substraktionsangiographie – diagnostische Bereicherung oder technische Spielerei? – Standortbestimmung und Ausblick. Herz Gefäße 2: 742–757
18. Staple TW (1968) Modified catheter for percutaneous transluminal treatment of arteriosclerotic obstructions. Radiology 91: 1041
19. van Andel GJ (1976) Percutaneous transluminal angioplasty. Excerpta Medica, Amsterdam
20. Zeitler E (1974) Leistungsfähigkeit der perkutanen Beseitigung arterieller Obliterationen mit der Dotter-Technik. In: Ehringer H (ed) Angiologie 24: Fortschritte der konservativen Therapie der peripheren arteriellen Verschlußkrankheit. Huber, Bern, pp 70–86
21. Zeitler E, Müller R (1969) Erste Ergebnisse mit der Katheter-Rekanalisation nach Dotter bei arterieller Verschlußkrankheit. ROEFO 111/3: 345–352
22. Zeitler E, Reichold J, Schoop W, Loew D (1973) Einfluß von Acetylsalicylsäure auf das Frühergebnis nach perkutaner Rekanalisation arterieller Obliterationen nach Dotter. Dtsch Med Wochenschr 98: 1285–1288
23. Zeitler E, Grüntzig A, Schoop W (1978) Percutaneous vascular recanalization. Springer, Berlin Heidelberg New York
24. Zeitler E, Richter E-I, Roth F-J, Schoop W (1983) Results of percutaneous transluminal angioplasty. Radiology 146/1: 57

19. Angioplasty of the Iliac and Inguinal Arteries

F.-J. Roth and G. Cappius

Angioplasty of the iliac arteries has become an accepted routine method for the treatment of peripheral occlusive vascular disease [3, 8, 9, 11, 13, 15–19, 21, 24–26].

In cases of single atherosclerotic lesions in the iliac arteries or of inoperability in a patient with atherosclerotic disease, angioplasty seems to be the therapy of choice. The technique, the primary results, and the complications of this important therapeutic principle are discussed in this chapter.

Technique

In the last 5 years we have achieved 659 angioplasties of the iliac arteries, the common as well as the external (Table 1). Usually, the balloon catheter is introduced by means of the common femoral approach [4–6, 20, 23, 24]. In our material the ipsilateral technique was used in 72.7% and in 27.3% the crossover technique had to be employed. In rare cases, the axillary approach may be necessary. The latter approach is the most complicated one, and should only be choosen when no other technique can be used. We successfully attempted angioplasty of the iliac arteries using this approach in three patients.

If angioplasty is attempted using a retrograde technique, measurement of the systolic blood pressure proximal and distal to the stenosis should be performed [7, 17, 22, 24]. This is done for two reasons. First, the hemodynamic effect of the stenosis is then well outlined, and secondly, the success of the angioplasty is

Table 1. Technique and primary results of angioplasty of the iliac artery

	n	+	–
Ipsilateral approach	479	416 (87%)	63 (13%)
Contralateral approach	180	151 (84%)	29 (16%)
	659	567	92

n = number of treatments
\+ = technically succesful
– = technically failed

Percutaneous Transluminal Angioplasty
(ed. by C. T. Dotter, A. Grüntzig, W. Schoop, E. Zeitler)

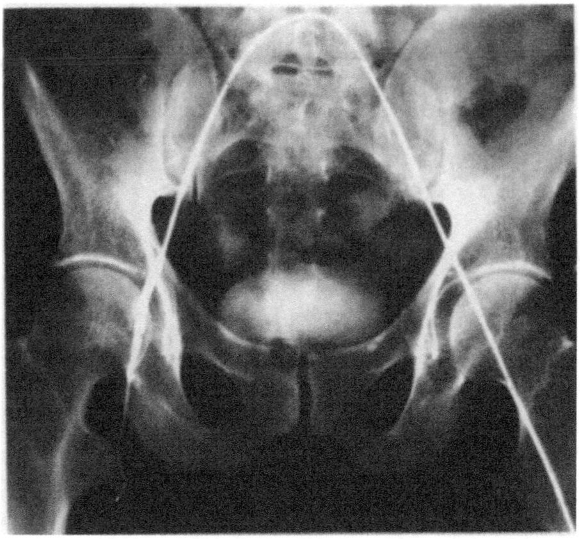

Fig. 1. Crossover technique: the left common femoral artery is punctured, the balloon inflated for the purpose of dilating the stenosed contralateral common femoral artery

reliably documented. If no pressure gradient is recorded after angioplasty, normalized blood supply should be expected. Should there be a slight residual stenosis but relief of the pressure gradient, no repeated dilatation of the stenosis is necessary. On the other hand, repeated dilatation is indicated if both a residual stenosis and a pressure gradient are demonstrated. In cases of significant intimal or medial damage (Fig. 2c) in the arterial segment combined with a residual pressure gradient, a repeated dilatation is without further benefit for the patient in most instances. Often an additional splitting of the intima and media is observed under these circumstances.

Crossover Technique

When angioplasty is performed by the crossover technique [2, 14], the balloon catheter has to be introduced from the contralateral side and advanced over the aortic bifurcation to widen a stenosis of the distal iliac or groin arteries (Fig. 1). Furthermore, the right and left iliac arteries (Fig. 2) or the iliac and femoral arteries of the ipsilateral side (Fig. 3) may be treated simultaneously in one procedure.

Special Technique

In very selected cases a combination of angioplasty with fibrinolytic therapy may be used. On principle, cases of acute reocclusion are treated with systemic fibrinolytic therapy, or low-dose fibrinolytic therapy is added to routine angioplasty. The latter has to be accomplished by the crossover technique in

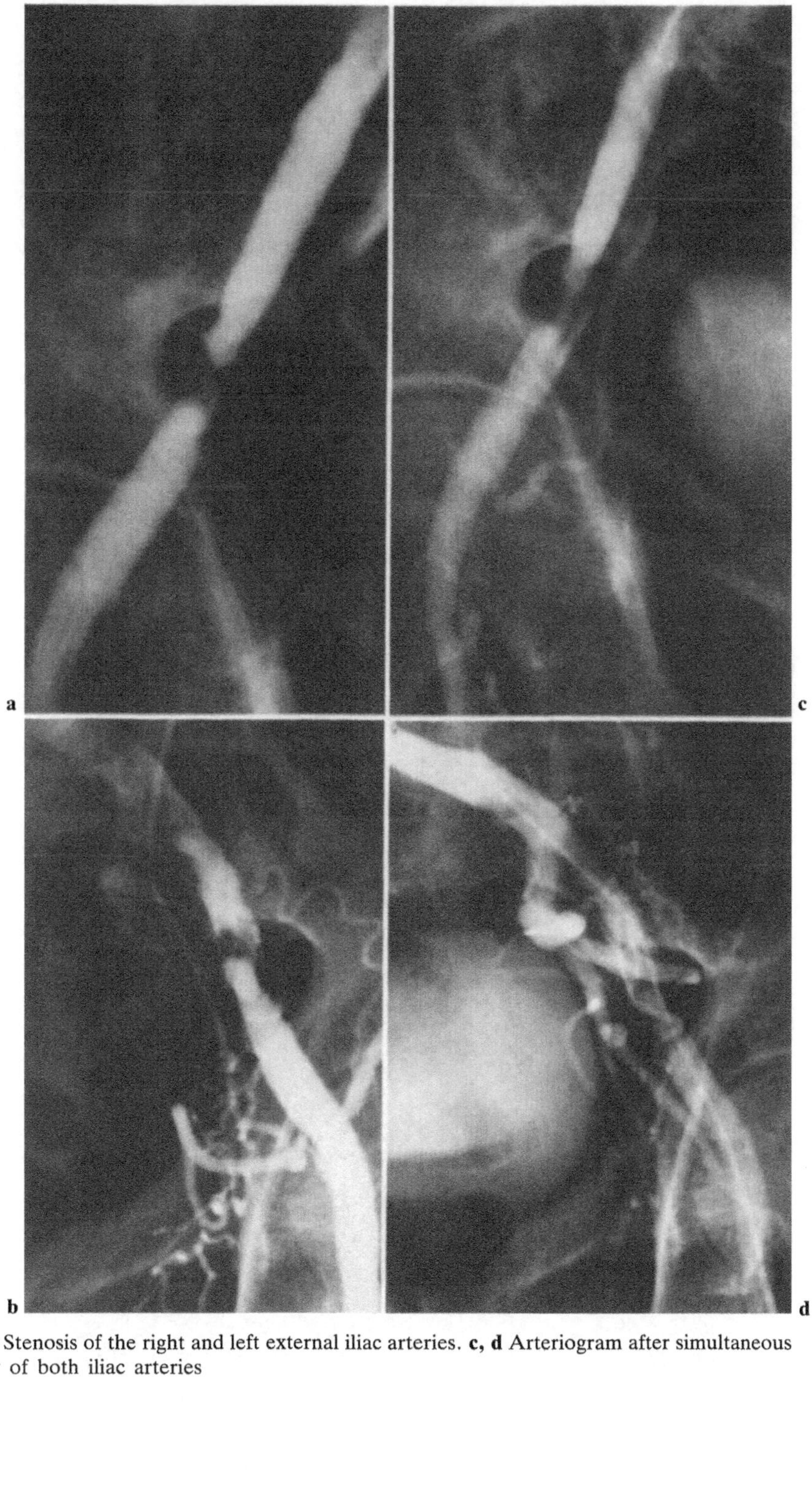

Fig. 2. a, b Stenosis of the right and left external iliac arteries. **c, d** Arteriogram after simultaneous angioplasty of both iliac arteries

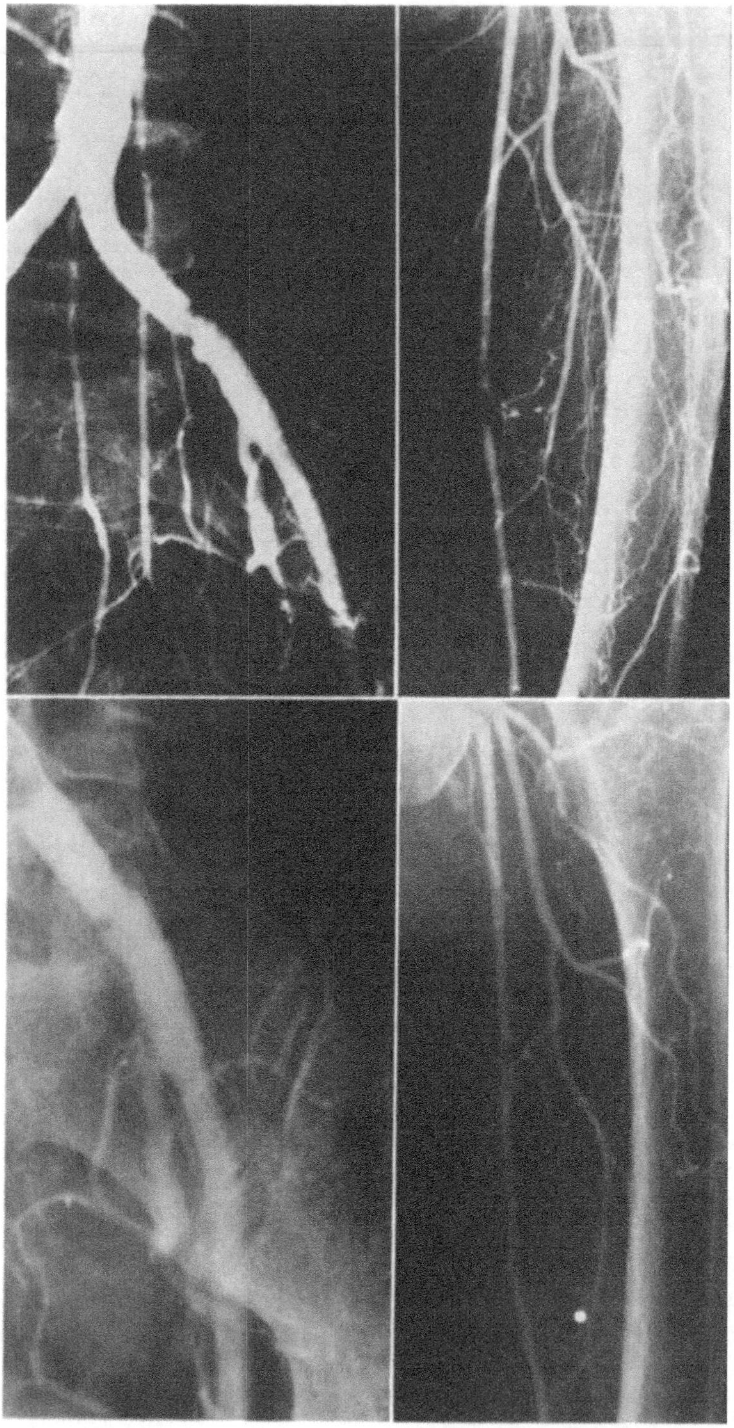

a b c d

Fig. 3. a, b Stenosis of the left common iliac and left superficial femoral arteries. **c, d** Arteriogram after dilatation of the superficial and the common iliac arteries in the same procedure

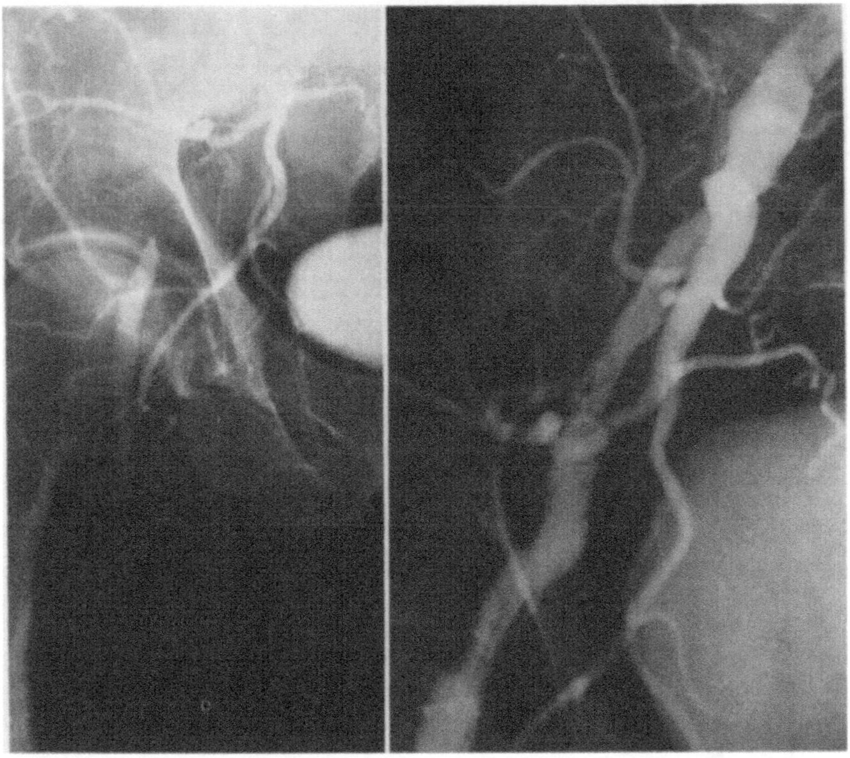

a b

Fig. 4. a Acute occlusion of the external iliac artery following routine angioplasty of a stenosed external iliac artery at its origin. **b** Recanalization of the acute occlusion by means of low-dose fibrinolytic therapy and crossover technique

most cases (Fig. 4). The combination of angioplasty with fibrinolytic therapy may be used if angioplasty of an occluded iliac artery is considered. In our experience, an acute reocclusion often occurs following recanalization of an occluded iliac artery.

Primary Results

We have attempted angioplasty of the iliac artery in 659 patients and have been successful in 86% (Table 2). The primary results are a little better with the ipsilateral approach than with the contralateral one (Table 1). The average pressure gradient of 75 consecutive cases was reduced from 60 to 12 mm Hg by means of the dilating balloon. A comparison of 20 eccentric with 24 concentric iliac stenoses shows that the primary results are better in the latter. On average, the residual stenoses of eccentric stenoses are of a higher degree than in the concentric ones. The relief of the pressure gradient is consistent with this finding (Table 3).

Table 2. Initial results of angioplasty of stenosed iliac arteries and complications requiring surgery [7]

	n	+ (%)	− (%)	Complication requiring surgery (%)
Seven clinics (up to 1976)	206	92	8	3
Aggertalklinik (1976–1982)	659	86	14	0.5

n = number of treatments
+ = technically succesful
− = technically failed

Table 3. Comparison of residual stenosis and pressure gradient in angioplasty of iliac arteries with eccentric and concentric stenosis

Stenosis	n	Average percentage stenosis		Pressure gradient (mm Hg)	
		Before PTA	After PTA	Before PTA	After PTA
Concentric	24	76	28	51	6
Eccentric	20	75	38	55	13
Total	44	76	33	53	9

n = number of patients

Table 4. Primary results of angioplasty of the groin arteries

	n	+	−
Distal external iliac artery	18 (13%)	15 (83%)	3
Common femoral artery	58 (41%)	40 (69%)	18
Proximal superfical femoral artery	24 (17%)	21 (88%)	3
Deep femoral artery	41 (29%)	34 (83%)	7
Total	141	110 (78%)	31 (22%)

n = number of treatments
+ = technically succesful
− = technically failed

We treated 141 patients with occlusive vascular disease of the groin arteries (Table 4), in most cases using the crossover technique. In our definition of groin arteries we include the distal external iliac, the common femoral, the proximal superficial, and the deep femoral arteries (Table 4). The distal external iliac artery starts at the iliopectineal line and ends at the hip joint. The common femoral artery begins and ends at the femoral bifurcation (Fig. 5). If the

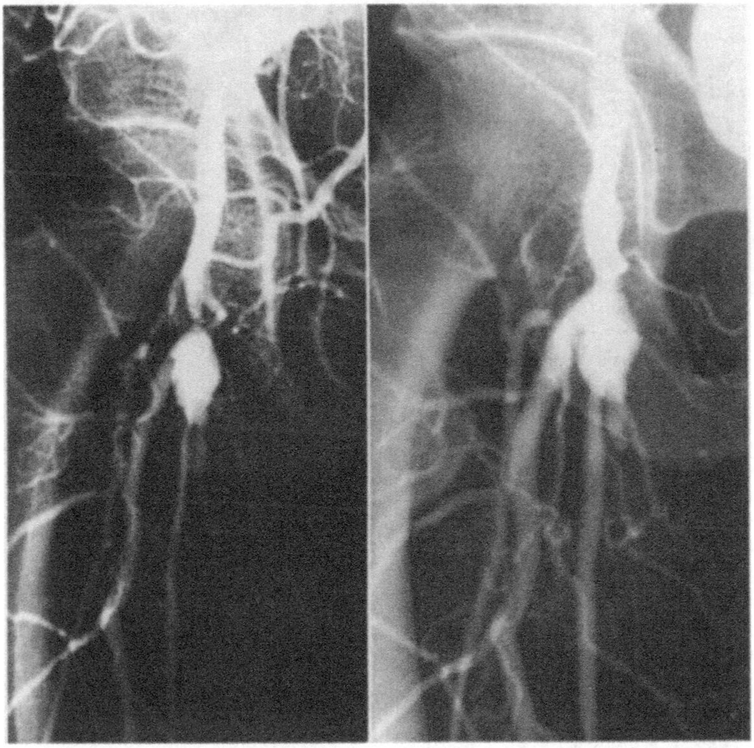

a b

Fig. 5. a Stenosis of the common femoral artery, an aneurysm of the superficial femoral artery at its origin following vascular surgery. **b** Postangioplasty arteriogram with widened stenosis of the common femoral artery

proximal superficial femoral artery was treated, a stenosis of its origin was the lesion typically widened (Fig. 6).

The overall primary success rate (Table 4) of the 141 Dotter procedures of the groin arteries was 78%. It is of note that angioplasty of the occluded common femoral arteries failed in 9 of 19 patients (47%). In 39 treatments of common femoral artery stenoses the average degree of the stenosis was reduced from 69% to 18% (Table 5).

Complications

Angioplasty of the iliac artery has a low complication rate [7, 22]. In the experience of seven clinics up to 1976 and in our own (Table 2), severe complications requiring surgery occur in about 2% of cases. We lost one 80-year-old patient in stage IV (Fontaine), who had acute occlusion of the iliac artery following routine angioplasty of a stenosis of the iliac artery and then required surgery. The patient suffered cardiac arrest at the end of the operation a 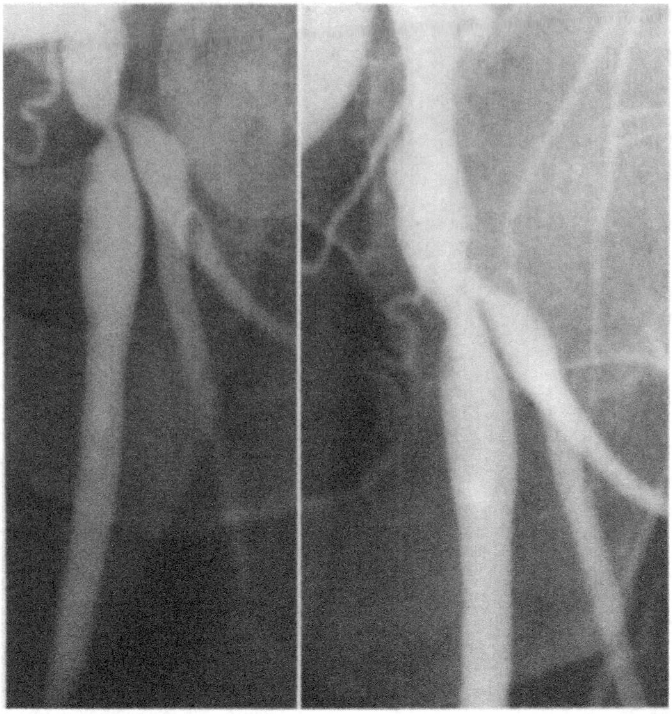 b

Fig. 6. a Stenosis of the superficial and deep femoral arteries at their origins. **b** Postangioplasty arteriogram showing both stenoses widened with a residual stenosis of the deep femoral artery

Table 5. Primary results of angioplasty of the common femoral artery

	n	+	–	Average percentage stenosis of arteries	
				Before PTA	After PTA
Stenosis	39	31 (80%)	8 (20%)	69 (range 50–90)	18 (range 0–54)
Occlusion	19	9 (47%)	10 (53%)	4,5 cm (range 1–11 cm)	36 (range 0–66)
Total	58	40 (69%)	18		27

n = number of treatments
\+ = technically succesful
– = technically failed

Table 6. Complications of 659 angioplasties of the iliac artery

Dissection	6 (0.9%)
Embolization	7 (1.1%)
Occlusion	7 (1.1%)
Occlusion of the internal iliac artery	5 (0.75%)
Huge hematoma	3 (0.5%)
Surgery	3 (0.5%)
Stroke 1 day after PTA	1 (0.15%)
Death	1 (0.15%)

and died (Table 6). Another patient had a stroke 1 day after angioplasty (Table 6).

Angioplasty of the iliac arteries may also be complicated by a dissection, peripheral embolization, an acute occlusion, or a huge hematoma at the puncture site (Table 6). These above-mentioned complications are mostly without important clinical evidence. In cases of failed angioplasty, our patients did not significantly deteriorate clinically. Where surgery was needed as alternative therapy because of failed angioplasty, the operation was made only slightly more difficult.

After angioplasty in 141 inguinal arteries using the crossover technique, no severe complications were observed except in one patient who suffered an occlusion of the iliac artery in the healthy leg 3 weeks after treatment. Surgery was required. One iatrogenic occlusion of the deep and one of the superficial femoral artery occurred in two other patients. These remained without clinical consequences.

Discussion

The primary results of angioplasty of the iliac arteries are good (Tables 1 and 2), success rates being as high as 92% in the literature [7, 16] and 86% in oure own series. The stress for the patient during angioplasty is small compared to that attending vascular surgery. The risk and the complication rate [3, 7, 17, 19, 24, 25] of this therapeutic principle are low. Therefore, in cases of isolated iliac artery stenosis angioplasty should be considered before surgery is recommended. The initial results of angioplasty of occlusions of the iliac artery are not as good as for stenoses, however, so surgery should be considered before a Dotter procedure is attempted.

The recording of the pressure gradient during angioplasty is necessary because the pressure readings before angioplasty of the iliac artery outline the hemodynamic effect of the stenosis. After treatment a residual stenosis with hemodynamic effect can easily be discovered, and an additional dilatation may be attempted to improve the therapeutic effect [22, 24].

With the crossover technique, the main difficulties arise when the catheter encounters resistance at its tip. Because of the indirect power transmission, the catheter has the tendency to slide back into the aorta, and it is then impossible to pass the balloon catheter through the stenosis for the purpose of dilatation. The most important disadvantage of the crossover technique is the risk of a complication in the healthy leg. Reasons for technical failure are tortuosity of the iliac arteries, an acute angle of the aortic bifurcation, and the indirect power transmission in handling the balloon catheter.

On the other hand, the achievements of this therapeutic principle are high. Angioplasty may be extended to the groin arteries (Figs. 1, 5, and 6). The Dotter procedure is possible in cases of obesity or postoperative scar in the inguinal area. The right and left iliac arteries or the iliac and femoral arteries of the ipsilateral side may be managed in the same procedure.

In spite of the technical difficulties, the overall success rate of angioplasty of the groin arteries using the crossover technique is 78% (Table 4). In the treatment of stenoses, a good initial success of almost 85% (Table 4) is observed. In recanalization of occluded arteries, the primary success rate drops down to 47% (9 out of 19 cases). The main reason for our low success rate with occlusions of the groin arteries is the technical difficulty of directing the guide wire into the patent deep femoral artery past the occlusion. In most instances the guide wire engaged the likewise occluded superficial femoral artery. Therefore, it is recommended that patients with occlusions, especially of the common femoral artery, should be treated surgically. However, if a patient cannot withstand an operation, angioplasty of the occluded groin artery may represent the only remaining means of possibly salvaging the limb.

If angioplasty of the deep femoral artery is attempted, the superficial femoral artery is most often likewise occluded [10, 12, 19]. In these circumstances the deep femoral artery is the only vessel which supplies the leg. One should beware of attempting angioplasty of the only collateral vessel of an extremity, and the indications for angioplasty must be very strong. The radiologist should work closely with a vascular surgeon in such instances.

Summary

Angioplasty of the iliac and groin arteries is discussed on the basis of experience gained during 659 treatments of the iliac and 141 of the groin arteries. Angioplasty of the groin arteries requires use of the crossover technique in most cases. The primary results of the iliac artery stenoses show a success rate as high as 92% in the literature and 86% in our own series. The initial results of angioplasty of the groin arteries are not quite as good (78%). It is obvious that the crossover technique involves a drop in the initial success rate because of technical difficulties. On the other hand, the crossover technique makes possible angioplasty of the groin arteries. It also allows the left and right iliac arteries or the iliac and femoral arteries of the ipsilateral side to be treated in the same procedure.

Severe complications requiring surgery occur in about 2%. Since angioplasty gives good primary and late results in the treatment of stenosis of the iliac and groin arteries, it is recommended for such cases. On the other hand, in occlusions of the iliac and groin arteries angioplasty gives relatively poor initial results. Surgery is therefore recommended in these circumstances. Only when a patient cannot withstand an operation should such a procedure be undertaken, as a last possible means of limb salvage.

References

1. Alter M, Kieffer S, Resch J, Ansari K (1972) Cerebral infraction. Clinical and angiographic correlations. Neurology 22: 590–601
2. Bachmann DM, Casarella WJ, Sos TA (1979) Percutaneous iliofemoral angioplasty via the contralateral femoral artery. Radiology 130: 617–621
3. Dotter CT (1980) Transluminal angioplasty: a long view. Radiology 135: 561–564
4. Dotter CT, Judkins MP (1964) Transluminal treatment of arteriosclerotic obstruction. Description of a new technic and a preliminary report of its application. Circulation 30: 654
5. Grüntzig A (1976) Die perkutane Rekanalisation chronischer arterieller Verschlüsse (Dotter-Prinzip) mit einem neuen doppellumigen Dilatationskatheter. ROEFO 124: 80
6. Grüntzig A, Hopff H (1974) Perkutane Rekanalisation chronischer arterieller Verschlüsse mit einem neuen Dilatationskatheter. Modifikation der Dotter-Technik. Dtsch Med Wochenschr 99: 2502
7. Grüntzig A, Zeitler E (1978) Cooperative study of results of PTR in twelve different clinics. In: Zeitler E, Grüntzig A, Schoop W (eds) Percutaneous vascular rekanalization. Springer, Berlin Heidelberg New York, pp 118
8. Hess H (1981) Differentialtherapie zur Wiederherstellung der peripheren arteriellen Strombahn. Vasa [Suppl] 8: 43
9. Katzen BT, Chang J, Knox WG (1979) Percutaneous transluminal angioplasty with the Grüntzig balloon catheter. Arch Surg 114: 1389–1399
10. Mahler F, Grüntzig A, Schlumpf M (1978) Transluminal dilatation of a stenosis in the deep femoral artery. In: Zeitler E, Grüntzig A, Schoop W (eds) Percutaneous vascular rekanalization. Springer, Berlin Heidelberg New York, pp 141
11. Motarjeme A, Keifer JW, Zuska AJ (1980) Percutaneous transluminal angioplasty of the iliac arteries. AJR 135: 937–944
12. Motarjeme A, Keifer JW, Zuska AJ (1980) Percutaneous transluminal angioplasty of the deep femoral artery. Radiology 135: 613–617
13. Olbert F, Kumpan W, Ogris E, Denck H, Weidinger P, Jonas M, Hugeneck J, Russe O (1975) Die perkutane transluminale Dilatation nach Dotter – eine radiologische Methode zur Wiederherstellung der arteriellen Strombahn. Kongreßbericht der Österreichischen Gesellschaft für Chirurgie, 16. Tagung 5.–7. 6. 1975
14. Roth F-J (1978) Die Dilatation von Stenosen der A. femoralis communis nach der Dotter-Technik von der Gegenseite aus. Vortrag: Deutsche Gesellschaft für Angiologie, Jahrestagung Heidelberg, 21.9.–23. 9. 1978
15. Schmidtke I, Roth F-J, Schoop W, Cappius G (1980) Perkutane transluminale Katheterbehandlung bei Kranken mit arteriellen Durchblutungsstörungen im Stadium III und IV. In: Müller-Wiefel H, Barras J-P, Ehringer H, Krüger M (eds) Mikrozirkulation und Blutrheologie, Therapie der peripheren arteriellen Verschlußkrankheit. Witzstrock, Baden-Baden, pp 411–420
16. Schoop W, Levy H, Cappius G, Mansjoer H, Zeitler E (1978) Early and late results of PTD in iliac stenosis. In: Zeitler E, Grüntzig A, Schoop W (eds) Percutaneous vascular recanalization. Springer, Berlin Heidelberg New York, pp 111
17. van Andel GJ (1976) Percutaneous transluminal angioplasty. The Dotter procedure. A manual for the radiologist. Excerpta Medica, Amsterdam
18. van Andel GJ (1980) Transluminal iliac angioplasty: long-term results. Radiology 135: 607–611

19. Waltman AC (1980) Percutaneous transluminal angioplasty: iliac and deep femoral arteries. AJR 135: 921–925
20. Zeitler E (1972) Die perkutane Rekanalisation arterieller Obliterationen mit Katheter nach Dotter (Dotter-Technik). Dtsch Med Wochenschr 97: 1392
21. Zeitler E (1974) Leistungsfähigkeit der perkutanen Beseitigung arterieller Obliterationen mit der Dotter-Technik. In: Ehringer H (ed) Fortschritte der konservativen Therapie der peripheren arteriellen Verschlußkrankeit. Aktuelle Probleme in der Angiologie, vol 24. Huber, Bern, pp 70
22. Zeitler E (1978) Dilatation technique of iliac artery stenosis with balloon catheters. In: Zeitler E, Grüntzig A, Schoop W (eds) Percutaneous vascular recanalization. Springer, Berlin Heidelberg New York, pp 24
23. Zeitler E, Müller R (1969) Erste Ergebnisse mit der Katheter-Rekanalisation nach Dotter bei arterieller Verschlußkrankheit. ROEFO 111: 345
24. Zeitler E, Grüntzig A, Schoop W (1978) Percutaneous vascular recanalization. Technique, application, clinical results. Springer, Berlin Heidelberg New York
25. Zeitler E, Schmidtke I, Schoop W, Giessler R, Dembski J, Mansjoer H (1978) Ergebnisse nach perkutaner transluminaler Angioplastie bei über 700 Behandlungen. Röntgenpraxis 29: 78
26. Zorn-Bopp E, Ingrisch H, Mietaschk A, Frey KW (1981) Transluminale Gefäßdilatation der distalen Bauchaorta der Arteria iliaca communis und externa. ROEFO 134/5: 471–475

20. Percutaneous Transluminal Angioplasty in Cases of Stenosis in the Region of the Infrarenal Abdominal Aorta and the Aortoiliac Bifurcation

H. Ingrisch, W. Seyferth, and G. Küffer

In atheromatous occlusive disease, stenoses and occlusions of the infrarenal aorta are seldom found (in only 3%–4%) [4]. Usually the aortoiliac bifurcation is involved. A single stenosis in the aorta is rarely seen. Percutaneous transluminal angioplasty (PTA) [1] was not applied to the stenosis of the distal abdominal aorta until after the description of an inflatable dilatation catheter by Grüntzig [3]. Due to the low incidence of the disease, very little literature is available on this topic [2, 5, 6].

I shall describe first the technique and then the results of this therapy in ten patients.

Technique

Nine of the ten patients were treated using the "kissing balloon technique," and one patient with a very small aorta required only one dilatation catheter to compensate the pressure difference. In the kissing balloon technique a dilatation catheter is introduced into each femoral artery and advanced over a guide wire into the aorta. The balloons of both dilatation catheters are positioned adjacent to each other in the region of the stenosis. Before and after dilatation the mean intraarterial pressure difference is measured. An angiographic examination completes the procedure. An example of the PTA of a stenosed aorta using the kissing balloon technique is given in Fig. 1.

Patients

Ten patients were treated between October 1979 and September 1981. Seven of these patients had a single aortic stenosis and three an aortic stenosis with involvement of the bifurcation. The average age was 58.6 years (range 36–79); six were female and four male. The follow-up period extended over a minimum of 6 and a maximum of 30 months. Intermittent claudication as a clinical symptom before and after PTA was classified according to Fontaine.

Percutaneous Transluminal Angioplasty
(ed. by C. T. Dotter, A. Grüntzig, W. Schoop, E. Zeitler)

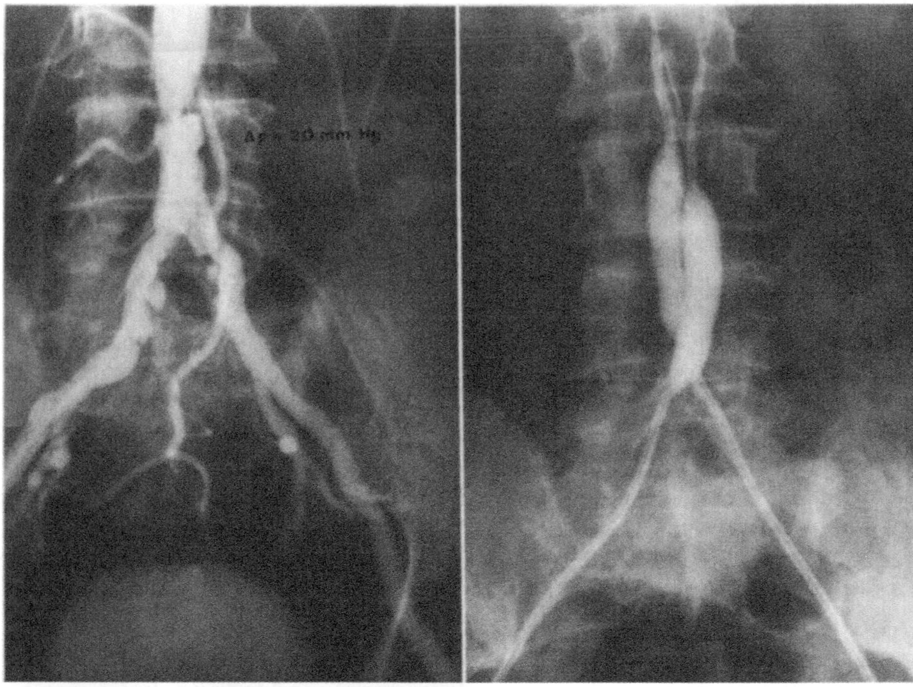

a b

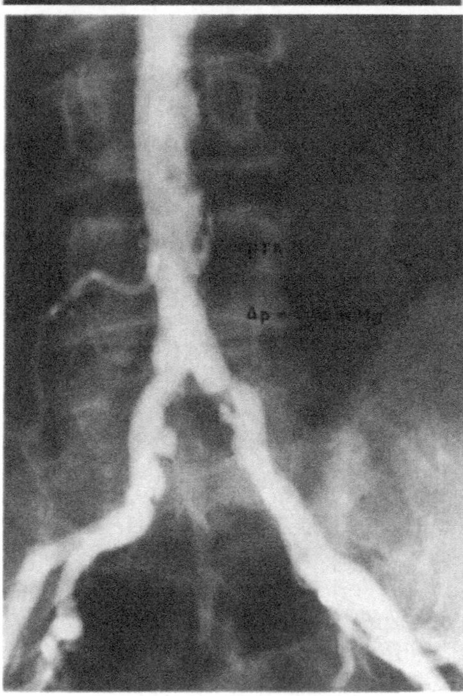

c

Fig. 1. a A 71-year-old male with aortic stenosis and intermittent claudication stage IIb; **b** PTA with two dilatation catheters: kissing balloon technique; **c** angiographic control 13 months later: walking distance was clinically unlimited

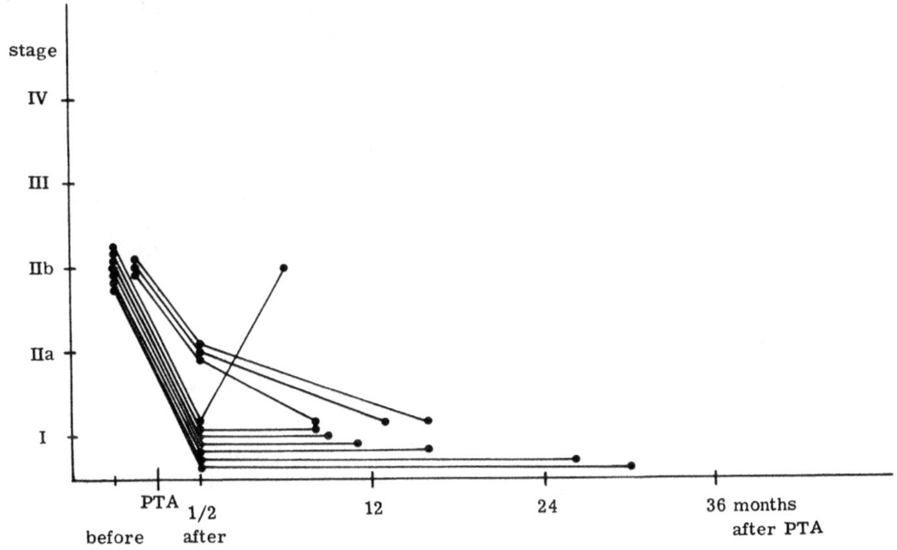

Fig. 2. Clinical stage (Fontaine) in 10 patients with aortic stenosis before and after PTA related to the individual follow-up period

Results

The clinical stage (Fontaine) before and after PTA with regard to the individual follow-up period is demonstrated in Fig. 2. Before PTA all ten patients were classified as stage IIb (walking distance less than 200 m). By the day after therapy seven of the patients could be classified as stage I and the remaining three as stage IIa (walking distance limited but more than 200 m).

After the individual follow-up period all patients except one could be classified as stage I (Fig. 2). One patient who had been free of complaints for 6 months developed a severe iliac stenosis below the level of the previously dilated area.

Intraarterial pressure difference before PTA was found to be between 20 and 50 mm Hg. After PTA five patients showed no pressure difference and the other five a pressure difference of up to 10 mm Hg.

In three patients the procedure produced complications, but these were without later consequences. Two were cases of peripheral embolism; in one we had to use a Fogarty catheter to remove it. The third case was a dissection of the aortic wall.

Discussion

A stenosis in a narrow abdominal aorta can be treated using a single dilatation catheter, as can an iliac stenosis. When the aorta is somewhat larger in diameter the kissing balloon technique is sufficient to achieve an adequate dilatation. In the choice of catheter the diameter of the aorta above the stenosis should be

Table 1. Various diameters and cross-sectional areas of aorta and some combinations of balloon diameters necessary to obtain the required cross-sectional area of aorta

Diameter (mm) of vessel	8	10	12	14	16	18	20
Cross section (mm^2)	50.2	78.5	113.0	153.9	200.9	254.0	314.0
Outer diameter of balloon (mm) needed to achieve the cross section above	1 × 8	1 × 10	1 × 12	2 × 10	1 × 10 + 1 × 12	3 × 10	so on
			2 × 3	3 × 8	4 × 8 2 × 10 + 1 × 8	2 × 12	so on

taken into consideration. Table 1 shows diameters and cross-sectional areas of aorta and the diameters of the various dilatation balloons necessary to fill the cross-sectional area of the aorta. It should be ensured that the two adjacent-lying balloons have a smaller combined diameter than that of the aorta. However, it can be an advantage to use three small-diameter dilatation catheters simultaneously (two from the femoral and one from the axillary approach) because the more cylindrical form will fill out the lumen of the aorta better than two catheters with a larger balloon (Table 1). Our results have shown that this treatment of aortic stenosis provides a successful result for a longer period. This should encourage the discussion and if possible the use of this method before surgical intervention.

Despite the good surgical results after localized aortic endarterectomy or aortoiliac bypass, it is necessary to take into consideration the possibility of complications such as post-surgical impotence due to damage to the paraaortic nerves, and the surgical lethality, even though this is a small percentage.

Acknowledgements. We are very grateful to Dr. Theiss and Dr. Kramann, Klinikum r. d. Isar, Munich, for contributing one of the ten cases discussed.

References

1. Dotter CT, Judkins MP (1964) Transluminal treatment of arteriosclerotic obstruction. Circulation 30: 654–670
2. Freiman DB, McLean GK, Oleaga JA, Ring EJ (1981) Percutaneous transluminal angioplasty. In: Ring EJ, McLean GK (eds) Interventional radiology: principles and techniques. Little, Brown, Boston
3. Grüntzig A, Hopff H (1974) Perkutane Rekanalisation chronischer arterieller Verschlüsse mit einem neuen Dilatationskatheter. Dtsch Med Wochenschr 99: 2502
4. Münster W, Wierny L, Porstmann W (1966) Lokalisation und Häufigkeit arterieller Obliterationen der unteren Extremitäten. Analyse von 952 Aortoarteriographien. Dtsch Med Wochenschr 91: 2073
5. Velasquez G, Castaneda-Zuniga W, Formanek A, Zollikopfer CH, Barreto A, Nicoloff D, Amplatz K, Sullivan A (1980) Nonsurgical aortoplasty in Leriche syndrome. Radiology 134: 359–360
6. Zorn-Bopp E, Ingrisch H, Mietaschk A, Frey KW (1981) Transluminale Gefäßdilatation der distalen Bauchaorta, der Arteria iliaca communis und externa. Fortschr. Röntgenstr 134 (5): 411–475

21. Relapse Treatment by Percutaneous Transluminal Dilatation

I. Schmidtke and F.-J. Roth

An advantage of percutaneous transluminal dilatation (PTD) lies in the repeatability of this method in the same vascular section, insofar as the local conditions have not changed. During the 12 years of application of this method by the Aggertalklinik, the frequency of repetition of treatment has clearly been on the increase. In the following, we report the results of repeated treatment in the period between 1 January 1977 and 31 December 1981.

Patients and Procedure

Patients

The study was carried out on 98 treated extremities in 97 patients, 65 of which were men and 32 women. Forty-seven cases were in stage II, 20 in stage III, and 31 in stage IV (Table 1). Disease was primarily localized to the femoropopliteal region ($n = 87$); 11 cases exhibited iliac stenoses. Table 1 includes information on the risk factors. Worth special notice is the frequency of diabetes in stage IV.

Time Interval

The time interval between the first and second and/or third interventions varied considerably. Quite frequently, the procedure was repeated within a very short time, i.e., during the same hospitalization period, if the first treatment had yielded only a short-term success.

Procedure

The treatments were performed using the Andel and the Grüntzig balloon catheters. Apart from puncture problems due to pronounced scar formation in the inguinal region, no difficulties other than those prevailing during the first treatment were encountered.

Percutaneous Transluminal Angioplasty
(ed. by C. T. Dotter, A. Grüntzig, W. Schoop, E. Zeitler)

Table 1. Groups of patients classified by time interval, age, and risk factors

Localization	Stage	Extremities (*n*)	Men (*n*)	Women (*n*)	Time interval	Average age (years)	Risk factors		
							Nicotine (%)	Diabetes (%)	Hypertension (%)
Diac artery stenosis	II–IV	11	8	3	1 day to 5 years	59.4	91	36	44
Femoropopliteal artery	II	40	33	6	1 month to 11 years	56.7	90	33	40
Femoropopliteal artery	III	20	11	9	1 month to 6 years	66.5	65	45	55
Femoropopliteal artery	IV	17	8	9	2 days to 2 years	70.0	59	76	35
Femoropopliteal artery (three treatments)	IV	10	5	5	2nd PTD 5 days to 5.5 months 3rd PTD 6 days to 12 months	67.6	40	80	40
Total		98	65	32					

Assessment of Success

An intervention was regarded as successful from a radiological viewpoint when redilatation or recanalization was achieved, mostly confirmed by the control angiogram, whereas cases in which sphygmopalpation and oscilloscopic and Doppler readings improved were classified as successful from a clinical viewpoint. A differentiation between residual stenosis and entirely free vascular system was not made in this case.

Pre- and Posttreatment

Prior to PTD, most patients were given an acetylsalicylic acid preparation (ASSD); 69 patients also received ASS after the first treatment, 13 patients heparin; 15 patients did not get any prophylactics for various reasons. After the second treatment, 57 patients were given ASS, 20 patients anticoagulants, 1 patient heparin, and 15 patients no prophylactic at all; 5 patients were subjected to a vascular operation.

Findings

Iliac Stenosis

Eleven patients (eight men and three women) between 39 and 80 years of age underwent repeated treatment for iliac stenosis after periods ranging from 1 day to 5 years. In ten cases dilatation of the iliac stenosis was determined by radiological findings and in nine cases by clinical findings (Table 2). The time interval had no influence on the success. However, posttreatment prognosis for lesions of the common iliac artery seems to be more favorable than for stenoses of the external iliac artery.

Table 2. Iliac stenoses

Localization			*n*	Success	
1st PTD		2nd PTD		R (*n*)	Cl (*n*)
IC	→	IC	6	6	6
IC	→	IE	1	1	1
IE	→	IE	4	3	2
Total			11	10	9

IC, common iliac artery; IE, external iliac artery; R, radiological; Cl, clinical

Table 3. Femoropopliteal obliterations classified according to length and type

Localization			Total (*n*)	Success		Same length		Shorter		Longer	
1st PTD		2nd PTD		R (*n*)	Cl (*n*)	Total (*n*)	Success (*n*)	Total (*n*)	Success (*n*)	Total (*n*)	Success (*n*)
FO	→	FO	17	12	8	10	6	1	1	6	5
FO	→	FSt	5	5	4	2	2			3	3
FSt	→	FSt	10	10	10	7	7	1	1	2	2
FSt	→	FO	4	1	0	3	0			1	1
PO	→	PO	2	2	2	1	1			1	1
PO	→	PSt	2	2	1	2	2				
Total			40	32 (80%)	25 (62.5%)	25	18 (72%)	2	2 (100%)	13	12 (92%)

FO, femoral occlusion; FSt, femoral stenosis; PO, popliteal occlusion; PSt, popliteal stenosis

Femoropopliteal Section

Eighty-seven extremities were subjected to a relapse intervention in the femoropopliteal section; 40 cases were stage II, 20 stage III, and 27 stage IV. Ten patients were treated three times. Due to the varying initial conditions, such as obliteration length and vascular condition, the findings were classified by their clinical stage.

Stage II

Of 40 extremities investigated, 32 (80%) exhibited success in radiographic terms; however, clinically only 25 cases (62.5%) could be classified as successful. As becomes evident from the analysis of the angiographic findings prior to the first and second catheter treatments (Table 3), the constellation had changed in many cases by the second intervention. Reocclusions/stenoses were either longer or shorter; what had been obliterations during the first PTD had turned into stenoses; in a few cases, the previous stenoses had developed into outright occlusions. Also the occlusion or stenosis length had changed in 15 cases. Amazingly, evaluation of the control angiogram revealed better results (92%) for the occlusions and stenoses that had become longer (n = 13 cm) than for the 25 obliterations that had maintained their lengths, where only 72% showed any success. The least success was observed with the femoral occlusions resulting from femoral stenoses (one case out of four).

Of the cases of femoral occlusion subjected to one repeat treatment, 71% showed success from a radiological viewpoint, but only 47% showed clinical success. Analysis of these 17 cases by the lenght of occlusion (Table 4) revealed least success in the range 4–6 cm; only 28% of these could be treated from a clinical point of view.

Classification by time interval (Table 5) does not reveal any remarkable variations within the first 2 years in terms of clinical success (50%–67%). The results after 2–9 years are amazingly good, clinical success rates being 75% and 100% respectively.

Table 4. Femoral occlusions remaining after the first treatment, classified by length at second intervention

Length	n	Success	
		R (n)	Cl (n)
1–3 cm	3	2 (67%)	2 (67%)
4–6 cm	8	5 (63%)	3 (28%)
7–9 cm	1	1 (100%)	1 (100%)
>9 cm	5	4 (80%)	2 (40%)
Total	17	12 (71%)	8 (47%)

R, radiological; Cl, clinical

Table 5. Stage II femoropopliteal obliterations classified by time interval

	Total (*n*)	< 1 month (*n*)	1–3 months (*n*)	4–6 months (*n*)	7–12 months (*n*)	1–2 years (*n*)	2–3 years (*n*)	3–9 years (*n*)
n	40	7	5	6	10	4	4	4
Success								
R	32	5	3	5	7	4	4	4
Cl	25	4	3	4	5	2	3	4
		(57%)	(60%)	(67%)	(50%)	(50%)	(75%)	(100%)

R, radiological; Cl, clinical

Table 6. Stage III femoropopliteal obliterations classified by localization and type

Localization			*n*	Success	
1st PTD		2nd PTA		R	Cl
FO	→	FO	5	4	4
FO + PO	→	FO + PO	5	4	2
F/PO	→	F/PSt	3	3	3
F/PSt	→	F/PSt	3	2	2
PO	→	PO	4	4	2
Total			20	17 (85%)	13 (65%)

F, femoral; P, popliteal; O, occlusion; St, stenosis

Stage III

For 20 patients, stage III existed at the time of the second treatment, and in most of these cases already at the time of the first treatment. The patency of the vascular system was much worse than in the stage II cases. Only four patients had all three lower leg arteries patent. Of the patients in this group 45% were women.

As shown in Table 6, 17 patients (85%) were treated with radiological success, 13 patients (65%) with clinical success. This success rate is identical to that for the treatment in stage II.

The worst results occurred in once-repeated treatments of the femoropopliteal occlusions and the popliteal occlusions with poor distal runoff in stage III. The legs of two patients had to be amputed after an unsuccessful second treatment.

Stage IV, Once-Repeated PTD

Seventeen patients showed stage IV disease both at the first and the second treatments, the interval ranging between 2 days and 2 years. The proportion of diabetics (56%) was much higher than among patients in stage II and stage III, and the percentage of women slightly higher than of men. The vascular systems

Table 7. Second PTD in cases of stage IV femoropopliteal obliteration: localization and success

Localization			Length (cm)	n	Success	
1st PTD		2nd PTD			R (n)	Cl (n)
FO	→	FO	10, 18	2	2	2
FPO	→	FPO	17, 24, 25	3	1	1
FO	→	FSt		1	1	1
F/PSt	→	F/PSt		2	2	1
PO	→	PO	3, 12	2	0	0
PO	→	PSt		2	1	1
PSt	→	PO + FSt		1	1	1
FSt/O	→	PO/St/lower leg		4	2	1
Total				17	10 (58.8%)	8 (47.1%)

F, femoral; P, popliteal; FP, femoropopliteal; O, occlusion; St, stenosis

were largely bypassed (two lower leg arteries were occluded in eight patients and all three in five patients). Most femoropopliteal occlusions were quite long (up to 25 cm), the stenoses often of a filiform nature. This lowered the expectations of success right from the beginning, surgical intervention being performed in the hope of saving the leg.

As Table 7 shows, the second PTD was radiologically successful in ten cases (58.5%), but from a clinical viewpoint only in eight (47.1%).

The table further reveals that there is a great diversity of radiological findings, the cases with popliteal occlusions, either isolated or in combination with femoral occlusions or distal occlusions, yielding the worst results.

Stage IV: Twice-Repeated PTD

Ten patients (five men and five women) with stage IV disease (not included in the evaluation in the previous section were subjected to PTD three times. The second catheterization took place at an interval of 5 days to 5.5 months after the first PTD, the third treatment between 6 days and 12 months after the second PTD.

The caracteristic feature of this group is again the high share of diabetics and of women. After the second treatment in stage IV patients, the preconditions for another PTD were very adverse because of the poor condition of the vascular system and the long, particularly distal, occlusions. Remarkable progression of obliterations occurred in the time intervals between treatments, especially in the lower leg arteries and the distal popliteal artery. Table 8 lists each case indicating the length of occlusion and the results. From a radiological point of view, the first PTD was successful in all cases, the second treatment in nine, but the third in only five cases. The first PTD was clinically successful in seven cases, the second in six, and the third in only two. At discharge, two patients were in stage

Table 8. Cases of stage IV femoropopliteal obliterations treated three times by PTD: classification according to localization, type length and success

Localization					Length (cm)			1st angioplasty		2nd angioplasty		3rd angioplasty	
1st PTD		2nd PTD		3rd PTD	1st	2nd	3rd	R	Cl	R	Cl	R	Cl
FO	→	FO	→	FO	6	10	12	+	0	0	0	+	0
FO	→	FO	→	FPO	4	2.5	15	+	0	+	+	+	0
FO	→	FO	→	FO	18	18	18	+	+	+	0	0	0
FO	→	FPSt	→	PO	12	St	6	+	+	+	+	+	+
FPSt	→	FPSt	→	FPSt				+	+	+	0	+	0
PO	→	PO	→	PO	7	7	4	+	+	+	+	0	0
PO	→	FO	→	PO	3.5	10	14	+	+	+	+	0	0
PO	→	FPO	→	PO	25	28	4	+	+	+	+	0	0
PO	→	FPSt	→	FO	10	St	8	+	+	+	+	+	+
Total								10	7	9	6	5	2

F, femoral; P, popliteal; FP, femoropopliteal; O, occlusion; St, stenosis

Table 9. Summary of the results of multiple treatment according to localization and stage

Localization	Stage	Extremities (*n*)	Succesful after the 2nd or 3rd PTD	
			R (*n*) (%)	Cl (*n*) (%)
ISt	II/IV	11	10 (91)	8 (82)
F/P	II	40	32 (80)	25 (63)
F/P	III	20	17 (85)	13 (65)
F/P	IV 2 × PTD	17	10 (59)	8 (47)
	IV 3 × PTD	10	5 (50)	2 (20)
Total		98	74 (76)	57 (58)

ISt, iliac stenosis; F, femoral; P, popliteal

II; a partial amputation (toes or forefoot) had to be performed in two cases; five patients underwent amputation at the knee or upper leg; one patient died before amputation.

With such poor results (only 20% clinical success), a third PTD in stage IV must be regarded dubiously. It must be remembered that treatment brings great stress to these patients because of the severe rest pain they suffer when lying flat for a long period of time.

Summary

The best results for treatment of a recurrene at the same vascular level (Table 9) were observed for the iliac stenoses, namely 82% from a clinical viewpoint. Quite similar (63%–65%) were the findings in the area of the femoropopliteal artery. Much worse were the results in stage IV: 47% of these cases were improved from a clinical point of view after once-repeated treatment, 20% after twice-repeated treatment. The reasons for the poor results in stage IV were mainly the length of occlusions and the poor general condition of the vascular system. The majority of the patients were diabetics, the high proportion of women being characteristic. Upon reocclusion after a second PTD in stage IV, another catheterization is rarely successful.

VI. Percutaneous Transluminal Angioplasty in Combination With Fibrinolysis

22. Fibrinolysis and Transluminal Catheter Treatment: A Multistage Approach for the Removal of Chronic Arterial Occlusions

M. Martin, B. J. O. Fiebach, and T. Godula

Introduction

Results of percutaneous transluminal angioplasty (PTA) followed by fibrinolytic therapy have already been reported. Another therapeutic scheme using lytic and catheter methods is established by the sequence: clearance by fibrinolysis → widening of a remaining arterial stenosis by PTA. The present study deals with ten cases in which this multistage treatment was performed.

Method

In all ten cases fibrinolytic removal of chronic arterial occlusions was feasible. Fibrinolytic agents used were either streptokinase or activator (streptokinase-human plasminogen complex). The treatment period varied between 1 and 3 days. After lysis one or more residual narrowings persisted. In terms of clinical examination this correlated with peripheral pulses not fully normalized, arterial bruits, improved but not normalized ankle pressure values, and oscillographic recordings indicating a residual obstruction in the arterial segment cleared by fibrinolytic therapy. In the case of four combined femoroiliac locations both diminished pulse and systolic bruit in the groin were indicative of a residual narrowing.

Patients

In all ten patients a fibrinolytic treatment had led to the removal of chronic arterial occlusions but with a residual stenosis persisting. Five occlusions were located in the femoral artery and five in the iliac artery (four times in combination with a long-standing femoral occlusion). Patient age varied between 45 and 73 years. The male/female ratio was 9 : 1. The femoral occlusions were estimated to thave been present for between 5 days and 4 weeks, the iliac occlusions for between 4 weeks and 6 months (Tables 1 and 2).

Percutaneous Transluminal Angioplasty
(ed. by C. T. Dotter, A. Grüntzig, W. Schoop, E. Zeitler)

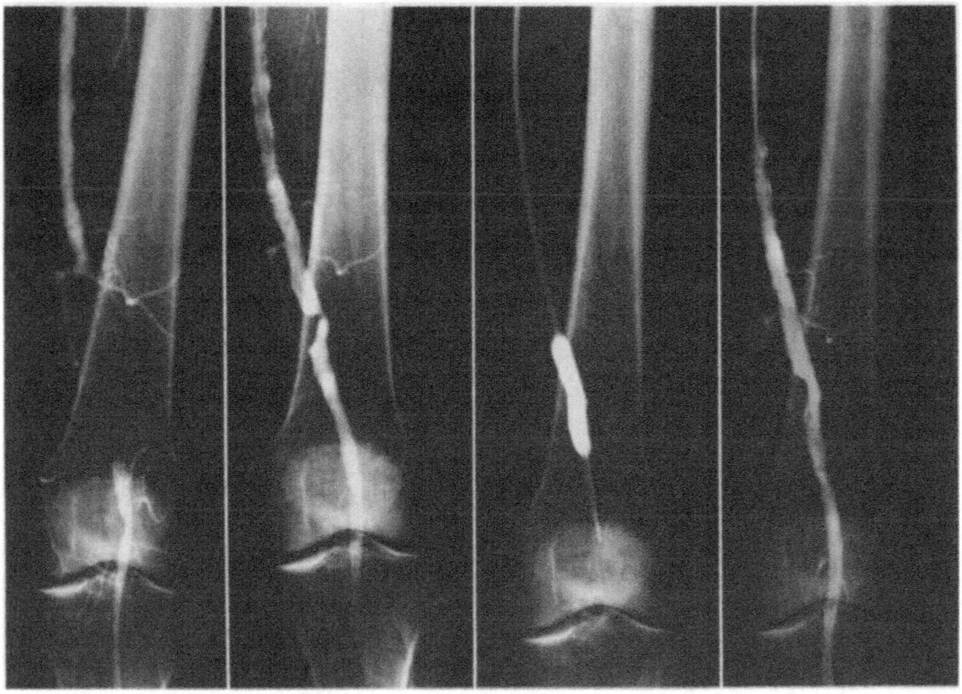

a b c d

Fig. 1a–d. Patient A.R. **a** left-sided femoral occlusion prior to treatment; **b** residual stenosis after lytic therapy; **c** PTA procedure using Grüntzig catheter; **d** stenosed segment after dilatation

Table 1. Five chronic femoral occlusions in which fibrinolytic clearance was feasible and where a subsequent PTA dilatation of residual stenoses was performed

Patient	Age	Duration of occlusion	Period between lysis and PTA	Follow-up investigation
J. S.	58	4 weeks	10 days	Reocclusion after 3 months
A. R.	71	3 weeks	12 days	Still patent after 7 months
E. Z.	68	8 days	1 day	Still patent after 1 month
D. M.	45	5 weeks	4 days	Still patent after 1 week
F. W.	59	12 days	1 day	Reocclusion 1 day after PTA. Definite clearance by second PTA 8 days later

Results

In all cases fibrinolytic treatment was successful in that the arterial segment of interest was cleared. However, a residual narrowing of hemodynamic importance persisted in each case and PTA was subsequently carried out 1 day to $2^1/_2$ weeks later.

Table 2. Five chronic iliac occlusions in which fibrinolytic clearance was feasible and where a subsequent PTA dilatation of residual stenoses was performed

Patient	Age	Artery of interest	Duration of occlusion	Accompanying occlusion	Period between lysis and PTA	Follow-up investigation
T. R.	51	Ext. iliac	4 weeks	Femoral a.	1 day	Still patent after 9 months
H. J.	52	Comm. iliac	6 weeks		1 week	Still patent after 2 years
P. Z.	68	Comm. iliac	6 months	Femoral a.	$2^1/_2$ weeks	Still patent after 2 years
E. R.	47	Comm. iliac	3 months	Femoral a.	1 week	Early reocclusion
H. M.	73	Ext. iliac	8 weeks	Femoral a.	6 days	Still patent after 8 months

Table 4. Ankle pressures and pressure gradients in five patients with iliac occlusions in which fibrinolytic clearance was feasible and where subsequent PTA was performed for residual stenoses

Patient	Artery of interest	Accompanying occlusion	Pressure gradient (mm Hg)			Ankle pressure (mm Hg)		
			Prior to lysis	After lysis	After PTA	Prior to lysis	After lysis	After PTA
T. R.	Ext. iliac	Femoral a.	90	80	50	50	70	100
H. J.	Comm. iliac		75	55	25	60	65	105
P. Z.	Comm. iliac	Femoral a.	110	75	65	30	40	55
E. R.	Comm. iliac	Femoral a.	120	50	30	0	80	90
H. M.	Ext. iliac	Femoral a.	115	105	75	20	40	55
Mean			102	73	49	32	59	81

Table 3. Ankle pressure and pressure gradients in five patients with femoral occlusions in which fibrinolytic clearance was feasible and where subsequent PTA dilatation of residual stenoses was performed

Patient	Artery of interest	Pressure gradient (mm Hg)			Ankle pressure (mm Hg)		
		Prior to lysis	After lysis	After PTA	Prior to lysis	After lysis	After PTA
J. S.	R. femoral	140	40	30	0	80	90
A. R.	L. femoral	65	0	−25	85	110	140
F. W.	R. femoral	75	50	− 5	45	50	125
D. M.	R. femoral	30	20	− 5	90	100	125
E. Z.	R. femoral	80	35	−15	70	125	165
Mean		78	29	− 4	58	93	129

Femoral Occlusions

Treatment by PTA was successful in widening the residual stenoses and thus raising the ankle pressure. In one patient (not receiving anticoagulants after treatment) an early reocclusion occurred. Although local urokinase infusion (1.2 million IU i.v. over 20 min) opened up a narrow canal, no hemodynamic improvement in terms of raised ankle pressure was demonstrable. Therefore, 2 weeks later a second PTA attempt was performed, leading to a definite vessel clearance. There was no reocclusion during a follow-up period of 4 weeks in this patient. The average ankle pressure in the femoral occlusion group rose by 35 mm Hg (from 58 to 93 mm Hg) and after PTA by another 36 mm Hg (from 93 to 129 mm Hg) (Table 3).

Iliac Artery

The iliac occlusion groups was made up by one single iliac and four combined femoral and iliac obstructions, which were removed by fibrinolytic treatment. After conclusion of lytic procedures, three residual common iliac artery and two external iliac artery stenoses were recorded and subsequently treated by PTA (Table 4). As a result of fibrinolysis the average ankle pressure rose by 28 mm Hg, and in response to PTA by another 22 mm Hg (from 59 to 81 mm Hg) (Table 4).

Discussion

The combination of fibrinolytic therapy and PTA is a useful multistage approach in the treatment of chronic arterial occlusion disease. Formerly occluded arteries cleared by fibrinolytic therapy but still showing a hemodynamically significant residual narrowing are prone to reocclusion processes. The dilatation of these stenoses reduces the tendency to reocclusion.

Changes in ankle pressure in cases of combined iliac and femoral occlusions were of special interest. In these cases iliac clearance was feasible but femoral occlusion persisted. The residual iliac stenoses were then dilated by PTA. Even in these iliofemoral blockages an average ankle pressure gain of 50 mm Hg was achieved by applying the lysis-PTA combination.

Summary

In ten patients with femoral and/or iliac occlusions fibrinolytic therapy was performed. In all cases the vessel of interest was cleared but residual narrowings of hemodynamic importance persisted. Next these nonlysable narrowings were dilated by PTA, leading to a significant secondary rise in ankle pressure. Besides blood flow improvement the combined lysis-PTA multistage approach might equally well reduce reocclusion tendencies in arterial segments cleared by fibrinolytic therapy but still displaying high-grade stenoses.

References

1. Martin M, Zeitler E (1978) Percutaneous transluminal recanalization (PTR) and fibrinolysis: fibrinolytic treatment of femoral reocclusions subsequent to PTR procedures. In: Zeitler E, Grüntzig A, Schoop W (eds) Percutaneous vascular recanalization. Springer, Berlin Heidelberg New York, pp 152–156

23. Clot Lysis in Peripheral Arteries

H. Hess

Fibrinolysis

Principles

There is no longer any doubt that platelet adhesion and coagulation on the vessel wall are processes essential to the beginning and the progression of every kind of obliterative arteriopathies [8–10, 14, 15, 20]. The material for complete occlusion of an artery is always predominantly thrombotic. As long as this thrombotic material is not already organized, it can be lysed and changed back to normally flowing blood by thrombolytic therapy [4, 19]. If obliterative arteriopathy leads to symptoms within a few days after occurrence – and this happens when total occlusion of an artery develops rapidly – this arteriopathy may be completely cured by thrombolytic therapy [13]. Similarly, an embolic occlusion of an artery can be lysed completely within the first weeks after its occurrence. More patients seek treatment because chronic arteriopathy is symptomatic for weeks or months or becomes worse within this time. These progressive obliterative arteriopathies can be fully reversed by systemic thrombolytic therapy or by local low-dose thrombolytic therapy.

To dissolve an arterial stenosis or a short occlusions by means of systemic thrombolytic therapy, treatment for 24 h is usually sufficient, whereas a longer segmental occlusion requires 2–5 days or even more. The usual daily dose amounts to 2–2.5 million units streptokinase [3, 6, 16–18]. Systemically administered streptokinase stimulates circulating plasminogen, which after conversion to plasmin acts on the surface of the thrombus, leading to exogenous lysis. It also leads to a more or less considerable alteration in the coagulating system, which enhances the risk of bleeding. Only a relatively small amount of streptokinase penetrates the thrombus and activates plasminogen present in the clot, causing endogenous lysis, and this appears to be the most effective mechanism of thrombolysis [5]. Because of the considerable risk of bleeding, the list of contraindications is long. Therefore, only a small percentage of all patients with dissolvable arterial occlusions can be treated by systemic thrombolytic therapy.

Local thrombolytic therapy was first performed by Dotter et al. [2] and later by Dembski and Zeitler [1] in selected patients with acute arterial occlusions. Their method involves the placing of a catheter into an occluding arterial lesion and the continuous "blind" infusion of streptokinase in dosages between 1,000

Percutaneous Transluminal Angioplasty
(ed. by C. T. Dotter, A. Grüntzig, W. Schoop, E. Zeitler)

and 100,000 units/h, up to a total dose of 100,000 to 1.6 million units streptokinase for periods ranging from less than 1 day to up to 2 weeks.

On the basis of the assumption that the small amount of streptokinase penetrating the clot in particular would lead to endogenous lysis, we developed a method which primarily infiltrates the intraarterial clot with small concentrations of steptokinase, achieving a complete lysis even of large clots within a few hours [11–13].

Method

As in the case of PTA, a Grüntzig catheter is introduced into the femoral artery and is first placed approximately 1 cm into the occluding clot. The clot is then infiltrated with 1 ml streptokinase solution (containing 1,000 units/ml). Afterward the catheter is advanced centimeterwise into the clot under fluoroscopic monitoring at intervals of 5–10 min; the clot is thus repeatedly infiltrated with the same amount of streptokinase.

The progressive softening of the occluding material usually allows the advancement of the smooth catheter alone without the guidance of a wire, thus diminishing the risk of the catheter taking an intramural route, which is the most frequent reason for failure of local thrombolytic therapy as well as of the original PTA.

The shorter a segmental occlusion is, the longer the time intervals should be for advancing the catheter. The intensive infiltration of the whole clot before recanalization occurs is the best way of preventing permanent macroembolization into distal open arteries, which is the most frequent and serious complication of this procedure.

When the catheter has reached the distal open lumen of the artery it is then retracted behind the original occlusion and the free passage is angiographically confirmed. This permits identification of possible local stenoses, remaining thrombi, or new peripheral occlusions from embolized thrombotic material. In these instances it is possible to enlarge the stenoses immediately by balloon dilatation, as well as to dissolve macroemboli by further infiltration with streptokinase.

The thrombotic material remaining within a recanalized segment has a good chance of being removed within the next few hours due to the aftereffects of thrombolysis, provided that the clot has been sufficiently infiltrated with streptokinase.

The total doses of streptokinase administered used to lie in the range of 4,000–180,000 units per patient. We now recommend a total of 70,000–120,000 units streptokinase.

To avoid rethrombosis and to decrease the risk of bleeding we omit heparin during and immediately after the procedure, and instead use platelet function inhibitors only. Since the combination of acetylsalicylic acid with dipyridamole apparently potentiates the vasodilating effect of the activated fibrinolytic system, and is followed eventually by a dangerous decrease in blood pressure, we use acetylsalicylic acid alone (3×0.5 g) 1 day before and for 3 days after the procedure [12]. Later on we administer a combination of acetylsalicylic acid and dipyridamole as long-term prophylactic therapy in cases of thrombotic occlusions, and anticoagulants if the occlusion was embolic.

PTA in Combination With Fibrinolysis

Different combinations of PTA and fibrinolytic therapy are possible and each one has its special indication.

Primary PTA With Secondary Systemic Thrombolytic Therapy

Stenoses and short arterial occlusions (< 4 cm) are the best indications for primary PTA. In cases of reocclusion within the first few days after the procedure, systemic thrombolytic therapy even 2 weeks later has a good chance of removing the fresh thrombus as well as the dissolvable material of the original occlusion. Therefore, under these circumstances systemic fibrinolytic therapy is indicated, provided that no contraindication exists.

Primary Systemic Thrombolytic Therapy With Secondary PTA

Primary systemic thrombolytic therapy should be considered for every thrombotic stenosis or occlusion of a peripheral artery where the time limit can be met and/or angiographic criteria fulfilled, and where there is a good chance of lysis with no contraindications. In cases where a stenosis remains, it can be removed by PTA within the next few days (Fig. 1).

Local Low-Dose Thrombolytic Therapy Potentially With Simultaneous PTA

Local low-dose thrombolytic therapy, possibly with simultaneous PTA, should be considered for every segmental occlusion longer than 4 cm, and especially for all femoropopliteal occlusions including the trifurcation which involve marked ischemia (stages IIb–IV) and probably contain still lysable material. Our 2-year experience with local low-dose thrombolytic therapy for peripheral arteries is as follows.

Out of the first 205 patients treated, 122 (59.5%) were male and 83 (40.5%) female, with ages ranging between 14 and 91 years. Most of our patients were older than 70 and therefore not suitable candidates for systemic thrombolytic therapy. The occlusive process was thrombotic in 186 patients and embolic in 19 patients. In all the embolic cases the vascular surgeon had rejected embolectomy. Table 1 summarizes localization of the occlusions and the early results obtained.

In 145 patients (70%) primary recanalization was achieved, and in 38 of these additional balloon dilatation was not necessary. In 36 patients (25%)

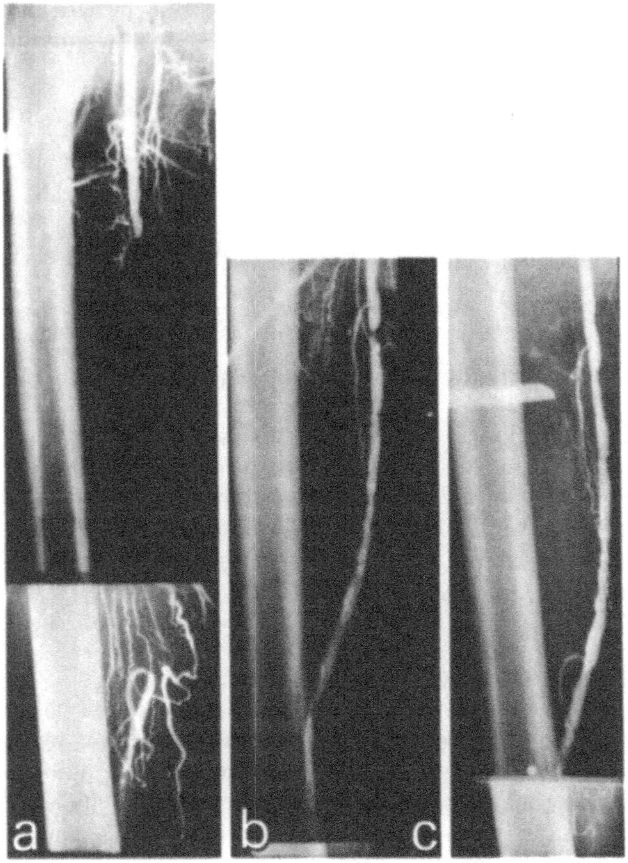

Fig. 1a–c. Arteriograms of a 63-year-old man who suffered for 6 weeks from a long occlusion of the right femoral artery **a** before and **b** after systemic thrombolytic therapy, and **c** after PTA for a residual stenosis

Table 1. Results of local low-dose thrombolytic therapy in 205 patients with peripheral arterial occlusions

Location of occlusion	No. of patients	No. of recanalizations	No. of early reocclusions	No. of recanalizations-lasting 2 weeks
Femoral and popliteal arteries with trifurcation open	145	110	27	83
Femoral and popliteal arteries involving trifurcation	45	32	9	23
Aortoiliac area	6	3		3
Total	205	145	36	109

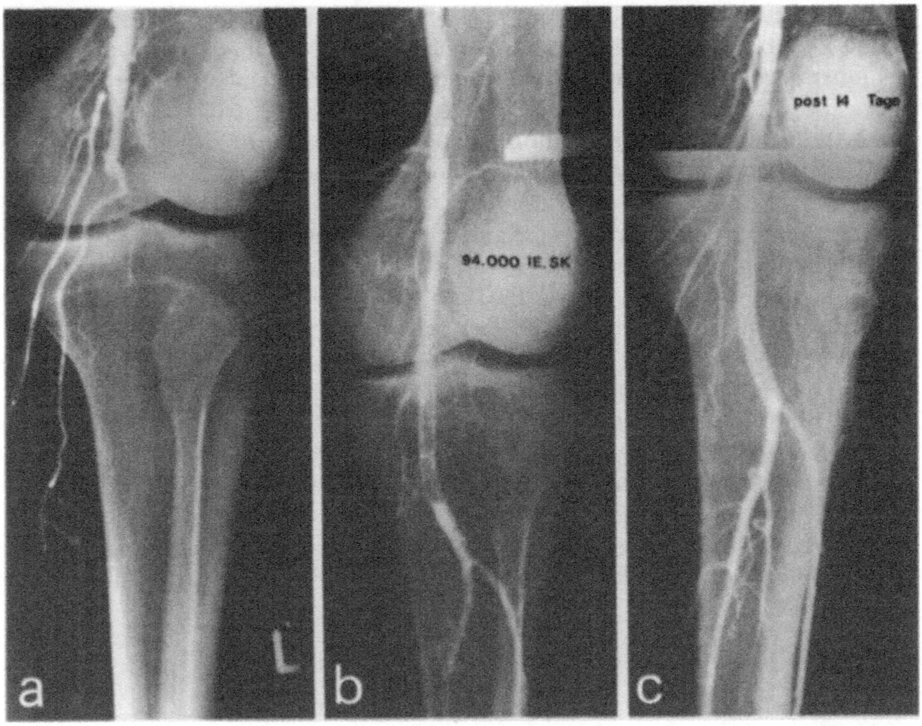

Fig. 2a–c. Arteriogram showing a 6-week-old thrombotic occlusion of the left popliteal artery involving the trifurcation in a 70-year-old woman. **a** before, **b** at the end of, and **c** 2 weeks after local low-dose thrombolytic therapy with 94,000 units streptokinase. Arteriogram *b* shows residual clots within the popliteal artery at the end of the procedure, disappearing 14 days later due to the aftereffect of lysis (*c*)

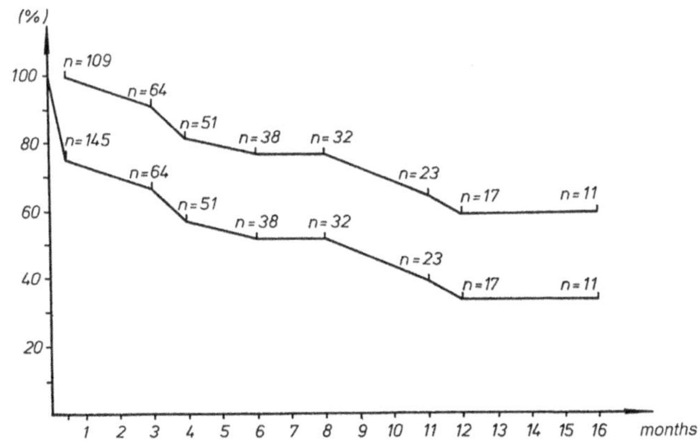

Fig. 3. Cumulative patency rate following recanalization with local low-dose thrombolytic therapy. The *lower curve* indicates the cumulative patency rate in all patients (n = 145). The *upper curve* illustrates this rate in patients (n = 109) who underwent recanalization, excluding those who had reocclusion within the first 2 weeks

reocclusion occurred within the first 2 weeks. Clinical improvement was evident in all 109 patients in whom there was permanent recanalization. Improvement was most impressive in cases with a femoropopliteal occlusion, including those where the trifurcation was involved (Fig. 2). In the 109 patients in whom the primarily achieved recanalization remained permanent for 2 weeks, the cumulative patency rate was still 60% during a follow-up period of 16 months (Fig. 3).

The chance of achieving a recanalization is indirectly correlated with the age of the occlusion as well as with its length. With occlusions up to 6 months of age the probability of permanent success is 60%, up to 11 months 40%, and even older occlusions still have a 20% chance (Fig. 4). Occlusions of the femoropopliteal segment with a length of up to 25 cm have a better chance both of primary and of long-term success than do the longer ones (Fig. 5).

The reasons for failures among the 205 local thrombolytic treatments are summarized in Table 2, and the complications in Table 3. Microembolisms were lysed without exception by the aftereffect of thrombolysis, whereas macroembolism in some cases was a serious complication. Most of the macroembolic lesions were dissolved completely or partially, either by local infiltration or by the aftereffects of thrombolysis. Nevertheless, one patient suffered a marked

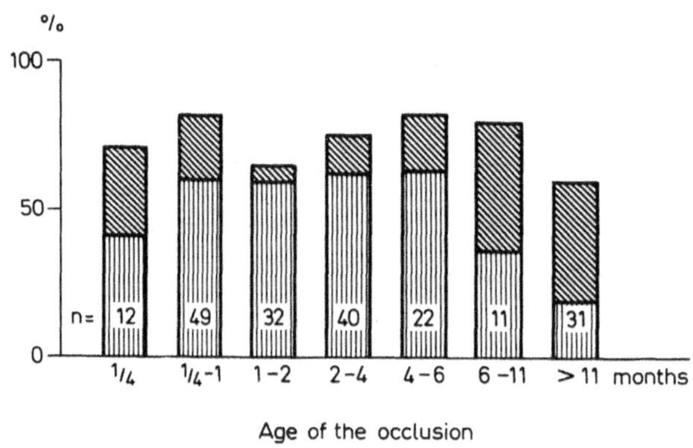

Fig. 4. Primary recanalization and early reocclusion as a function of the age of the occlusion. The *upper hatched* part of the columns indicates the reocclusions within the first 2 weeks

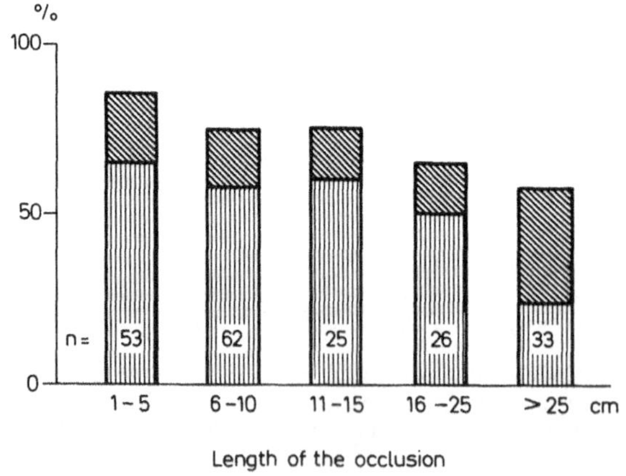

Fig. 5. Primary recanalization and early reocclusion as a function of the length of the occlusion. The *upper hatched* part of the column indicates the reocclusions within the first 2 weeks

deterioration in condition for some weeks and two suffered a moderate increase in ischemia.

Four hours after uncomplicated and successful local thrombolytic therapy of a femoropopliteal occlusion, a 73-year-old hypertensive patient developed symptoms of a dissecting aneurysm of the abdominal aorta and died. It is uncertain whether that single death within a series of 205 local thrombolytic treatments resulted from a complication associated with the method or if it occurred by chance.

Severe local hematomas never required surgical intervention. Slight bleeding from the site of venous puncture was seen in only one patient. In all cases the thrombolytic system was temporarily activated and consequently the coagulating system was moderately altered [12]. None of the patients treated locally suffered from side effects such as fever or a general feeling of malaise, which very often occur during systemic thrombolytic therapy with streptokinase. In all patients who successfully underwent thrombolytic therapy we observed local hyperemia lasting 1–2 days (Fig. 6).

Hemorrhagic diseases, a recent ischemic or hemorrhagic cerebral insult, and peptic ulcer were regarded as contraindications. Other potential contraindications, such as advanced age and hypertension, were not taken into consideration.

Table 2. Failures arising among 205 local thrombolytic treatments

Reasons	
Intramural route of the catheter	19%
Thrombus organized	7%
Puncture technically impossible	2%
Entreapment-Syndrom	1%

Table 3. Complications arising among 205 local thrombolytic treatments

Microembolism	16 %
Macroembolism	9 %
Excessive local hematoma	1,5%
Spasm of femoral-artery	0,5%

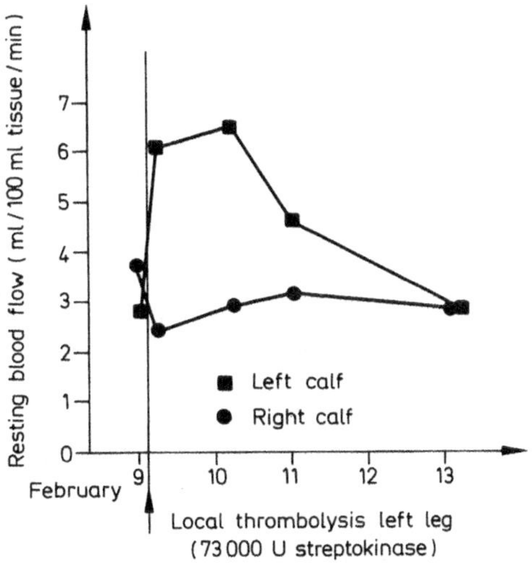

Fig. 6. Blood flow at rest in both calves before, immediately at the end of, and 1–4 days after local low-dose thrombolytic therapy of the leg with 73,000 units streptokinase

Thromboembolic Complications of Primary PTA and Subsequent Local Low-Dose Thrombolytic Therapy

Thromboembolic complications occurring during the primary PTA or reocclusions occurring during the first few days followed by severe ischemia requiring rapid recanalization can be treated effectively by immediate local low-dose thrombolytic therapy. Under these circumstances systemic thrombolytic therapy would involve a high risk of severe local bleeding.

Summary

In combination with PTA local low-dose thrombolytic therapy:

1. Facilitates the probing of the occlusion by softening the clot
2. Removes the lysable component of the occlusive material
3. Supports prevention of rethrombosis by the aftereffects of thrombolysis
4. Provokes local hyperemia lasting for 1–2 days
5. Is capable of rapidly dissolving early reocclusions.

Local low-dose thrombolytic therapy in combination with PTA has considerably extended the number of nonsurgical recanalizations of peripheral arterial occlusions in our clinic.

References

1. Dembski IC, Zeitler E (1978) Selective arterial clot lysis with angiography catheter. In: Zeitler E, Grüntzig A, Schoop W (eds) Percutaneous vascular recanalization. Springer, Berlin Heidelberg New York, p 157
2. Dotter CD, Rösch I, Seaman AJ (1974) Selective clot lysis with low-dose streptokinase. Radiology 111:31
3. Ehringer H, Fischer M (1968) Erfolgreiche thrombolytische Therapie bei subakuten arteriellen Thrombosen. Med Welt 19:1726
4. Gottlob R, Blümel G, Piza F, Brücke P, Böhmig HJ (1968) Die Lysierbarkeit operativ gewonnener menschlicher Thromben verschiedenen Alters in Streptokinase. Wien Med Wochenschr 118:1
5. Gross R (1964) Blutgerinnung und Fibrinolyse. Behring Werk Mitteilungen 44:1
6. Heinrich F (1975) Streptokinase-Therapie bei chronischer arterieller Verschlußkrankheit. Die Medizinische Verlagsgesellschaft mbH, Marburg
7. Hess H (1979) Akute und subakute akrale Ischämie-Syndrome. Münch Med Wochenschr 121:517
8. Hess H (1980) Por-Contra: Entstehung der Arteriosklerose, essentielle Bedeutung des strömenden Blutes und der Systeme der Blutgerinnung und Fibrinolyse. Internist 22:658
9. Hess H, Frost H (1969) Argumente für eine einheitliche Pathogenese arterieller Verschlußprozesse. Verh Dtsch Ges Kreislaufforsch 35:333
10. Hess H, Marshall M, Mallasch M (1974) Eine einheitliche Theorie der Morphogenese aller obliterierenden Angiopathien. VASA 3:373
11. Hess H, Mietaschk A, Ingrisch H (1980) Niedrig dosierte thrombolytische Therapie zur Wiederherstellung der Strombahn bei arteriellen Verschlüssen. Dtsch Med Wochenschr 105:787
12. Hess H, Ingrisch H, Mietaschk A, Rath H (to be published) Local low-dose thrombolytic therapy of peripheral arterial occlusions

13. Hess H (1982) Systemische und selektive Streptokinase-Therapie bei arteriellen Verschlüssen. Internist 23: 405
14. Mustard JF, Murphy EA, Rowsell HC, Downie HG (1964) Platelets and atherosclerosis. Atherosclerosis 4: 1
15. Ross R, Glomset JA (1976) The pathogenesis of atherosclerosis. N Engl J Med 295: 369
16. Schoop W, Martin M, Zeitler E (1968) Thrombolytische Therapie bei chronischer okklusiver Arteriopathie. Verh Dtsch Ges Kreislaufforsch 34: 287
17. Schoop W, Martin M, Zeitler E (1968) Beseitigung von Stenosen in Extremitätenarterien durch intravenöse Streptokinase-Therapie. Dtsch Med Wochenschr 93: 1629
18. Schoop W, Martin M, Zeitler E (1968) Beseitigung alter Arterienverschlüsse durch intravenöse Streptokinase-Infusion. Dtsch Med Wochenschr 93: 2312
19. Sherry S, Fletcher AP, Alkjaersing N (1959) Fibrinolysis and fibrinolytic activity in man. Physiol Rev 39: 343
20. Sinapius D (1968) Die Entstehung subendothelialer Lipophagenherde bei Coronarsklerose. Virchows Arch (Pathol Anat) 345: 169

24. Early Experience of Catheter Lysis

F.-J. Roth, G. Cappius, and I. Schmidtke

The purpose of catheter lysis – local low-dose fibrinolytic therapy – is to offer the benefit of lysis without the risks of systemic fibrinolytic therapy. The primary success of angioplasty is limited by the length of the occlusion. Acute reocclusion occurs in about 50% of the cases when the length is more than 10 cm [16]. The primary results of the routine Dotter procedure are occasionally complicated by acute reocclusions and in rare cases by embolism. The latter occurs if the occlusion is acute or of less than 3 months duration. In such instances the combination of angioplasty with fibrinolytic therapy is suggested [1, 2, 4–6, 9, 10, 12, 15]. Two different methods are possible: (a) treatment of an acute embolus or occlusion by means of systemic fibrinolysis; and (b) the application of low-dose fibronolytic therapy using an angioplasty catheter [3, 6, 10, 12, 14, 15]. In 1980 Hess [5] and co-workers described good results in local low-dose fibrinolytic catheter therapy for femoropopliteal artery occlusions (70% success with 136 treatments).

Method and Material

Basically, we perform an angioplasty under local anesthesia. By means of a guide wire, which usually has a catheter mounted over it, the occlusion is passed and dilated. This step makes damage to the clot possible and enlarges the area of contact between it and the lytic material. On fluoroscopy the beginning of the occlusion is located and the catheter is advanced into the core of the occluding substance in order to inject repeated single doses of streptokinase or urokinase. Every 10 min the catheter is pushed 1 cm further through the occlusion. The single dose ranges from 5,000 to 10,000 units. The total dose is limited to 250,000 units. To prevent acute rethrombosis heparin or aggregation inhibitors are applied after the catheter lysis.

We treated 56 patients – 40 males and 16 females. The average age was 65 years (range 29–86). Sixteen patients (29%) were clinically in stage II (Fontaine), 40 in stages III–IV (71%). Both the femoropopliteal area and the iliac artery were treated by this method (Table 1). In 11 cases (Table 2) a catheter lysis was performed because a routine Dotter procedure was complicated by an embolization into the distal popliteal artery (Fig. 1). Catheter lysis was achieved in clinically acute occlusions (Fig. 2) as well as in acute recurrence of a long occlusion after the Dotter procedure (Fig. 3) in 45 patients.

Percutaneous Transluminal Angioplasty
(ed. by C. T. Dotter, A. Grüntzig, W. Schoop, E. Zeitler)

Table 1. Distribution of 56 catheter lyses

External iliac artery	3
Common femoral atery	2
Deep femoral artery	2
Superficial femoropopliteal artery	49

Table 2. Indications for 56 catheter lyses

Thromboembolic occlusions following PTA	11
Occlusions longer than 10 cm	29
Subacute occlusions and acute reocclusions following angioplasty	16

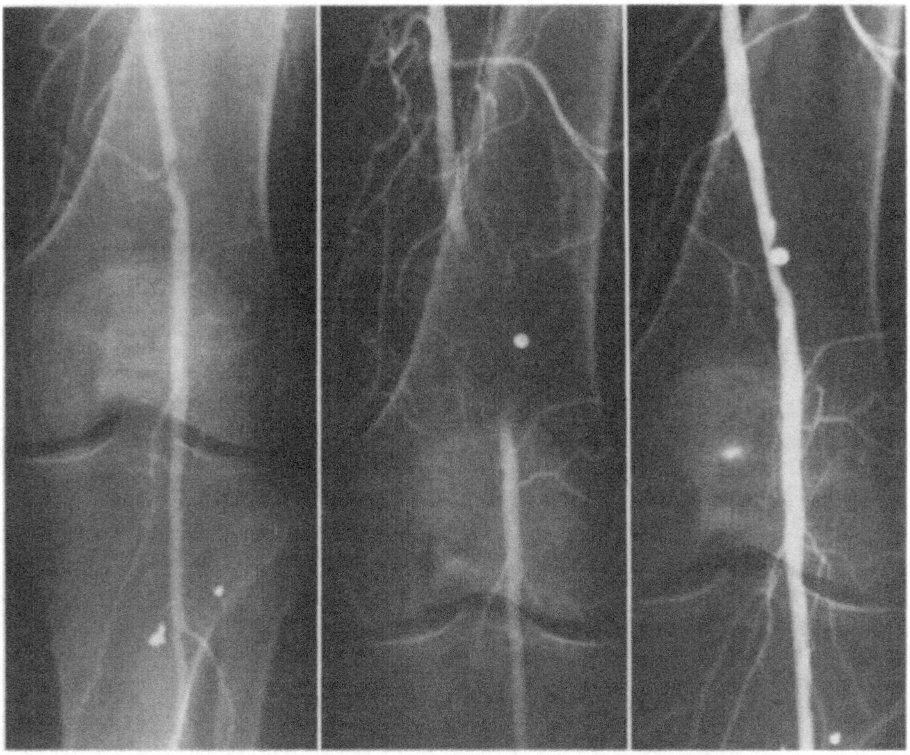

a b c

Fig. 1. a Stenosis of proximal popliteal artery. **b** Acute occlusion of popliteal artery during angioplasty. **c** Patent popliteal artery after catheter lysis

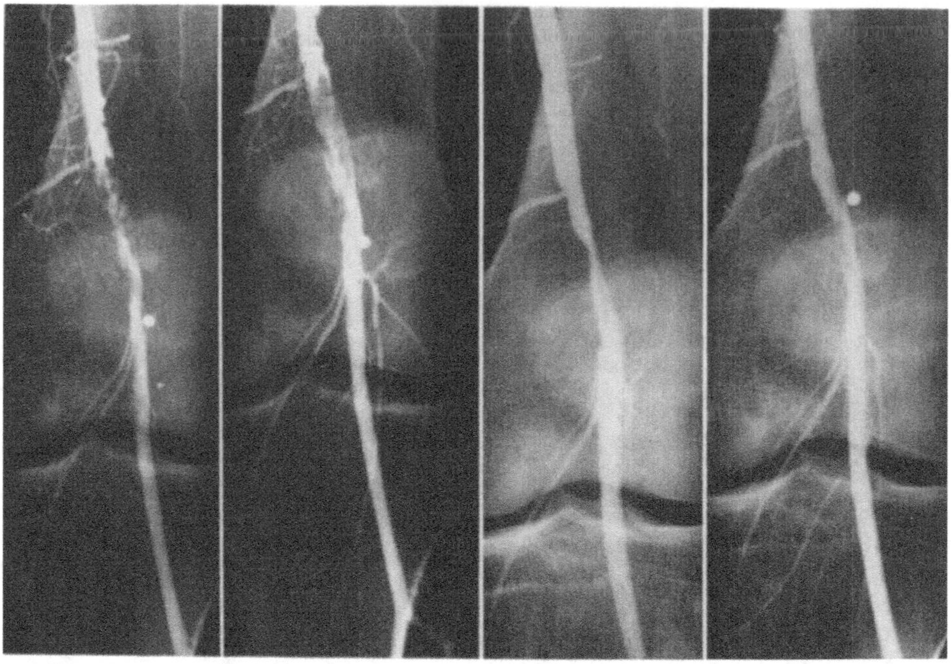

a b c d

Fig. 2. a Acute reocclusion of the popliteal artery following routine angioplasty. **b** Patent popliteal artery still with clot material in it after catheter lysis. **c** 10 months later stenosis of popliteal artery in the area of the former occlusion. **d** Patent popliteal artery with irregularities in the treated segment after routine angioplasty

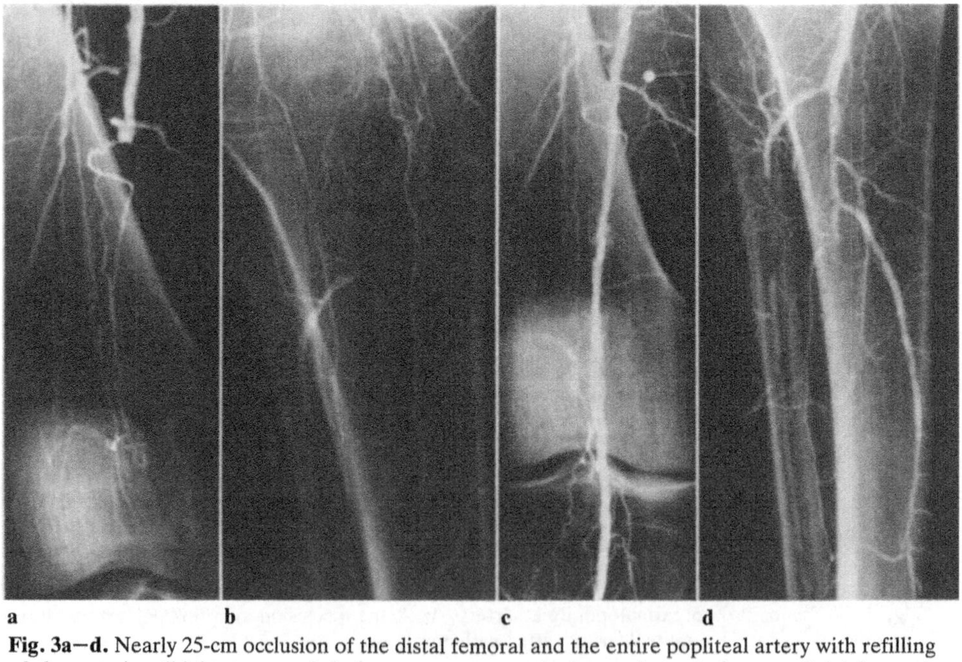

a b c d

Fig. 3a–d. Nearly 25-cm occlusion of the distal femoral and the entire popliteal artery with refilling of the anterior tibial artery. **a, b** before treatment; **c, d** after catheter lysis: superficial femoral, popliteal, and posterior tibial arteries patent, peripheral embolization into the anterior tibial artery

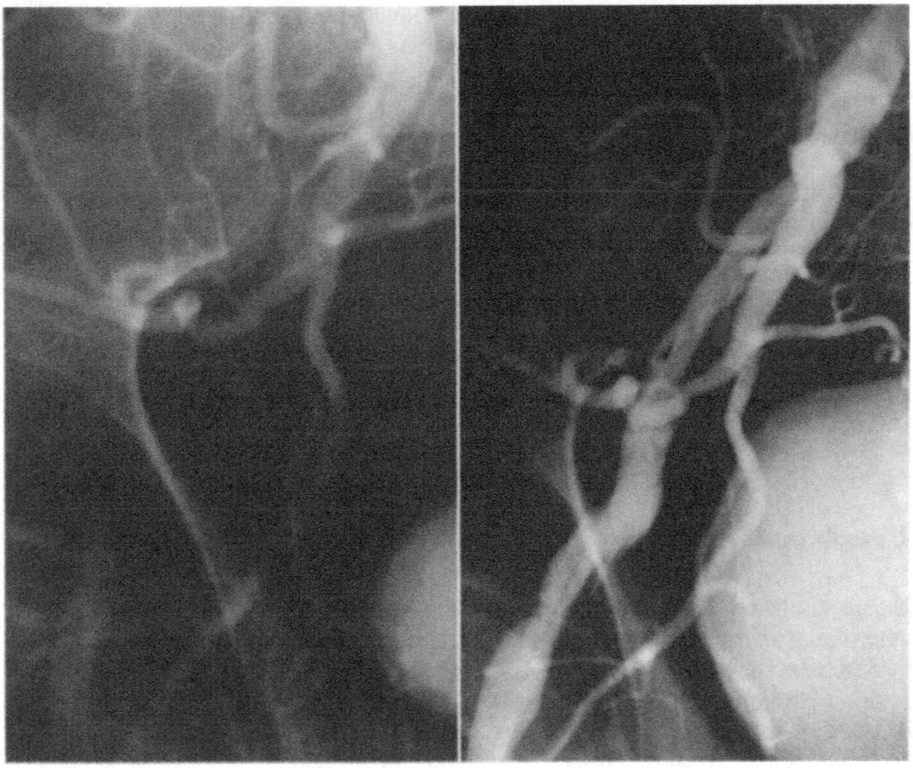

a b

Fig. 4. Occlusion of the distal external iliac artery. **a** before treatment; **b** after catheter lysis

Results

Three iliac artery occlusions were treated with good technical and clinical results (Fig. 4). Of 56 catheter lyses, 43 were performed successfully (Table 3). The overall success rate was 77%. The patients in whom the procedure failed did not suffer a deterioration in condition as a result of the maneuvring of the balloon catheter. A short-term (3 weeks to 3 months) follow-up of the 13 failures (all stages III–IV) showed that 9 patients underwent surgery and 4 were treated conservatively. In 6 patients amputation of the lower extremity could not be avoided. Following catheter lysis, a standard intravenous heparin therapy was employed in all patients. The catheter lysis was complicated (Table 4) by peripheral embolization and bleeding at the puncture site. The seven small emboli in the lower arteries (Fig. 3) were not accompanied by any clinical symptoms. There were two deaths from retroperitoneal bleeding, in a 76-year-old man and a 73-year-old woman; the bleeding began on the 1st and 3rd day following standard heparin therapy. I therefore now require all patients undergoing low-dose fibrinolytic therapy to be kept under intensive care for at least 2 days if heparin therapy is added.

Table 3. Primary results of 56 catheter lyses

Localization	*n*	Success	Failure
Iliac	3	3	0
Femoropopliteal	53	40	13
Total	56	43 (77%)	13 (23%)

Table 4. Complications in 56 catheter lyses

Bleeding	5
Embolization in lower leg arteries	7
Death because of retroperitoneal bleeding	2

Conclusions

Because of the poor general condition of the patients and the potential risks, the complication rate attending catheter lysis is a little higher than in routine Dotter procedure. However, in our experience, low-dose fibrinolytic therapy (catheter lysis) is indicated in:

1. Acute occlusions (emboli)
2. Subacute occlusions (up to 3 months' duration)
3. Acute reocclusions following routine angioplasty
4. Occlusions longer than 10 cm
5. Acute embolization during routine angioplasty.

Catheter lysis may be used as a last therapeutic trial before amputation. Six of 13 patients referred to us for this reason lost their legs because angioplasty failed.

The disadvantages of catheter lysis are:

1. Treatment takes 1–4 h.
2. The patients may be moaning and restless (stages III–IV).
3. They are in poor general condition (stages III–IV).

Therefore, enough personnel must be available during treatment to take care of the patients.

On the other hand, the advantages of this therapeutic principle are high, and there is only a low risk to the patient.

1. Systemic reaction is minimal or nil.
2. Catheter lysis is possible in patients in whom systemic lysis is contraindicated.
3. Indications for routine angioplasty may be extended to cover:
   a) Acute and subacute occlusions (less than 3 months)
   b) Occlusions longer than 10 cm
   c) Acute reocclusions following routine angioplasty
   d) Embolization during routine angioplasty.

Catheter lysis is a therapeutic principle which should at least be used in stages III–IV when amputation is suggested. This treatment also allows the rare complication of peripheral embolization met during routine angioplasty to be dealt with satisfactorily.

Summary

Cather lysis – local low-dose fibrinolytic therapy – extends the indications of the Dotter procedure. Occlusions longer than 10 cm and younger than 3 months may be treated by this method. The main indication for this therapeutic principle is disease of stages III–IV (Fontaine). The complication of acute embolization or acute reocclusion during routine angioplasty can be handled satisfactorily by means of catheter lysis. The risks of catheter lysis, especially the bleeding at the puncture site and peripheral embolization, are higher than in routine angioplastic work, so the indications must be strong. When amputation is otherwise the last resort for the patient, this technique is strongly recommended.

References

1. Dembski JC, Zeitler E (1978) Selective arterial clot lysis with angiography catheter. In: Zeitler E, Grüntzig A, Schoop W (eds) Percutaneous vascular recanalization. Springer, Berlin Heidelberg New York, pp 157–159
2. Dembski JC, Zeitler E, Martin M (1978) Infusion into thrombus material via catheter. In: Martin M, Schoop W (eds) New concepts in streptokinase dosimetry. pp 65–69
3. Dotter CT, Rösch J, Seaman HI (1974) Selective clot lysis with low-dose streptokinase. Radiology 111: 31–37
4. Eie H, Ro J, Amundsen E (1972) Combined thrombotic and Dotter treatment in arterial occlusive disease. I. Oslo by Hosp. 22: 141
5. Hess H (1981) Differentialtherapie zur Wiederherstellung der peripheren arteriellen Strombahn. VASA [Suppl] 8: 43
6. Hess H, Mietaschk A, Ingrisch H (1980) Niedrig dosierte thrombolytische Therapie zur Wiederherstellung der Strombahn bei arteriellen Verschlüssen. Dtsch Med Wochenschr 105: 787–791
7. Hirsch J (1978) Local streptokinase treatment. In: Martin M, Schoop W, Hirsch J (eds) New concepts in streptokinase dosimetry. Huber, Bern, pp 63–64
8. Hirsch J, O'Sullivan EF, Gallus AJ (1969) Thrombosis in a patient with chronic thrombocytopenia: successful treatment with intraarterial infusion of streptokinase. Med J Amer. 1304
9. Klos J, Gottlob R, Denck H, Piza F (1972) Lysierbarkeit operativ gewonnener Thromben. Münch Med Wochenschr 114: 1927–1932
10. Martin M, Zeitler E (1978) Percutaneous transluminal recanalization (PTR) and fibrinolysis: fibrinolytic treatment of femoral reocclusion subsequent to PTR procedures. In: Zeitler E, Grüntzig A, Schoop W (eds) Percutaneous vascular recanalization. Springer, Berlin Heidelberg New York, pp 152–156
11. McNichol GP, Read W, Bain WH, Douglas AS (1963) Treatment of peripheral arterial occlusion by streptokinase perfusion. Br Med J 1: 1508
12. Mietaschk A, Hess H, Ingrisch H, Krämer U (1981) Früh- und Spätergebnisse lokaler niedrig dosierter thrombolytischer Therapie peripherer Arterienverschlüsse. VASA [Suppl] 8: 43

13. Müller-Fassbender H, Hess H (1978) Percutaneous transluminal recanalization combined with fibrinolysis. In: Zeitler E, Grüntzig A, Schoop W (eds) Percutaneous vascular recanalization. Springer, Berlin Heidelberg New York, pp 148–151
14. Rath H, Hess H, Engstle L, Gegenfurtner W, Mietaschk A (1981) Gerinnphysiologische Untersuchungen bei der lokalen thrombolytischen Therapie. VASA [Suppl] 8: 44
15. Rentrop P, Blanke H, Köstering H, Karsch KH (1980) Intracoronare Streptokinaseapplikation bei akutem Infarkt und instabiler Angina pectoris. Dtsch Med Wochenschr 105: 221
16. van Andel GJ (1970) Percutaneous transluminal angioplasty. The Dotter procedure. Excerpta Medica, Amsterdam
17. Zeitler E, Grüntzig A, Schoop W (1978) Percutaneous vascular recanalization. Springer, Berlin Heidelberg New York

VII. Complications

25. Complications During and After Percutaneous Transluminal Angioplasty

W. Seyferth, M. Ernsting, R. Grosse-Vorholt, and E. Zeitler

Local and general complications are possible during and after percutaneous transluminal angioplasty (PTA). Since the introduction of Grüntzig's [4–7] double-lumen balloon catheter, postprocedural bleeding, false aneurysm formation (Fig. 1), and embolization of the main arteries of the calf are seen less often than with the coaxial Dotter catheter employed previously [2, 10, 14, 19].

The complications observed in the cooperative study reported at the symposium in Nuremberg in May 1982 include 1963 PTAs of the femoro-popliteal artery and are listed in Table 1. The results of PTA should always

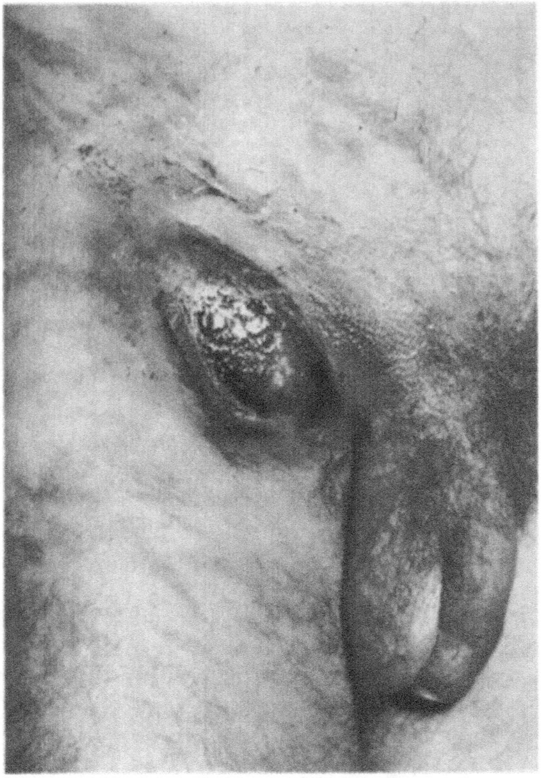

Fig. 1. Pulsating hematoma or spurious aneurysm after PTA in the right groin [18]

Percutaneous Transluminal Angioplasty
(ed. by C. T. Dotter, A. Grüntzig, W. Schoop, E. Zeitler)

Table 1. Complications with femeropopliteal PTA ($n = 1963$): Cooperative study 1982, Nuremberg

Puncture site	62 (3.2%)
Elsewhere	49 (2.4%)
Needing surgery	39 (2.0%)

Table 2. Complications of vascular surgery

Operation	Mortality	Patency at discharge	Patency at 5 Years
Bifurcation graft	2.9%	96.4%	86%
Aorta-/iliacofemoral bypass	0.7%	99.8%	89%
Femorofemoral	1.1%	96.6%	83%
Femoropopliteal bypass	1.2%	97.2%	73.6%
Femorotibial bypass	1.5%	89.6%	58.7%

Chir. Universitätsklinik, Erlangen
D. Raithel, M.D.

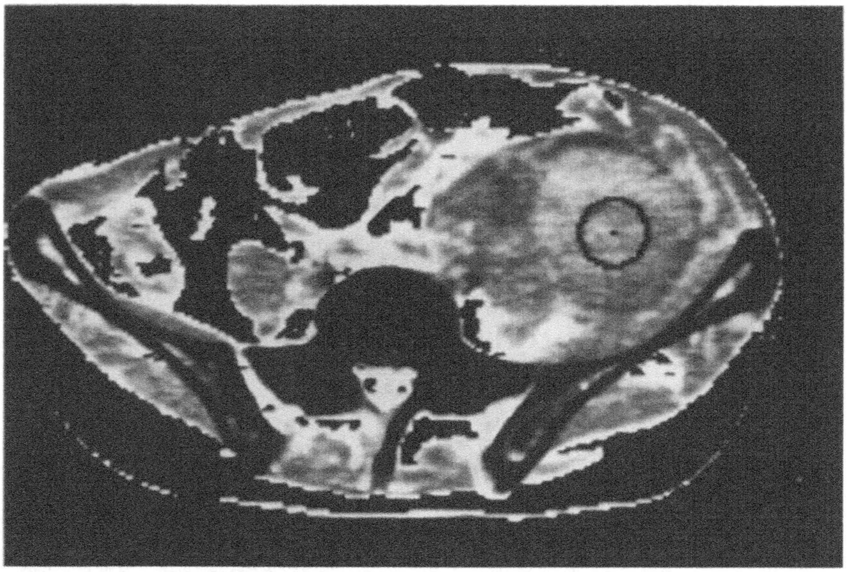

Fig. 2. Computer tomography scan of the pelvic area with a large retroperitoneal hematoma in the left iliac fossa. (75-year-old diabetic female with gangrene of the left foot and lower leg and superficial femoral artery obstruction. The hematoma occurred after orthograde puncture of the common femoral artery above the inguinal ligament)

be compared with the best results of vascular surgery and its attendant risks (Table 2).

Possible complications during and after percutaneous dilatation of iliac artery stenoses include subintimal dissection, retroperitoneal bleeding (Fig. 2),

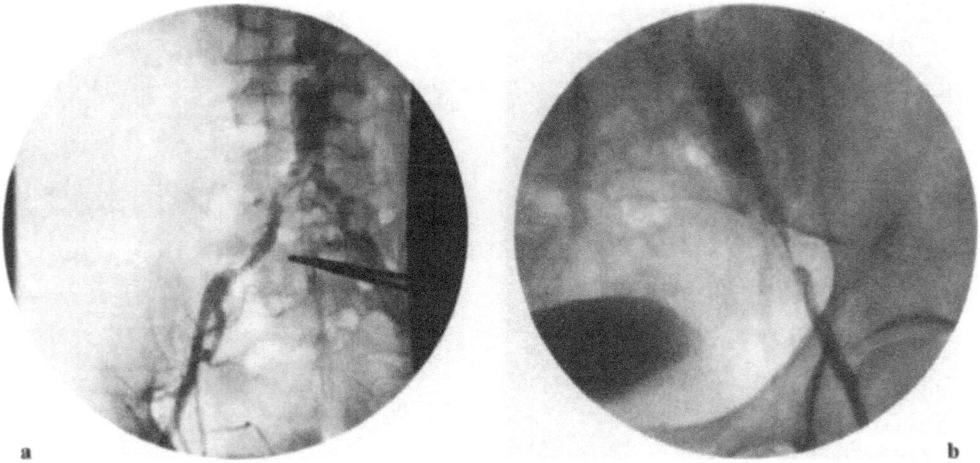

a b

Fig. 3a, b. Control angiogram after retrograde dilatation of multiple stenoses of the left iliac artery. Overstretching of the iliac artery and spasm behind the dilated segment. (63-year-old man with multiple iliac artery stenoses and a long superficial femoral artery occlusion on the left side.) **a** before PTD; **b** control angiogram after PTD

Table 3. Complications at and after PTA requiring vascular surgery (Klinikum Nürnberg, July 1976 – March 1982)

Obliteration	Stage II		Stage III-IV	
	n	Complications	*n*	Complications
Iliac a. stenoses	132	1 (0.76%)	40	1 (2.5%)
Femoropopl. obstructions	285	6 (2.1%)	245	8 (3.3%)

overstretching (Fig. 3), and early rethrombosis. Complications in this area needing vascular surgery can be seen more often in patients with multiple stenoses than in those with single stenosis, and in patients with gangrene or rest pain. Patients with gangrene (stage IV, Fontaine's classification) and the prospect of amputation should primarily be submitted to PTA as a limb-saving procedure (Table 3).

Analysis of complications in a 12-year period since the introduction of the Dotter procedure at the Aggertalklinik in Engelskirchen (1968) and in the Department of Diagnosis at the Radiologisches Zentrum of the Klinikum Nürnberg (1976) shows (Fig. 4a) that the complication rate is decreasing with experience [11, 18, 20].

The introduction of single Teflon catheters and the balloon catheter technique have considerably helped to diminish the arterial wall lesion at the puncture site and in the nonpathological arteries passed by the catheter before reaching the obstruction to be dilated.

a

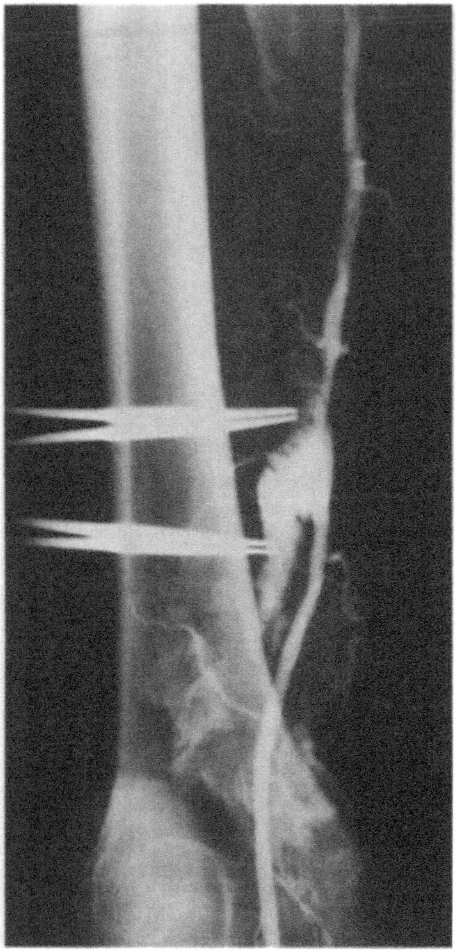

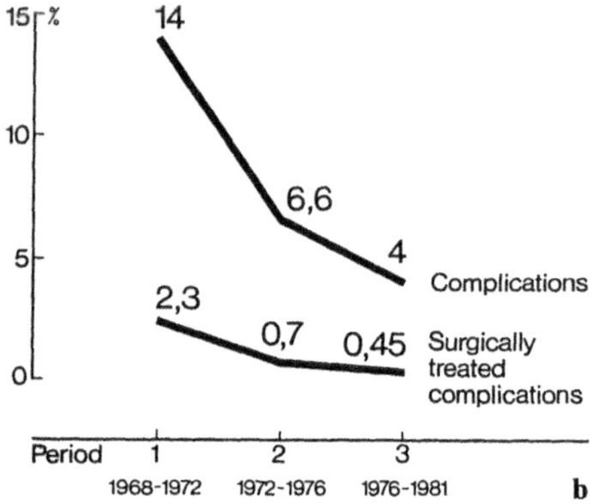

b

Fig. 4b. Development of the complications

Fig. 4a, b. Perforation of the superficial femoral artery at the site of the occluded segment. Control angiogram with patent superficial femoral artery and contrast extravasation

General Complications

General complications may occur during PTA and within the following 2 weeks. These may be related only to the procedure itself or to the underlying general arteriosclerosis as well. Myocardial infarction and cardiac insufficiency within the first 2 weeks may develop predominantly in correlation with coexisting severe coronary heart disease. This occurred twice out of 2,800 patients in the Aggertalklinik and the Klinikum Nürnberg.

Apoplectic shock can also occur, especially when the systemic blood pressure decreases due to postprocedural bleeding in a patient with coexisting carotid artery stenosis. However, we have not yet encountered such a case in our own patient series.

Posttherapeutic pulmonary embolism can be another systemic complication. One week after successful recanalization of a femoral artery occlusion, a

64-year-old female suffered pulmonary embolism although she had already been out of bed for several days. The patient died consequent to the embolism, and postmortem examination demonstrated the dilated arterial segment to be patent, although with some residual stenoses. However, the femoral vein was thrombosed up to the groin. Since that time, we routinely check the venous status before and after treatment in order to initiate thrombus prophylaxis with compression stockings and active foot exercises. Nevertheless, these tragic events must be compared with the risks and results of vascular surgery (Table 2). Published figures on operative mortality vary and depend on the experience of the examiner and the patient selection [8, 9, 16]. According to Bollinger [1] approximately 4.5% of the patients die as a consequence of surgical intervention in the femoral region.

Local Complications

One must differentiate between:
Misplaced puncture with ineffective PTA
Complications at the arterial puncture site
Complications beyond the puncture site.

Misplaced Puncture with Ineffective PTA

An orthograde puncture of the femoral artery is required to treat femoropopliteal obliterations. If during this procedure the deep femoral artery instead of the superficial femoral artery is punctured, the lesion obviously cannot be approached and a new puncture is required. If recanalization is not possible, the procedure should be stopped. Deterioration seldom occurs, but if it does, it stems from the extension of an occlusion or from the formation of a local thrombosis or hematoma at the puncture site. If the puncture is misplaced, in some cases one can change the position of the tip of the needle under fluoroscopic control from the deep into the superficial femoral artery. Particularly in obese patients it is advantageous to hyperextend the hips by placing a cushion beneath the buttocks, thus avoiding mispuncture of the deep femoral artery. Sometimes, ultrasound-B-scan is helpful in finding the best puncture site.

Complications at the Puncture Site due to Catheterization

The most frequent complication is a small hematoma and occasional posttreatment bleeding from the puncture defect. If compression is ineffectively applied or if posttreatment bleeding is not quickly perceived, a pulsating hematoma may develop (Fig. 1).

If the dilating catheter is introduced above the inguinal ligament, not only an inguinal hematoma but also retroperitoneal bleeding may result. This occurred in 5 cases out of 2,800 and surgical treatment was necessary in 3 of these patients. The recognition of postprocedural bleeding requires that the patients remain under ward observation for at least 24 h, especially if the puncture site was not definitely below the inguinal ligament.

A hematoma may also develop in the abdominal wall or the scrotum. This is not externally visible but can be demonstrated by computed tomography. We most often observed such large hematomas in the groin and anterior wall in obese women and in patients with hypertension in whom local compression was rather difficult. Afterbleeding occurs more frequently in heparinized patients or in those on warfarin therapy [5, 15].

We have also noted posttreatment bleeding after using the Grüntzig double-lumen balloon catheter, and have seen a large hematoma in one case. The hematoma was absorbed by 3 weeks. For this reason, manual compression after PTA must be done very carefully, particularly in women, and an optimal compression bandage must be applied. Moreover, in the prevention of postprocedural bleeding it is advantageous to have the patient laid directly onto his bed in the angiography room, thus avoiding undue repositioning and patient motion. For the first 24 h after treatment the patient should be kept lying quietly supine.

Nevertheless, compression after PTA must be done in such a way that the leg remains well perfused. A special help here is the monitoring of the pedal pulse with oscillography of the big toe. To allow adequate perfusion during manual compression, the following measures may be helpful:

1. Injection of a vasodilator (Laevadosin; Priscolin) before removing the catheter from the artery
2. Dependent positioning of the leg during manual compression
3. Warming the foot with an electric cushion or hot water bottle
4. Active foot movement

If, in spite of these measures, a spurious aneurysm develops from ineffective compression, vascular surgical treatment is indicated.

Complications Beyond the Puncture Site

One must differentiate between arterial perforation or dissection by the guide wire or catheter, peripheral embolization, thrombotic occlusion, and arterial spasm. Subintimal dissection of the iliac or femoral artery by the guide wire has no immediate consequences, but it may cause a thrombotic occlusion to develop. Perforation of the arterial wall by the guide wire can lead to a hematoma, but in most cases this has no practical consequences.

Perforation by the catheter, however, can cause major bleeding, and surgery becomes necessary. We were confronted with four perforations, two of them needing vascular surgical correction [18, D. Raithel, Ergebnisse gefäßchirurgischer Behandlung bei Becken- und Beinarterien, personal communication]. In one perforation bleeding could be controlled (Fig. 4) during the procedure and PTA was then successful [3].

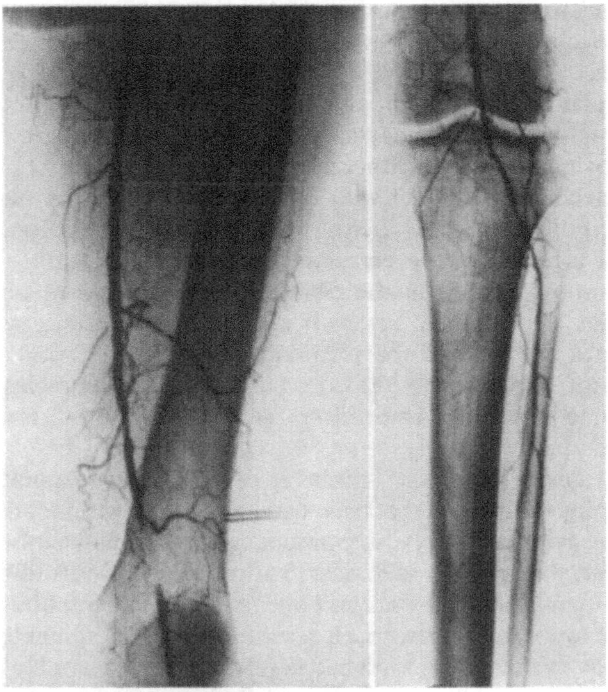

a

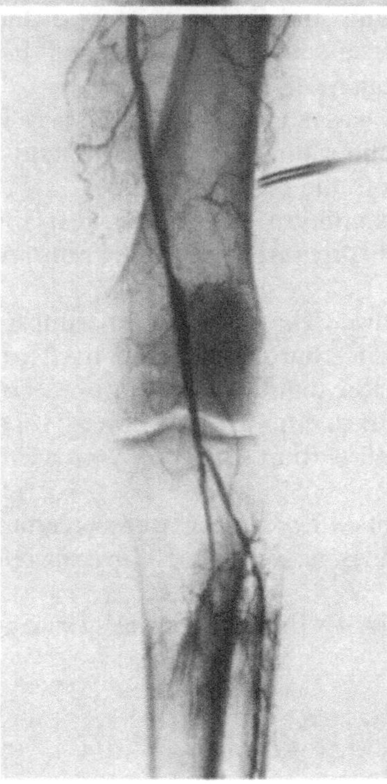

b

Fig. 5a, b. Overstretching of the popliteal artery and perforation of the tibiofibular trunk with contrast material extravasation. **a** distal femoropopliteal artery occlusion 3 cm in length, multiple stenoses of the mid-superficial femoral artery, and occlusion of the tibiofibular trunk in the lower leg arteries; **b** control angiogram after effective recanalization of the superficial femoral artery occlusion: overstretching of the proximal popliteal artery and extravasation distal to the recanalized tibiofibular trunk at the site of its bifurcation

High-risk areas for arterial perforation during PTA are:
1. The proximal end of the obstruction
2. The popliteal bifurcation

Prophylaxis against vascular spasm is an initial measure which helps prevent perforation in the popliteal region. It is only necessary when mechanical ablation of the popliteal bifurcation by guide wire or catheter is possible. Therefore, it is important to try to avoid mechanical contact with the popliteal artery. In all other cases, we inject 3 ml lidocaine 1% before passing the bifurcation. Perforation of the popliteal artery must be corrected by surgery.

However, such a perforation (Fig. 5) in the tibiofibular trunk cannot be attributed to spasm alone, as the popliteal artery is clearly patent. Contrast paravasation can be seen in a site beyond the recanalized tibiofibular trunk. Nevertheless, the gangrene of the fifth toe healed well during the following weeks. The patient has some residual claudication, but operation was not necessary.

Peripheral emboli may occur as a result of loosening of thrombi or plaques from the vessel wall or loosening of thrombi that have developed on or within the catheter. Embolization of the popliteal artery, in particular, can be followed by acute ischemia. We have seen this in three instances, and all were successfully operated on. Follow-up angiographic examinations have shown that even after only a few days emboli in the lower leg arteries often are no longer ascertainable [5, 12, 13, 18]. The reason for this may be spontaneous thrombolysis, as well as disintegration of the embolus into small fragments and their transport to the periphery. It seems that distal embolization occurs in less than 5% of the patients, and in general it is clinically asymptomatic [17].

The occurrence of complications that make vascular surgery necessary is dependent not only on the experience of the examiner, the selected instruments, and the auxiliary medical therapy, but also on the patient's clinical stage (Table 3) and the patient's general clinical condition. The latter can be influenced by factors such as hypercoagulability, hypertension, and reduced general mobility.

Another significant problem is balloon rupture. The potential for rupture depends on the pressure applied, the volume of contrast material used for inflation, and the size of the balloon in relation to the diameter of the artery. For prevention of this complication the following rules should be followed [17]:
1. The inflation pressure should be kept well within the safety margins recommended by the manufacturers.
2. Introduction of balloon catheters through groins with scars and fibrosis can be recommended only when carried out through a sheath of appropriate size.
3. The shape of the balloon should always be observed fluoroscopically during inflation.

Conclusion

Complications during PTA rarely occur. Nonetheless, it is necessary that all measures for diagnosis and treatment of arterial circulatory disturbances be immediately available during and after PTA. Close cooperation between the cardiovascular radiologist and vascular surgeon is a matter of course for the treatment of complications after PTA, just as for the follow-up of surgically treated patients.

References

1. Bollinger A (1979) Funktionelle Angiologie. Lehrbuch und Atlas. Thieme, Stuttgart
2. Dotter CT (1980) Transluminal angioplasty: a long view. Radiology 135: 561–564
3. Grosse-Vorholt R, Groos G (1981) Komplizierter Verlauf einer perkutanen Gefäßrekanalisation. Radiologe 21: 84–86
4. Grüntzig A (1976) Die perkutane Rekanalisation chronischer arterieller Verschlüsse mit einem doppellumigen Dilatationskatheter (Dotter-Prinzip). ROEFO 124: 80
5. Grüntzig A (1977) Die perkutane transluminale Rekanalisation chronischer Arterienverschlüsse mit einer neuen Dilatationstechnik. Witzstrock, Baden-Baden
6. Grüntzig A, Hopff H (1974) Perkutane Rekanalisation chronischer arterieller Verschlüsse mit einem neuen Dilatationskatheter. Dtsch Med Wochenschr 99: 2502–2505
7. Grüntzig A, Kumpe DA (1979) Technique of percutaneous angioplasty with the Grüntzig ballon catheter. AJR 312: 547–552
8. Hansteen V, Lorentsen E, Sivertsen E, Bergan F (1975) Long-term follow-up of patients with peripheral arterial obliterations treated with arterial surgery. Acta Chir Scand 141: 725
9. Heberer G, Rau G, Schoop W (1974) Angiologie. Grundlagen, Klinik und Praxis. Thieme, Stuttgart
10. Höhn P, Wagner R, Zeitler E (1975) Histologische Befunde nach der Katheterbehandlung arterieller Obliterationen nach Dotter und ihre Bedeutung. Herz/Kreislauf 7: 13–23
11. Horváth L, Illés I, Varró J (1978) Complications of the transluminal angioplasty excluding the puncture site complications. In: Zeitler E, Grüntzig A, Schoop W (eds) Percutaneous vascular recanalization. Springer, Berlin Heidelberg New York, pp 126–139
12. Mathias K, Spillner G, Staiger J, Strecker E-P (1979) Bedeutung der Kontrollangiographie nach der perkutanen transluminalen Angioplastik (PTA). In: Hild R, Spaan G (eds) Therapiekontrolle in der Angiologie. Witzstrock, Baden-Baden, pp 288–291
13. Mathias K, Schlosser V, Heiss HW, Staiger J (1980) Erfahrungen mit mehr als 350 Katheterangioplastiken der Becken-Beinarterien. Deutscher Röntgenkongreß, Cologne, May 1980 (Abstract no. 183)
14. Porstmann W, Wierny L (1967) Intravasale Rekanalisation inoperabler Obliterationen. Zentralbl Chir [Suppl] 92: 1586
15. van Andel GJ (1976) Percutaneous transluminal angioplasty. Excerpta Medica, Amsterdam
16. Vollmar J (1975) Rekonstruktive Chirurgie der Arterien. Thieme, Stuttgart
17. Waltman AC, Greenfield AJ, Athanasoulis CA (1982) Transluminal angioplasty: general rules and basic considerations. In: Athanasoulis CA, Pfister RC, Greene RE, Robertson GH (eds) Interventional radiology. Saunders, Philadelphia, pp 253–272
18. Zeitler E (1978) Complications in and after PTR. In: Zeitler E, Grüntzig A, Schoop W (eds) Percutaneous vascular recanalization. Springer, Berlin Heidelberg New York, pp 120–125
19. Zeitler E, Schoop W, Zahnow W (1971) The treatment of occlusive arterial disease by transluminal catheter angioplasty. Radiology 99: 19–26
20. Zeitler E, Richter E-I, Roth F-J, Schoop W (1983) Results of percutaneous transluminal angioplasty. Radiology 146: 57

26. Prevention of Complications in Percutaneous Transluminal Angioplasty

L. Horváth, I. Illés, and K. Fendler

No invasive medical treatment is without risk of complication, but the complication rate depends not only on the routine and skill of the operating team but also on the age and general condition of the patient, on the state of the whole vascular system and the blood itself, and partly on luck during and immediately after the procedure. Fortunately, fatal complications occur very seldom, but it must not be forgotten that the loss of a limb is drastic for a patient of, say, 40 or 45.

The prevention of complications is not a task for a single radiologist but for a team comprising internist, surgeon, and intensive care staff, and must be started long before the catheterization procedure itself. Failure to calculate the risk factors in advance invites trouble: these include smoking, unstabilized diabetes, hyperfibrinogenemia, and dehydration.

A minimum quantity of contrast agent given subintimally does not usually cause any harm, whereas a higher dosage of injected liquid may damage the origins of collaterals and may occlude the stenosis to be treated. Perforation by the guide wire happens quite frequently during angioplasty, but usually does not require any treatment. Perforation of the arterial wall by a catheter in the limb may cause mild hematoma, which can be prevented by a few minutes of local compression. Perforation of an iliac artery, however, can cause serious retroperitoneal hemorrhage. The increasing dislocation of the bladder is doubtless a sign of such a complication. The arterial wall can be perforated by a subintimal route or through a collateral vessel. Orientation by visualization on the screen during vascular catheterization is therefore indispensable if major hemorrhage is to be avoided. It is unadvisable to push the catheter when there is strong resistance. A hard cannula should be used to keep the catheter straight, not to make the catheter able to perforate the vessel wall: it is much better not to use the metal instrument. If perforation occurs while the balloon catheter is inflated in the hole in the vessel wall, it should be kept there until vascular suture has been performed (Tables 1 and 2). Arteriovenous fistula is a sort of perforation. When the opening on the two vessel walls is small, the job may be continued and the fistula will probably close. If it does not, a balloon catheter should be inflated inside the artery and the atheromatous material of the artery should be used to occlude the fistula. If this is unsuccessful, the patient must be operated upon.

Peripheral spasm of the small arteries happens especially in Buerger's disease [in which percutaneous transluminal angioplasty (PTA) is in any case not

Percutaneous Transluminal Angioplasty
(ed. by C. T. Dotter, A. Grüntzig, W. Schoop, E. Zeitler)

Table 1. Hematoma

Location	Prevention
Puncture site	Limited heparinization Proper selection of consectuive catheters Proper compression
Elsewhere	Compression of perforation site on the limb Insertion balloon into the perforation Neutralization of heparin

Table 2. Perforations

Cause	Prevention
Guide wire	Do not force into collaterals Stay in route Use double projection
Catheter	Do not move against hard resistance Do not use stiffening cannula

Table 3. Prevention of peripheral arterial spasm occuring during distal manipulation

Well-performed local anesthesia
Additional periarterial infiltration
2 ml Lidocaine 2% i.a.
Tolazoline i.a.
Rheomacrodex i.a.
Repetition of intraarterial lidocaine if manipulation below knee level is undertaken

advisable] and in relatively young patients. But this does not mean that it will not be encountered in elderly patients. Spasm is a serious state if not released within a few minutes, since it can cause extensive thrombosis in the limb. Lidocaine intraarterially and periarterially, tolazoline, papaverine, and similar drugs are useful means of forcing blood flow. Spasm often happens in smokers. If arterial spasm is to be avoided it is advisable not to manipulate below knee level with the guide wire or with the catheter (Table 3).

The most feared complication during transluminal angioplasty is thromboembolism, the likelihood of which is influenced by:

1. The preparation of the patient
2. The puncture technique
3. The length of time the wire and catheter remain in the vessel
4. The degree of compression after removal of the catheter
5. The general condition of the patient
6. The age of the patient
7. The hydration of the patient

8. Hematological parameters
9. Heart failure
10. The quantity of heparin used
11. Peripheral arterial spasm
12. The existence of pancreatic carcinoma
13. Nicotine intake (perhaps most important).

The usual premedication (as advised by Zeitler) with 0.5–1.0 g aspirin or its equivalent 3 days before PTA is essential; it is also essential that the patient stops smoking, preferably 4–6 weeks before PTA (Table 4) [1–3]. Where there is distal embolization a catheter may be used to suck the emboli out of the peripheral vessels [3] or infuse streptokinase at 5,000–10,000 units/h as close to the clots as possible [4, 5]. Heparin should be given during and anticoagulation after the procedure. Rheomacrodex during and after PTA has proved valuable in preventing thromboembolic complications and in increasing blood flow in the peripheral arteries [3]. SP 54, a heparin-like drug which is more effective in stimulating fibrinolytic activity and is less anticoagulant, is actually being tested for use in transluminal angioplasty and the preliminary results are more than encouraging [6, 7]. If SP 54 is not used in the long term, anticoagulation is indispensable, as Zeitler stated on the basis of experience with large series of patients. Anticoagulation is an integral part of PTA anyway: without it the long-term results are disappointing. The procedure should not be called PTA if anticoagulation is not included.

Drastic fall in blood pressure (circulatory collapse) is a rare entity in PTA, but one should be aware of it as it can be followed by coronary insufficiency and heart attack (Table 5). Its prevention need cause no difficulty.

Early reocclusion appears not to be as frequent as it might otherwise seem if we consider only the technically well-performed transluminal angioplasties. Every effort should be made to find the axis of the original lumen [3]. Common causes of early reocclusion are subatheromatous canalization and over compression (to say nothing of smoking). It is not as easy to find the right degree of compression to avoid the two extremes of bleeding and reocclusion. The Doppler probe is of help here. It should be compressed hard enough to stop blood flow and released gradually until the flowmeter records pulse strokes; this pressure should then be maintained. Compression should always be applied over a large area (see Table 6).

It is important not to damage the balloon of the Grüntzig catheter as it may be lost into the vascular system, and the rupture may damage the vessel to be dilated and can enlarge the puncture hole in the artery. There are several methods of preventing balloon rupture, but one of them is expensive (air pump) and the other one depends on the subject being operateur even if he sees a gauge. The most simple, safe, and inexpensive method is used in our department. The pressure limit of a Medrad IV injector is fixed at 5 atm. The volume of the balloon is evaluated beforehand and a little (1 ml) more liquid is injected slowly in the usual manner as with contrast injection (at only ca. 10–12 ml/min) and expirated afterwards. It may be repeated any number of times. The mechanism prevents the injection of much more liquid or a higher rate of flow.

Table 4. Thromboembolism

Cause	Prevention
Occurs with quick clotting and inhibited fibrinolytic activity, especially in smokers	Attend to hydration Do not do PTA in smokers Do not recanalize recently occluded vessels unless you are prepared for clot lysis Stop moving in subintimal route Use Aspirin, Heparin, SP 54, or Rheomacrodex; limit duration of PTA Apply proper compression

Table 5. Fall in blood pressure

Risk groups	Prevention	Action
Elderly patients	Hydration	Give oxygen
Patients with congestive heart disease	Strophanthin	Lift the legs
Patients with cardiac infarct	drip infusion	Quickly give infusion

Table 6. Early reoclussion

Risk factors	Prevention
Smoking	Hydration
Immobility	Exercise
Diabetes	Heparin
Intercurrent diseases	SP 54
Heart failure	Rheomacrodex
Major operations	Aspirin
	Dipyridamole
	Doxium
	Dicumarol
	Cessation of smoking
	Detection of the first sign of restenosis and immediate treatment

One way of preventing complications is to be ready to treat them. This requires physiological, hemodynamic, hemorrheological, pharmacologic, and other knowledge, but it is worth the trouble!

References

1. Astrup P, Kjeldsen K, Wanstrup J (1967) Enhancing influence of carbon monoxide on the development of atherosclerosis in cholesterol fed rabbits. J Atheroscler Res 1: 343
2. Schmidtke J, Zeitler E, Schoop W (1978) Late results of percutaneous catheter treatment (Dotter's technique) in occlusion of the femoropopliteal arteries, stage II. In: Zeitler E, Grüntzig A, Schoop W (eds) Percutaneous vascular recanalization, vol 15. Springer, Berlin Heidelberg New York, pp 96–110

3. Horváth L, Illés I, Varró J (1978) Complications of the transluminal angioplasty excluding the puncture site complications. In: Zeitler E, Grüntzig A, Schoop W (eds) Percutaneous vascular recanalization, vol 19. Springer, Berlin Heidelberg New York, pp 126–139
4. Dotter CT, Rösch J, Seaman AJ (1974) Selective clot lysis with low dose streptokinase. Radiology 111:31
5. Katzen BT, Van Breda A (1981) Low dose streptokinase in the treatment of arterial occlusion. Am J Roentgenol 136:117
6. Halse, T, Philipp K, Ruf F (1950) Tierexperimentelle Untersuchung über intravasale Thrombolyse mit Heparin und Thrombocid. Langenbecks Arch Chir 263:459
7. Horváth L (1980) Percutaneous transluminal angioplasty: importance of anticoagulant and fibrinolytic drugs. Am J Roentgenol 135:951

VIII. Percutaneous Transluminal Angioplasty: Late Results in Leg Arteries

27. Long-Term Patency Rates After Percutaneous Transluminal Angioplasty for Iliac and Femoropopliteal Obstructions

E. Schneider, A. Grüntzig, and A. Bollinger

In 1964 Dotter and Judkins introduced the transluminal catheter treatment for atherosclerotic occlusions [3]. Since then, long-term results after percutaneous transluminal angioplasty (PTA) with the coaxial catheter have been reported repeatedly [14, 18]. However, not until the catheter and the technique [8] had been improved (1974) was the method widely used in Europe and the United States.

The present chapter reports on early and late results after PTA of the iliac and femoropopliteal segments in 882 consecutive patients treated with the double-lumen balloon catheter.

Patients and Method

In the Polyclinic of the Department of Internal Medicine at the Universitätsspital, Zurich, 200 PTAs of the iliac and 682 of the femoropopliteal segment were performed between 1974 and 1981. The patients with atherosclerotic occlusive disease of the iliac arteries (mean age 58 ± 11.7 years) were on the average 10 years younger than those with femoropopliteal obstruction (mean age 67 ± 11.7 years). In both groups there was a majority of males. While there were 95% stenoses of the iliac segment and only 5% occlusions, in the femoropopliteal segment the ratio was 54%–46%. Intermittent claudication was present in 95% of the patients with iliac stenoses and in 82% with obstruction in the femoropopliteal segment. A pain-free walking distance exceeding 200 m (Fontaine stage IIa) was found in 12% of the patients in both groups [10]. Ischemic rest pain was present in 5% of the patients with iliac obstruction and in 18% of those with femoropopliteal involvement; for these patients there was a threat of amputation [15]. In these severely ischemic cases (Fontaine stages III and IV) multilevel arterial occlusive disease was always present.

Indications for PTA were based on the limitations and complaints of the patients and the angiographic findings. From a morphological view, hemodynamically significant iliac artery stenoses (22.6%) and singular or multiple stenoses and occlusions with a length of up to 10 cm of the femoropopliteal segment are suitable for transluminal angioplasty. However, in severely ischemic limbs (Fontaine stages III and IV) even longer occlusions were recanalized if vascular surgery would have involved a high risk or primary amputation seemed inevitable.

Percutaneous Transluminal Angioplasty
(ed. by C. T. Dotter, A. Grüntzig, W. Schoop, E. Zeitler)

The PTA was performed according to Grüntzig's technique [8], using double-lumen balloon catheters (Schneider Medintag, Zurich). Platelet inhibition was induced by means of aspirin 1 g/day prior to and during the procedure. Except where there were contraindications, the patients were treated with anticoagulant agents for 1–2 years. All patients had a clinical and noninvasive workup prior to and after PTA; follow-up studies were performed after 3, 6, 12, 24, and 60 months.

Besides a careful evaluation of pulse status and auscultation, pulse volume recordings at the thigh, below the knee and at big toe level, systolic ankle (Doppler) pressure measurements, and determination of the arm–ankle pressure gradients were performed as standard tests. In selected cases exercise pressure measurements were made after a standardized treadmill test or tiptoeing exercise, which guarantees the early detection of a hemodynamically significant stenosis. The criterion for a partial restenosis was a reduction by 50% of the pressure gradient improvement achieved by PTA, and a reduction of more than 75% was taken as an indication of complete recurrence of obstruction [8]. Restenoses and reocclusions requiring a further PTA or vascular surgery were verified angiographically.

Statistical evaluation was made according to the life table method. Therefore, patients undergoing bilateral PTA or simultaenous therapy of iliac and femoropopliteal obstruction are recorded twice, and new angioplasties for recurrences of obstruction are also separately recorded. Early reocclusions, recanalized the same or the following day, are recorded under primary successes.

Results

In the iliac segment PTA was primarily successful in 186 out of 200 cases (93%). In 14 cases (7%) the procedure was unsuccessful. Failure was due to early reocclusions in 5 cases (2.5%), and passage of the stenosis proved impossible in 9 cases (4.5%) (Table 1).

In 10.6% of the primarily successful procedures follow-up study showed partial or complete recurrence of obstruction during the 1st year. Subsequently, the reocclusion rate dropped distinctly. The cumulative patency rates after 1, 2, and 5 years are 89.4%, 86.5%, and 84.6% respectively (Table 2).

In the femoropopliteal segment at least one hemodynamically significant obstruction was recanalized in 602 out of 682 cases. The improvement was assessed by clinical findings and verified by noninvasive techniques. This corresponds to a primary success rate of 88.3%, or a failure rate of 11.7%. The main cause of PTA failure was unsuccessful passage of the occlusions (55 cases, 8%). Early reocclusions in the first 3 days after PTA occurred in 25 cases (3.7%) (Table 3).

The long-term results after PTA are summarized in Table 4. The greatest decrease in patency (26%) occurs in the first 12 months. For the following 4 years the recurrence rate was 6%. The cumulative patency rates 1, 2, and 5 years after PTA are 74.0%, 69.3%, and 68.0% respectively.

Table 1. Initial results in 200 consecutive PTA procedures for iliac artery obliterations (1974–1981)

	n	%
Primary success	186	93.0
Obliteration not passed	9	4.5
Early reocclusion	5	2.5
Total	200	100.0

Table 2. Follow-up results after 186 primary successful PTA procedures for iliac artery stenoses (1974–1981)

Period (mos.)	*n* pts.	*n* pts. at risk	Occlusion and stenosis	Interval patency rate (%)	Cumulative patency rate (%)
0–12	186	169.5	18	89.4	89.4
13–24	115	94	3	96.8	86.5
25–60	66	47.5	1	97.9	84.6

Table 3. Initial results after 682 consecutive PTA procedures for femoropopliteal obstructions (1974–1981)

	n	%
Primary success	602	88.3
Failure	80	11.7
Obstruction not passed	55	
Early reocclusion	25	
Total	682	100.0

Table 4. Follow-up results after 602 primary successful PTA procedures for femoropopliteal obstruction (1974–1981)

Period (mos.)	*n* pts.	*n* pts. at risk	Occlusion and stenosis	Interval patency rate (%)	Cumulative patency rate (%)
0–12	602	547.5	142	74	74.0
13–24	297	266	17	93.6	69.3
25–50	182	166	3	98.2	68.0

No deaths were related directly to the PTA. A total of 22 patients (2.5%) required a surgical correction of complications: 2 embolic occlusions of the popliteal trifurcation and 2 superficial femoral artery emboli after PTA of the femoral and iliac arteries (0.5%). The embolization of smaller arteries is clinically not relevant and the emboli are mainly lysed spontaneously. The main complications were inguinal hematomas or false aneurysms at the puncture site (2.0%).

Of the patients who underwent iliac PTA, 81% received warfarin for 1–2 years as secondary prophylaxis and 19% aspirin (1 g/day). After femoropopliteal PTA 70% of the patients were treated with anticoagulants and 30% with platelet inhibitors. For patients with diffuse atherosclerotic disease and cardiac indications anticoagulants were prescribed for a longer period.

Discussion

Percutaneous transluminal angioplasty with the double-lumen balloon catheter is the least invasive intervention for reopening an occluded leg artery, given a suitable morphology. This is the case with isolated high-grade stenoses of the iliac artery, and this explains the high primary success rate of 93%. The present study confirms our own earlier results [7–9] and corresponds to the later results of other authors [4, 5].

The patency rate after 1, 2, and 5 years, at 89.4%, 86.5%, and 84.6%, is comparable with the results of surgical revascularization of these segments. However, PTA is a lower-risk intervention with a 2.5% complication rate. The perioperative mortality after surgical iliac reconstructions is 4.5% [1].

In a subgroup of patients with a free walking distance of more than 200 m and angiographically verified arterial occlusive disease (Fontaine stage IIa), 96.1% of arterial stenoses morphologically ideal for treatment by PTA and dilated by this procedure were patent after 2 years [10]. The different 2-year patency rates, recorded by other authors, ranging from 70% to 100%, probably mean that their criteria for selecting patients were different.

In the femoropopliteal segment PTA was performed for almost 50% of the occlusions of up to 10 cm and a few that were even longer. The primary success rates with the Grüntzig balloon catheter and the coaxial Dotter system were identical. In our patient group the primary success rate was 83%. The figures quoted in the literature range from 63% to 100% [5, 6, 11, 12, 18]. The differences from the results for the iliac segment are probably due to the different criteria for selecting patients. The success rate declined rapidly where occlusions exceeded 10 cm [8].

The complication rate was higher with the Dotter technique (23%) than with the Grüntzig procedure (10%). In our series the frequency of complications requiring surgical correction was between 1.4% and 5% and depended on the experience of the therapist. There are also significant differences between the two procedures with respect to long-term results. After 2 years only 51% of the segments treated by the Dotter technique in 48 consecutive angioplasties were patent, compared to 73% after use of the balloon catheter [8]. After 2 and 5 years only 40% and 26% of the segments recanalized for intermittent claudication (Fontaine stage II) were patent [14]. However, the percentage of patency in that study cannot be compared directly with ours, because the follow-up patients were selected at random. The patency rates after 1, 2, and 5 years of 74.0%, 69.3%, and 68.0% are only somewhat lower than the corresponding results after autogenous femoropopliteal vein grafting [13, 16]. However, one has to consider that venous grafts normally bypass longer occlusions than those recanalized by PTA. PTA shows even better results when compared to thromboendarterectomy. Higher patency rates (80%) after 2 years can only be achieved by means of this surgical procedure if it is followed by secondary prophylaxis with aspirin [2].

Contrary to the case with thromboendarterectomy, with PTA the therapeutic value of platelet-active substances is established only with respect to the prevention of early reocclusion [17]. There are no prospective randomized studies comparing aspirin to placebo and warfarin. In the present series the majority of the patients were treated with anticoagulants, as patients in whom anticoagulation is contraindicated have a higher late failure rate [18]. There appears to be considerable potential for medical prophylaxis of reocclusion: An improvement in the late results after PTA by means of new antithrombotic drugs and platelet active substances may be expected in the future.

Summary

Primary and late results after PTA of the iliac and femoropopliteal segment using a double-lumen balloon catheter are presented; the data are taken from 882 consecutive and prospectively controlled cases. Two hundred iliac artery stenoses and 682 stenoses or short (< 10 cm) occlusions of the femoropopliteal segment were treated: 82% of the patients suffered from intermittent claudication and 18% from ischemia at rest. In 93% of the iliac and 88.3% of the femoropopliteal obstructions the procedure was primarily successful. In the majority of failures the occlusion could not be passed. Complications requiring surgical correction occurred in 2.5% of all procedures: 4 distal embolectomies (0.5%) and 18 sutures of the artery at the puncture site (2.0% were necessary).

For iliac artery stenoses the cumulative patency rates (life table method) 1, 2, and 5 years after PTA were 89.4%, 86.5%, and 84.6% respectively, and for the femoropopliteal segment 74.0%, 69.3%, and 68.0%. Thus PTA using balloon catheters is established for treatment of iliac artery stenoses, whereas in femoropopliteal obstructions the results are not yet optimal. An improvement in long-term patency rates may be expected if new drugs are employed for secondary prophylaxis of atherosclerosis.

References

1. Bollinger A (1979) Funktionelle Angiologie. Thieme, Stuttgart
2. Bollinger A, Schneider E, Pouliadis G, Brunner U (1980) Thrombozytenfunktionshemmer und Antikoagulantien nach gefäßrekonstruktiven Eingriffen im femoro-poplitealen Bereich: Resultate einer prospektiven Studie. In: Thrombose und Atherogenese, Pathophysiologie und Therapie der arteriellen Verschlußkrankheit. Witzstrock, Baden-Baden, p 276

3. Dotter CT, Judkins MP (1964) Transluminal treatment of arteriosclerotic obstruction. Description of a new technique and the preliminary report of its application. Circulation 30: 654
4. Freimann DB, Spence R, Gatenby R, Gertner M, Roberts B, Berkowitz HD, Ring EL, Oleaga JA (1981) Transluminal angioplasty of the iliac and femoral arteries: follow-up results without anticoagulation. Radiology 141: 347
5. Gallino A, Mahler F, Probst P, Nachbur B (1982) Early and late results of 250 percutaneous transluminal dilatations (PTD) of the lower limbs. VASA 11 (4): 319
6. Grüntzig A, Mahler F, Kumpe D, Brunner U, Meier W (1976) Die Erfahrung mit der perkutanen Rekanalisation chronischer arterieller Verschlüsse nach Dotter. Schweiz Med Wochenschr 106: 422
7. Greenfield AJ (1980) Femoral, popliteal, and tibial arteries: percutaneous transluminal angioplasty. AJR 135: 927
8. Grüntzig A (1977) Die perkutane transluminale Rekanalisation chronischer Arterienverschlüsse mit einer neuen Dilatationstechnik. Witzstrock, Baden-Baden
9. Grüntzig A (1980) Rekanalisation stenosierter Arterien mit dem Dilatationskatheter. Consilium Akzente No. 4, CEDIP Verlag, Munich
10. Jäger K, Schneider E, Grüntzig A, Bollinger A (1982) Perkutane transluminale Angioplastie (PTA) im frühen Stadium II der peripheren arteriellen Verschlußkrankheit. VASA 11 (4): 332
11. Katzen BT, Chang J, Know WG (1979) Percutaneous transluminal angioplasty with the Grüntzig balloon catheter. Arch Surg 114: 1389
12. Motarjeme A, Keifer JW, Zuska AJ (1980) Percutaneous transluminal angioplasty of the iliac arteries: 66 experiences. AJR 135: 937
13. Reichle FA, Rankin KP, Tyson RR, Finestone AJ, Shuman C (1979) Long-term results of 474 arterial reconstructions for severely ischemic limbs: a fourteen-year follow-up. Surgery 85: 93
14. Schmidtke I, Zeitler E, Schoop W (1978) Spätergebnisse (5–8 Jahre) der perkutanen Katheterbehandlung (Dotter-Technik) bei femoro-poplitealen Arterienverschlüssen im Stadium II. VASA 7 (4): 4
15. Schneider E, Grüntzig A, Bollinger A (1982) Die perkutane transluminale Angioplastie (PTA) der Beinarterien im Stadium III und IV der peripheren arteriellen Verschlußkrankheit. VASA 11 (4): 336
16. Szilagyi DE, Hageman JH, Smith RF, Elliott JP, Brown F, Dietz P (1979) Autogenous vein grafting in femoro-popliteal atherosclerosis: the limits of its effectiveness. Surgery 86: 836
17. Zeitler E, Reichold J, Schoop W (1973) Einfluß von Acetylosalicylsäure auf das Frühergebnis nach perkutaner Rekanalisation nach Dotter. Dtsch Med Wochenschr 98: 1285
18. Zeitler E, Grüntzig A, Schoop W (eds) (1978) Percutaneous vascular recanalization. Springer, Berlin Heidelberg New York

28. Ten-Year Results of Percutaneous Catheter Treatment in Cases of Femoropopliteal Arterial Occlusion in Stage II*

I. Schmidtke

Material and Methods

The method of transluminal catheter treatment first introduced in 1964 by Dotter and Judkins was introduced at the Aggertalklinik in 1968 by Zeitler. At the inception of this new mode of treatment, we raised the question of the likelihood of success of this therapy, not only with regard to the early stages but also in the long term. We therefore began relatively early with follow-up examinations. The results of a group of cases of treatment for femoropopliteal occlusions have already been published on several occasions, most recently in 1978 [1–4]. The present compilation is based on the long-term observation of the same group over 10 years, with the posttreatment observation phase lasting over 12 years in the case of some patients.

Number of Cases

Of the many patients treated by the catheter method, those coming to us through the State Insurance Institute (called below by its German initials LVA) of the Rhine Province and Westphalia and those paying for their treatment themselves were chosen for reasons of space. Furthermore, the evaluation was limited to a particular period, i.e., to the treatments given between 1 December 1968 and 30 November 1971. In addition, only those patients were examined subsequently in whom the dilated femoropopliteal artery was still patent at the time of their release from the clinic [for further details see 3, 4]. We are thus concerned with 79 patients (72 men and 7 women aged 41–71 years at the time of treatment, average age 55.5 years), 81 extremities having been treated. Forty patients came via the LVA Rhine Province and 21 via the LVA Westphalia, and 18 patients were received as private patients.

Technique of Treatment

In 21 cases the recanalization was carried out using a simple straight Teflon catheter of 7 or 8 Charrière with four lateral holes from the firm of USCI (listed

* With the support of the Association for the Fight Against Vascular Diseases

Percutaneous Transluminal Angioplasty
(ed. by C. T. Dotter, A. Grüntzig, W. Schoop, E. Zeitler)

"Seldinger technique"). Fifty-nine occlusions were treated using the coaxial recanalization catheter system according to Dotter; in the case of one occlusion an expansion using the Fogarty balloon catheter was performed following the recanalization with the Seldinger catheter.

Pre- and Postoperative Drug Therapy

For at least 2 days prior to surgery, 66 patients received 1 tablet of Colfarit three times a day. In one case this was preceded by a streptokinase treatment. In 33 cases Colfarit was continued following surgery, in 14 cases a 48-h heparin infusion (1,000–1,500 E/h) was prescribed, and 32 times a combined treatment using heparin and Colfarit was employed. Thirty-one patients were given long-term anticoagulant therapy. The decision to institute long-term therapy was based partly on the primary results, partly on the framework of an alternating study, and partly on the wishes of the patient.

Assessment of the Results of the Treatment

The immediate results were assessed angiographically and clinically-angiographically. In the follow-up examinations, which were carried out ambulatorily either in the clinic or in the patient's home, the findings were based mainly on the clinical-angiological examination; in about half the cases a control angiography was performed in the course of the years.

A fully open vascular system was assumed if, in addition to the pulse, the stress oscillogram was normal. Those cases were judged to be constricted in which a weakening of the pulse, a stenotic murmur, and a negative reaction in the stress oscillogram were found. Those cases were considered to be reobliterated in which no popliteal pulse was to be felt and no stenotic murmur was audible, and in which, in addition, a corresponding deterioration was present in the oscillogram.

In one female patient the vascular system was open after 11 years, both clinically and angiographically, and the findings had improved considerably over the years. In the 5-year results this patient had been listed as occluded.

We classified as doubtful those cases in which the exact time of the reobliteration could not be determined with certainty at the next checkup. We further registered those cases as doubtful in which the patient had still had an open artery at the last checkup but had died in the meantime.

Those cases in which either a new catheter treatment in the same vascular area ($n = 11$; due to stronger occurrence of stenoses $n = 7$, or reobliteration $n = 4$) or a vascular operation was performed were listed as operated upon.

Deceased Patients

Within the 10-year observation period 31 patients died, and by the deadline date, 1 March 1972, altoghter 35 patients had died (see Table 1).

Table 1. Ten-year mortality following transluminal catheter treatment

Cause of death	*n*
Coronary, etc.	13
Bronchial/laryngial cancer	8
Apoplexy	3
Pulmonary embolism	2
Miscellaneous	4
Unknown	5
Total	35

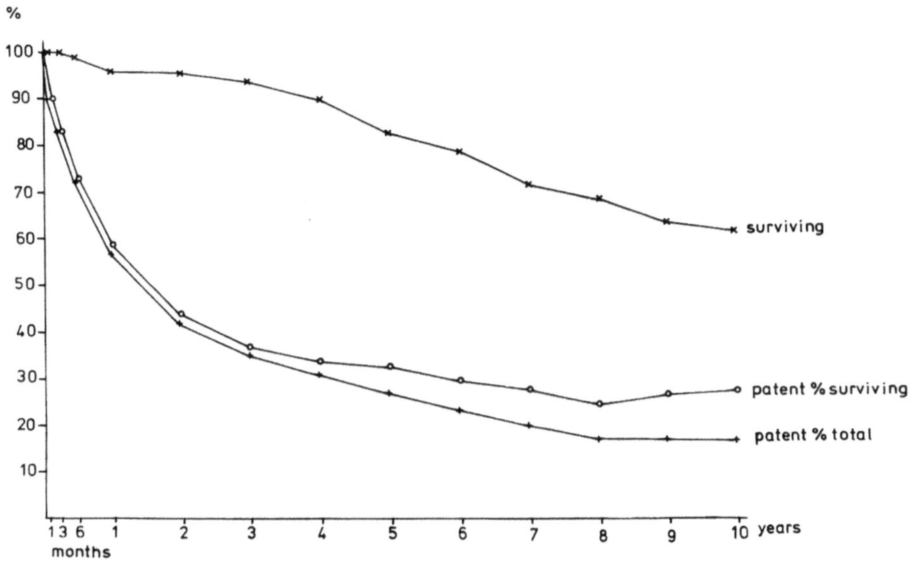

Fig. 1. Results of transluminal catheter treatment as percentages of total and surviving numbers of patients

Amputation

In six patients the treated leg had to be amputated due to reobliteration and the appearance of necroses, sometimes despite follow-up vascular surgery (7.4%).

Long-Term Results

In Fig. 1 the proportion of patent cases is shown by two curves, in terms both of the percentage of the total of 81 cases and of the percentage of those still living. The steepest downturn in the curves, representing an early reobliteration, renewed catheter treatment, or operation, corresponds to the first 2 years

(44%/42%). The curve relating to the total number of cases declines to a level of 17% by the 8 year and remains constant thereafter, while for that relative to the surviving patients these values lie between 30% and 25%. After 10 years, the recanalized artery is still patent in 28% (14 out of 50 surviving patients). As the postoperative examination comprises a treatment period of 3 years, the follow-up observation period is in some cases 11–13 years (see Table 2).

In Fig. 2 the total results, including those for the cases operated upon, and the finding in question for each point in time are shown in the form of bar graphs. Furthermore, in this figure we have differentiated between a free patency and a partial stenosis. The number of those undergoing a second operation (second PTD or vascular operation) no longer increased after 4 years. The proportion of stenoses and constrictions was about one-third in the month after the treatment, in the later periods just under one-half.

Table 2. Follow-up observation over 11–13 years

Years	*n*	Patent	Occluded	Operated upon	Deceased
11	60	10	18	5	27
12	37	4	12	3	18
13	4		2		2

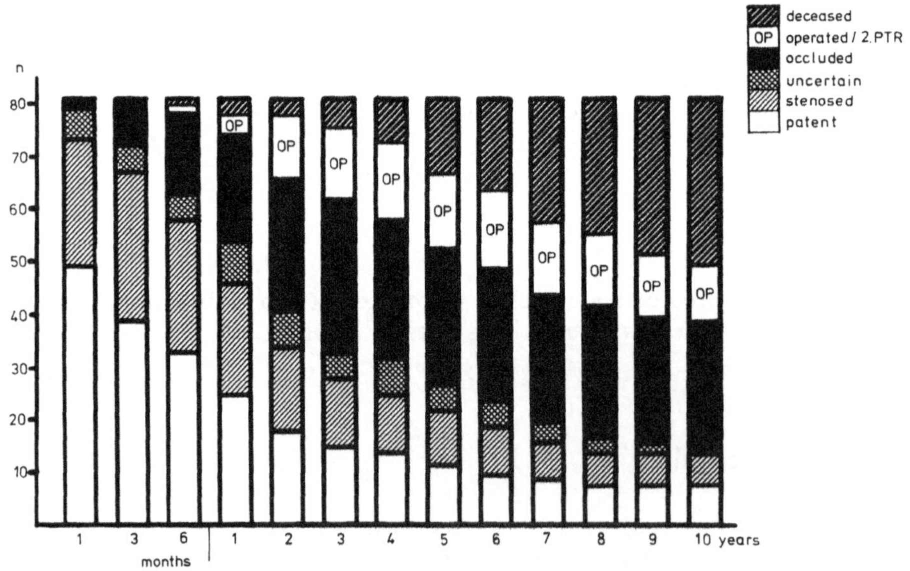

Fig. 2. Results of transluminal catheter treatment in terms of patent, stenosed, occluded, and reoperated arteries

Permanent Anticoagulation

The effect of the permanent anticoagulation has already been reported on in the first publication on the same group of patients [1]. In the 1st month following surgery the obliteration quota was about the same for those patients receiving anticoagulants as for those not receiving anticoagulants, but after the 6th month recurrences occurred far more seldom in the group receiving the anticoagulants. In about 80% of those cases in this group that could be evaluated, the treated arteries remained patent for 30 months (statistically highly significant), while an almost continuous downward curve is to be seen for those patients who did not take anticoagulants.

At the late observation an evaluation of the effects of the treatment with anticoagulants was no longer of great significance, as only very few patients had maintained this therapy. An evaluation of treatment with acetylsalicylic acid was not possible, as a large proportion of the patients had stopped taking it because of gastric intolerance.

Length of Occlusion

In Fig. 3 the results according to the length of the occlusion are illustrated in a bar graph. As was to be expected, the cases with very long occlusions (13–27

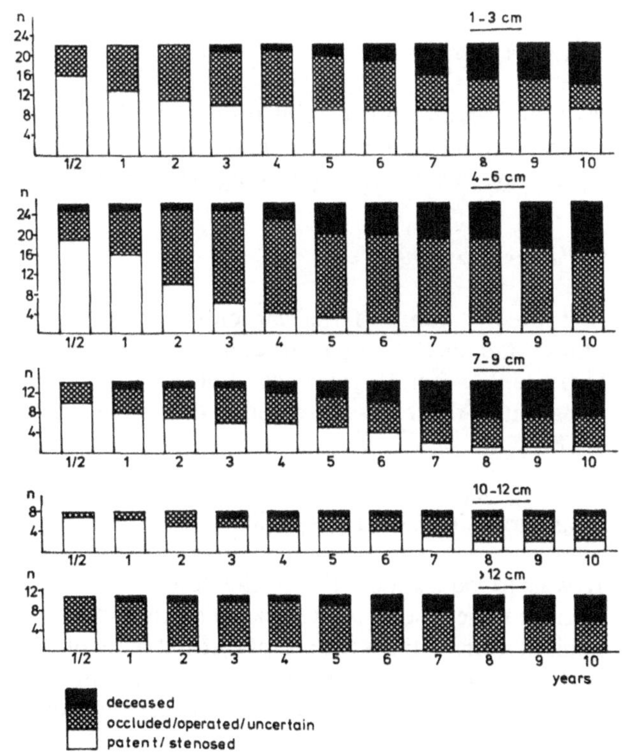

Fig. 3. Follow-up study of transluminally treated arterial occlusions in relationship to the length

Table 3. Lower leg arteries still patent: (percentage of cases)

Years	3 patent ($n = 42$)	2 patent ($n = 26$)	1 patent ($n = 13$)
1/2	72	73	69
1	60	50	62
2	38	42	54
3	33	31	46
4	29	27	46
5	24	23	46
6	19	19	46
7	17	15	38
8	14	15	31
9	14	15	31
10	14	15	31

cm) show a tendency toward early reobliteration. After 5 years, all of these were blocked again. The group with 4–6-cm-long occlusions came off relatively badly in comparison to the 7–9- and 10–12-cm-long occlusions, but the failure quota was largest in this group because of renewed catheter treatment or operation. The long-term result for the short occlusions of 1–3 cm was the most favorable. After 10 years, 9 of the 22 cases treated still had patent arteries (9 of the 14 survivors, 64.3%).

Outward Flow

As follows from our interim results of 1975 and 1978, the long-term result for recanalized femoral occlusions was best in the group with only one patent lower leg artery, the percentage being 31% as opposed to 14%–15% (Table 3).

Catheter Technique

In the early years of the catheter treatment at the Aggertalklinik, both the Dotter and the Seldinger catheter were used. Table 4 shows the long-term results in percent. After 10 years, as after 5 years, a better permanent result becomes apparent in those cases treated with the Seldinger catheter: 24% as opposed to 15%.

Angiographic Primary Results

It was to be expected that the long-term results would reflect the primary angiographic findings after catheter treatment. The results according to three angiographic definitions are presented in Table 5. The best result (22% after 10 years) is shown in the group without remaining stenosis; astonishingly, 11% (2 out of 18 cases) in the group with severe stenoses were still patent after 10 years.

Table 4. Catheter technique (patent cases in percent)

Years	Seldinger ($n = 21$)	Dotter ($n = 60$)
1/2	81	69
1	62	55
2	58	37
3	48	30
4	43	27
5	38	23
6	33	20
7	29	17
8	24	15
9	24	15
10	24	15

Table 5. Angiographic primary results (patent cases in percent)

Years	No stenosis ($n = 37$)	Little stenosis ($n = 26$)	Severe stenosis ($n = 18$)
1/2	76	69	67
1	68	50	44
2	49	35	39
3	43	27	28
4	41	23	22
5	35	19	22
6	30	15	22
7	24	15	17
8	22	15	11
9	22	15	11
10	22	15	11

Table 6. Influence of smoking: patent cases as percentages of the group and of the survivors

Years	Cigarettes ($n = 36$)	Pipes/cigars ($n = 7$)	Nonsmokers ($n = 38$)
1/2	64	72	79
1	39	72	71
2	25	43	58
3	17	43	50
4	14	43	45
5	14	29	42
6	11	14	37
7	5.6	14	34
8	5.6	14	29
9	5.6	14	29
10	5.6	14	29
10[a]	11[a]	20[a]	42[a]

[a] Referred to the number of survivors

Table 7. Results in private patients and LVA patients (patent cases in percent)

Years	Private patients ($n = 18$)	LVA patients ($n = 63$)
1/2	78	70
1	78	51
2	67	35
3	56	29
4	56	24
5	50	21
6	39	19
7	28	17
8	22	16
9	22	16
10	22	16

Smoking Habits

In assessing the results in relation to smoking habits (Table 6), we evaluated the patient data recorded 10 years after treatment; in the cases of deceased patients we fell back on the earlier data.

The group of nonsmokers had, as in earlier evaluations, the best long-term results; nonsmokers surviving after 10 years represented 29% of the total patient sample and 42% of the survivors. The cigarette smokers had the worst results (5.6% and 11%), while the pipe and cigar smokers had a result that was worse than that of the nonsmokers but better than that of the cigarette smokers (14% and 20%).

Patient Selection

As mentioned above, among those treated there were both patients who were admitted through the LVA and private patients paying for their treatment themselves. The previous results had shown a better result for the private patients. In Table 7 the findings up to the 10th follow-up observation year are listed. This still indicates a better result for the private patients (22% of the toal patient sample) than for the LVA patients (16%). Relative to the surviving patients, the percentages are 40% for the private patients and 25% for the LVA patients.

Length of Case History

In Table 8 the results are listed according to the duration of the complaint as stated by the patients. As was the case in the interim result after 5 years, the group with a case history of 1–2 years comes away worst, while the collectives with a shorter or longer case history are equal after 10 years.

Table 8. Duration of case history (patent cases in percent)

Years	1 year ($n = 34$)	1–2 years ($n = 32$)	2 years ($n = 15$)
1/2	77	72	60
1	56	59	53
2	44	41	40
3	38	34	27
4	38	28	20
5	38	19	20
6	29	19	20
7	26	13	20
8	21	13	20
9	21	13	20
10	21	13	20

Table 9. Date of treatment (patent cases in percent)

Year	1 Dec. 1968 to 31 Apr. 1970 ($n = 37$)	1 June 1970 to 30 Nov. 1971 ($n = 44$)
1/2	73	71
1	54	59
2	41	43
3	30	39
4	24	36
5	22	32
6	19	27
7	16	23
8	14	20
9	14	20
10	14	20

Date of Treatment

When the numbers of patients with arteries still patent at follow-up are listed according to the date of treatment (Table 9), a better long-term result can be recognized for the patients in the second treatment group. This corresponds to the 5-year result, and the cause is to be sought in an improved technique of treatment rather than in a more specific diagnosis.

Conclusion

Of patients undergoing catheter treatment at the Aggertalklinik during the initial years, 79 with 81 successfully treated segmental occlusions in the femoropopliteal segment (stage II) were selected and subsequently examined several times for up to 10–13 years.

The results largely confirm the earlier results of this group. One essential difference from the results of the 5-year analysis is due to the death rate. After 10 years, 17% of the recanalized arteries were still patent (28% of those of the survivors).

To summarize the results analyzed according to various parameters: the best results were in the cases with the short occlusions (1–3 cm), those with good angiographic primary results, the nonsmokers, and the privately insured patients. In addition, long-term success appears to depend on the choice of catheter and the experience of the person performing the therapy.

References

1. Zeitler E, Schmidtke I, Schoop W (1973) Die perkutane Behandlung von arteriellen Durchblutungsstörungen der Extremitäten mit Katheter. VASA 2: 401
2. Schmidtke I, Zeitler E, Schoop W (1975) Langzeitergebnis der perkutanen Katheterbehandlung (Dotter-Technik) bei femoropoplitealen Arterienverschlüssen im Stadium II. VASA 4: 210
3. Schmidtke I, Zeitler E, Schoop W (1978) Spätergebnisse (5–8 Jahre) der perkutanen Katheterbehandlung (Dotter-Technik) bei femoropoplitealen Arterienverschlüssen im Stadium II. VASA 7: 4
4. Schmidtke I, Zeitler E, Schoop W (1978) Late results of percutaneous catheter treatment (Dotter's technique) in occlusion of the femoropopliteal arteries, stage II. In: Zeitler E, Grüntzig A, Schoop W (eds) Percutaneous vascular recanalization. Springer, Berlin Heidelberg New York, pp 96–110

29. Late Results of Percutaneous Transluminal Angioplasty of Leg Arteries With Special Reference to the Popliteocrural Region

W. Ostheim-Dzerowycz

Between June 1978 and December 1980 percutaneous transluminal angioplasty (PTA) was performed in 194 patients with stenosis and/or occlusions of the femorocrural axis; it was primarily successful in 181. After 1 year there were 160 survivors, in 143 (89.4%) of whom the affected arteries were patent. A group with special problems and difficulties were those patients suffering from arterial occlusive disease in the popliteocrural region.

In 40 of these patients (45% men, 55% women) PTA was successfully performed. The mean age was 66 ± 11 years (42–81). Of this group, 75% had one or more calf arteries occluded, and 65% suffered from pain and necrosis. For the latter there was little chance of avoiding amputation, so that PTA was employed even in hopeless situations. In 29 of the 34 survivors (85.3%), the treated arteries were still patent after 1 year (Fig. 1), 2 lost the calf, 2 had reocclusions which were successfully redilated, and 1 patient was lost to follow-up. None of the 29 in whom the arteries remained patent had rest pain or necrosis, so that the result was a more or less well-compensated claudication. Ten (34.5%) had no more symptoms and an unlimited walking distance. The

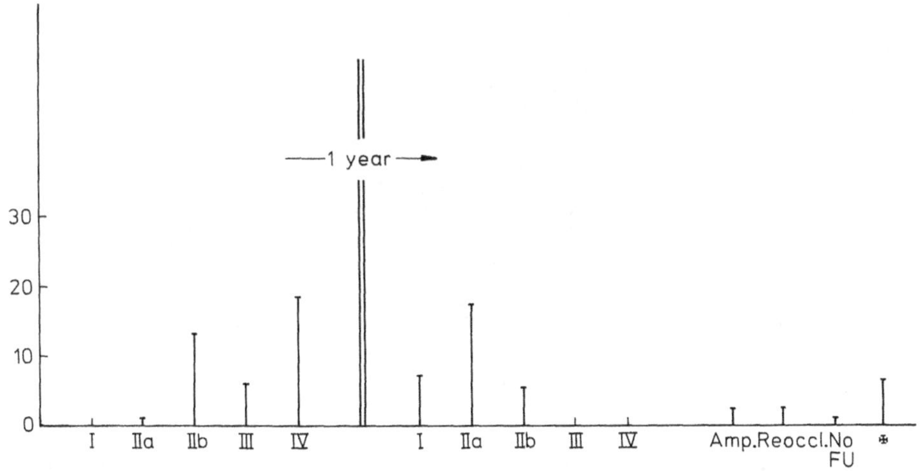

Fig. 1. One-year success rates following PTA of popliteocrural arteries ($n = 40$); the arteries were still patent in 29 (72.5%; 85.3% of the survivors). *Amp.*, amputated; *Reoccl.*, reoccluded; *No FU*, lost to follow-up

Percutaneous Transluminal Angioplasty
(ed. by C. T. Dotter, A. Grüntzig, W. Schoop, E. Zeitler)

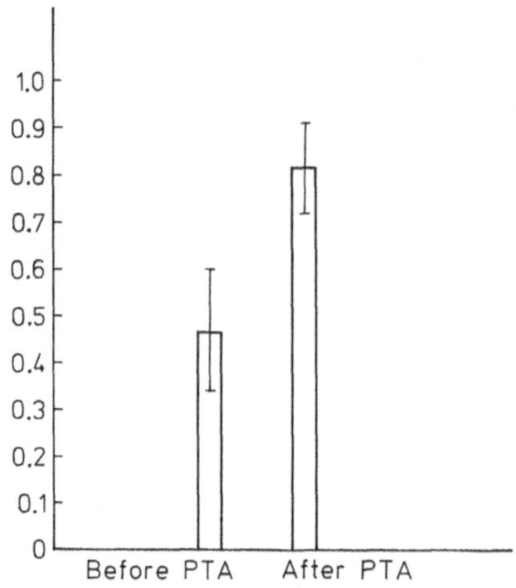

Fig. 2. PTA of popliteocrural arteries: ankle pressure index after 1 year ($n = 29$)

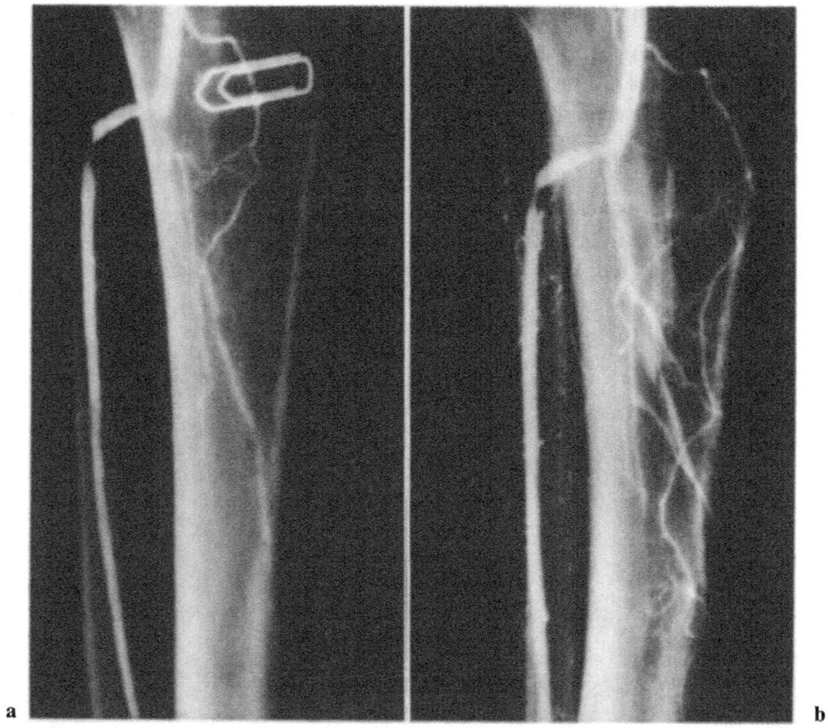

Fig. 3a, b. A 65-year-old woman with stenosis of common trunk and anterior tibial artery; **a** predilatation and **b** postdilatation angiogram

Doppler ankle pressure index rose from 0.46 ± 0.25 before therapy to 0.81 ± 0.19 after 1 year (Fig. 2).

This result convinced our team that PTA is an acceptable treatment alternative for this problematic group of patients, especially when it is combined

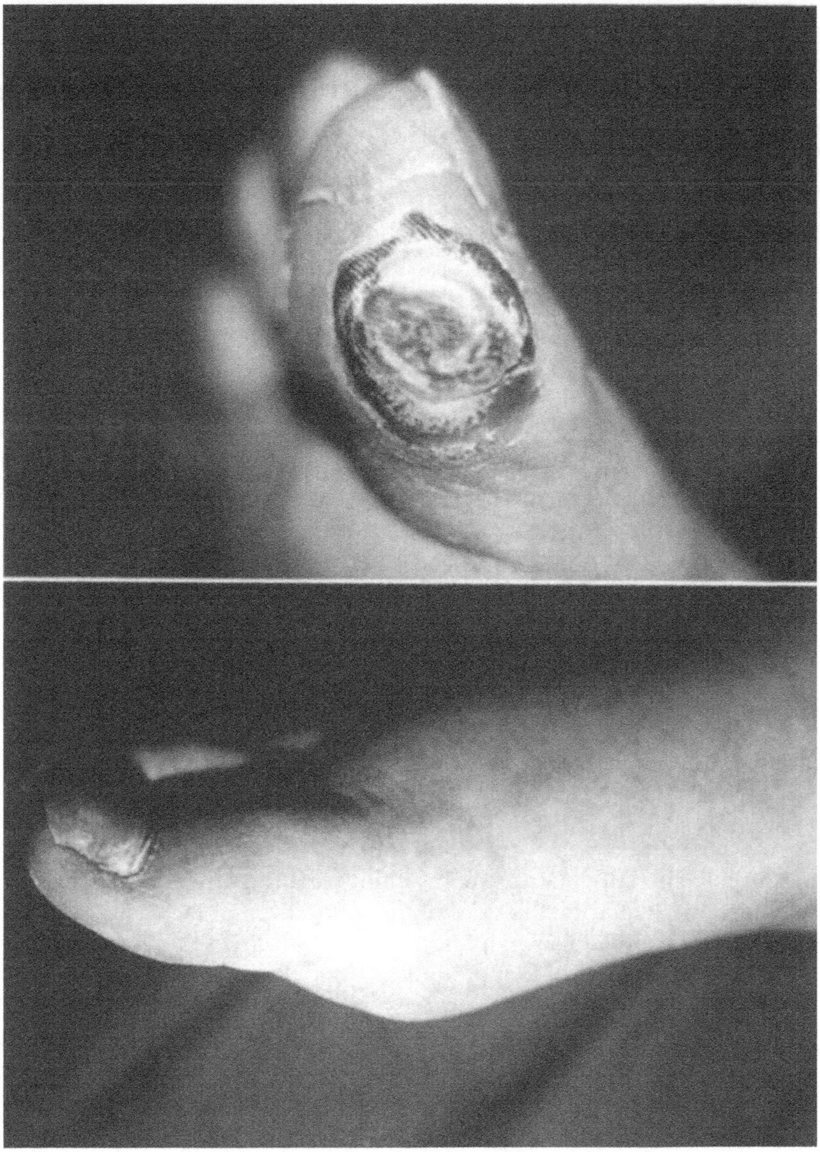

a

b

Fig. 4. **a** Necrotic first toe before dilatation. **b** Good results after 2 years. Same patient as in Fig. 1

with a conservative follow-up treatment and care of necrosis. Consequently, the indication for PTA of the popliteocrural region increased to about 30 patients in 1981, with good primary results.

An example of a good result of this technique is shown in Fig. 3. Figure 4 shows the necrosis before dilatation and the 2-year result in the necrotic first toe.

30. Late Results of Percutaneous Catheter Treatment in Iliac Stenoses – A Retrospective Study

H. Rieger*, F.-J. Roth, E. Zeitler, T. Palden,
M. Wegner, and W. Schoop

Introduction

Between the beginning of 1973 and the end of 1979 attempts were made to dilate a total of 306 iliac stenoses by Dotter's procedure in 292 inpatients. The inauguration and performance of the method have been described elsewhere [1, 3]. Early in 1982 we tried to reexamine as many patients as possible. The purpose of the study was to find out the rate of long-term patency 2–9 years after successful catheter treatment, and to assess the clinical benefit not only immediately after dilatation but also many years later. Finally, it was of some interest to see to what extent the vascular risk factors or risk conditions might influence the patency rate.

Methods of Examination

Apart from reports on the walking distance, means of pharmacologic prophylaxis (anticoagulating or antiaggregating drugs), and the development of vascular risk factors, the state of the treated vessel segment was checked with the help of careful pulse palpation, auscultation, oscillography at rest and after knee-bendings, and Doppler ultrasound technique. In cases with additional peripheral occlusions (femoral artery, lower leg artery) the evaluation of the inguinal pulse was of particular importance. The information thus obtained usually made it possible to state the degree of patency of the iliac vessel segment formerly dilated. The designations used are as follows: if the test results were similar to those obtained immediately after successful dilatation or even better, the vessel was assumed to be patent. The same holds true if there was a certain tendency toward restenosis but the hemodynamic and clinical situation were clearly better than prior to the therapeutic intervention. However, if the findings were approximately the same as before catheter treatment or if a deterioration had occurred, with missing or low pulses, the vessel was classified as restenosed or occluded.

* Supported by grants from the Verein zur Bekämpfung von Gefäßkrankheiten e.V., 5250 Engelskirchen, FRG

Percutaneous Transluminal Angioplasty
(ed. by C. T. Dotter, A. Grüntzig, W. Schoop, E. Zeitler)

Table 1. Primary analysis of cases according to year of treatment. There were 306 stenoses in 292 inpatients: 14 patients suffered from a double stenosis (4.8%). The numbers in the table refer to stenoses

Year	All stenoses		Successful treatments					Controlled stenoses		
	1 Total	2 Success	3 Con-trolled	4 Surg.	5 Lost	6 Far	7 Died	8 Patent	9 Resten.	10 Occlus.
1973	31	28 (90.3%)	10	3	4	3	8	6	1	3
1974	28	25 (89.2%)	11	1	4	1	8	9	0	2
1975	24	20 (83.3%)	11	1	0	0	8	8	1	2
1976	33	31 (93.9%)	17	1	2	1	10	14	0	3
1977	42	36 (85.7%)	25	0	3	3	5	19	2	4
1978	63	59 (93.6%)	37	2	7	6	7	30	4	3
1979	85	70 (82.3%)	53	1	3	5	8	46	4	3
Sum	306	269 (88.3%)	164 (60.9%)	9 (3.3%)	23 (8.6%)	19 (7.0%)	54 (20.0%)	132 (80.4%)	12 (7.3%)	20 (12.1%)

Col. 1: total no. of patients in whom treatment was attempted; col. 2: radiologically and clinically successful treatments; col. 3: patients who were actually reexamined; col. 4: patients who underwent operation; col. 5: patients who could not be located for follow-up; col. 6: patients who had moved to more than 300 km away and were therefore not available for reexamination; col. 7: no. of patent stenoses; col. 8: no. of treated stenoses found to be restenosed or occluded

Analysis of the Number of Cases

Analysis of the number of cases is presented in Table 1. In column 1 all stenoses treated between 1 January 1973 and 31 December 1979 and in column 2 all successful dilatations – divided according to the year of treatment – are listed. In 269 out of 306 cases the procedure was successful, usually both from the radiological and the clinical point of view. That means an average early success rate of 88.3%. Further data on successfully treated patients – again arranged by year of treatment – are shown in columns 3–7: besides those patients who could be reexamined (column 3), there remained a group consisting of patients who had meanwhile undergone surgical treatment (column 4), become lost to follow-up (column 5), moved away (column 6), or died (column 7). In the 164 patients followed up, it was found that 132 treated iliac vessels were apparently patent (column 8), 12 were restenosed (column 9), and 20 were apparently occluded (column 10).

Statistical Evaluation

Because of the fact that the study reported here is a retrospective one with a large number of dropouts, the life table method is not practicable. Thus the crucial question arises to which basic totality or reference group the number of patent cases should be referred. Among those patients who were followed up ($n = 164$), the patency rates over 2–9 years were excellent. Of course, this method

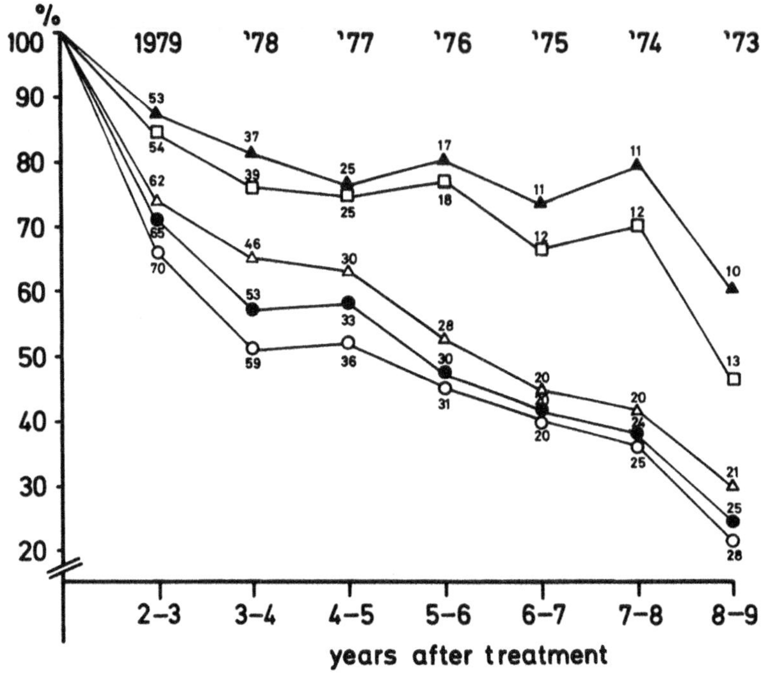

Fig. 1. *Upper abscissa,* years of treatment; *lower abscissa,* years after treatment; *ordinate,* percentage of patency. The *numbers of stenoses* corresponding to the percentages are given next to the symbols. ○——○ represents all successfully treated stenoses; ●——● represents this total minus the number of patients who had moved away; △——△ represents the former total with the additional exclusion of those who could not be located for follow-up; □——□ represents this total with the additional exclusion of patients who had died; ▲——▲ represents the total remaining after the exclusion of patients who had undergone operation, and thus the final total of patients who were reexamined

of interpretation must lead to an overestimation of the true situation. On the other hand, we come to a strong underestimation of long-term results if we take the totality of all successfully treated patients as 100%. We therefore decided simply to give the number of patent iliac segments (column 8 in Table 1) and to relate them to different reference groups, as can be seen in Fig. 1. Let us start from the lowest curve, symbolized by the open circles. This curve represents the largest reference group, which means all successfully treated patients ($n = 269$). In this case all successfully treated iliac vessels which – for whatever reason – could not be followed up must be regarded as occluded. Under these conditions the patency rate after 4–5 years is around 55%. Now we reduce the reference group stepwise for those patients who are listed in columns 4–7 of Table 1, excluding first those patients who had moved and lived farther than 300 km away. The patency rate after 4–5 years would then amount to 60%. After additional exclusion of patients who could not be located, the patency rate is 65%. After further exclusion of those patients who had died and had undergone operation the patency rate increases to nearly 80%.

Table 2. Number of patients (not stenoses) who showed a change in clinical stage at the time of reexamination

Change	: n =	128 (80%)
II → I	: n =	60 (47%)
IIa → IIa	: n =	35 (27%)
IIb → IIa	: n =	23 (18%)
III → II	: n =	6 (5%)
IV → II	: n =	4 (3%)
Uncertain	: n =	26 (20%)

From the clinical standpoint and in terms of everyday work, of particular interest is what one should tell a patient suffering from severe iliac stenosis who asks for a medical opinion on the late result he can expect – after successful Dotter procedure. In other words: which of the statistical reference groups described above represents best the real probability of patency? In our opinion reference should be made to that number of patients alive at the time of follow-up examination (including those having undergone surgery). We may therefore assume a probability of patency of nearly 80% 5–6 years after treatment.

Two to nine years after treatment, 73.3% (n = 128) of all patients followed up (n = 154) showed a definite improvement in clinical stage (see Table 2). In the remaining patients (26.7%) it was not possible to make any statement for various reasons (reduction in walking distance because of additional peripheral occlusions, general physical handicaps such as Parkinson's disease or lumbago). Most patients (49.0%) demonstrated a countinuous change from clinical stage II (claudication with a more or less limited painless walking distance) to stage I (symptom-free). These patients had usually suffered only from a single iliac stenosis without any additional peripheral flow impediment. In a second group (29.0%) a considerable enhancement of walking distance within stage II could be assessed. Usually in these cases a further occlusion of the ipsilateral femoral artery was present which, however, it was not necessary to remove in view of the clinically successful dilation of iliac stenoses. In some patients (15.0%) walking distances (200 m, clinical stage IIb) could be increased to much more than 200 m (so-called stage IIa). Only eight patients (7.0%) had suffered from rest pain or ischemic skin lesions (clinical stages III and IV respectively), and these were cured by the Dotter procedure. In cases of long-standing clinical stage III, rest pain was promptly alleviated. In stage IV cases the skin lesions had usually healed by a couple of months later.

Risk Factors Related to Reocclusion

As shown in Table 3 the percentage of those patients who had not received continuous antiaggregation or anticoagulation treatment was nearly twice as high in the reocclusion group as among the successful cases. Moreover, patients who had not stopped smoking were more highly represented in the reocclusion group, as were patients suffering from diabetes mellitus. We are all aware that the simple retrospective comparison of percentages does not meet the needs of a

Table 3. Percentage coordination of risk conditions to patent group and occlusion group

Risk factors	Group	
	Patent ($n = 132$)	Occlusion/restenosis ($n = 32$)
No continuous prophylaxis	48.4%	81.8%
Continued smoking	34.0%	70.0%
Hypertension	34.0%	24.2%
Diabetes	6.0%	12.0%
Hyperlipoproteinemia	26.5%	21.0%

complete statistical evaluation. This, in fact, is hard to do because of the different n-numbers (122 versus 32) and many other factors more or less influencing the occlusion rate. For the time being we may only take these results to indicate a certain tendency, which must be interpreted cautiously.

Conclusions

In confirmation of earlier results [2] we found the Dotter procedure to be the method of choice in patients suffering from isolated iliac stenoses or from stenoses combined with peripheral occlusions. Following successful treatment of isolated iliac stenoses most patients become symptom-free or have few symptoms. In cases with additional occlusions beyond the iliac stenosis, dilatation of the latter leads in many patients to a considerable and long-term improvement of the clinical picture. The procedure involves relatively little risk and is economical in terms of time and money.

References

1. Dotter CT, Judkins MP (1964) Transluminal treatment of arteriosclerotic obstruction. Description of a new technique and a preliminary report of its application. Circulation 30: 654
2. Schoop W, Levy H, Cappius G, Mansjoer H, Zeitler E (1978) Early and late results of PTD in iliac stenosis. In: Zeitler E, Grüntzig A, Schoop W (eds) Percutaneous vascular recanalization. Springer, Berlin Heidelberg New York, p 111
3. Zeitler E, Hüring HG, Schoop W, Schmidtke I (1971) Mechanische Behandlung von Beckenarterienstenosen mit der perkutanen Kathetertechnik. Verh Dtsch Ges Kreislaufforsch 37: 402

31. Factors Influencing Early and Late Follow-up Results After Percutaneous Transluminal Angioplasty of the Lower Limb Arteries

F. Mahler, A. Gallino, P. Probst, and B. Nachbur

Patients and Technique

Between 1977 and 1982 a total number of 305 percutaneous transluminal angioplasties (PTAs) of the lower limbs were performed in 254 patients using Grüntzig balloon catheters [1]. Of these 252 were carried out for stenoses or occlusions in the femoral or popliteal artery and 53 for isolated iliac artery stenoses. In 15 patients (9 femoral, 6 iliac) PTA was performed on both sides; in 36 patients (30 femoral, 6 iliac) it was carried out because of a reocclusion after an initially successful PTA. Follow-up examinations including clinical evaluation, Doppler ultrasonic pressure measurement, and segmental oscillography were performed prospectively 3, 6, 12, 24, 36, and 48 months after PTA. A criterion for the success of PTA was that it reduced arm-ankle pressure difference by half 1–2 days after PTA. Beginning 2 days before PTA, all patients received acetyl salicylic acid 1.0 g/day until peroral anticoagulation, started the day after PTA, was therapeutically effective, and no contraindications to anticoagulation (55 patients) were present.

Results

Initial Results

Of the 53 PTA performed on the iliac level only two attempts failed. The initial results for the femoropopliteal region are indicated in Table 1 with regard to different factors possibly influencing primary success or failure. Out of the 51

Table 1. Predictive factors for early results after PTA of femoropliteal arteries

Early result	n	Rest pain/ gangrene	Diabetes	Length of occlusion > 3 cm	≤ 1 patent calf artery
Failure (intra/postoperative)	51 (14)	61%	65%	60%	57%
Primary success	201	33%[a]	40%	13%[a]	36%[a]

[a] $p < 0.05$

Percutaneous Transluminal Angioplasty
(ed. by C. T. Dotter, A. Grüntzig, W. Schoop, E. Zeitler)

cases of primary failure, 14 were attempted in connection with vascular surgery (intra- or postoperatively). The remainder of the failures amount to 15% of the femoropopliteal PTAs performed. The presence of rest pain or gangrene, diabetes, occlusions longer than 3 cm, and poor runoff ($\leq$ 1 patent calf artery) was significantly more frequent among the primary failures.

Complications

In 20 cases (8%) the following complications were observed: 8 cases with dissection at the dilated site, 5 cases with peripheral emboli, 6 cases with hemorrhage at the puncture site in the groin, and 1 case with popliteal artery spasm. In 6 cases (2%) a surgical intervention for the repair of the complication was necessary.

Long-Term Results

Long-term results were calculated according to the life table method [1]. Two and four years after PTA of stenosed iliac arteries, 89% remained patent, while PTA of femoropopliteal arteries resulted in a patency rate of 71% and 69% respectively. When patency rate is related to all cases attempted (except for the 14 intra- or postoperative cases mentioned above) rather than to the primarily successful cases only, an overall treatment success rate 2 years after PTA of 85% in iliac and of 60% in femoropopliteal arteries is yielded. Inclusion of partial reocclusions in the occluded group (arm-ankle pressure difference increased but not up to the value prior to PTA) reduced the patency rate to 62%. The symptoms of the patients improved in accordance with the technical success of treatment: the percentage of patients with claudication was reduced from 61% to 22% and that with rest pain and/or gangrene from 39% to 8%; the remainder were asymptomatic after 2 years.

Prognostic Factors

Patency rates for different patient groups are given in Table 2. With the exception of the functional stage prior to PTA the same factors appear important

Table 2. Predictive factors for long-term patency rate after PTA of femoropopliteal arteries

Follow-up time (months) Number of patients (n)	7–12 (n = 100)	13–24 (n = 78)	37–48 (n = 10)
Patency rate (%)			
Total	72	71	69
Rest pain/gangrene	20	70	68
Occlusion > 3 cm	45	45	42
Diabetes	43	47[a]	44
$\leq$ 1 patent calf artery	37	37[a]	37

[a] Difference in patency rate from total statistically significant ($p < 0.05$)

for the late patency rate: 47% in patients with occlusions longer than 3 cm, 43% in diabetics, and 37% in patients with poor runoff were significantly lower values than the patency rate of 71% for the whole patient population ($p < 0.05$).

Discussion

The patency rates in our prospective follow-up study are of the same magnitude as the values given in previous reports working with similar methods [1, 3]. Without the patients with intra- or postoperative PTA, who are included in our primary failures, the primary failure rate of 15% also corresponds to the reported values [1, 2, 3]. Obviously the primary failure rate depends largely on the patient selection. The following conditions are significantly more frequent in primary failures: rest pain and/or gangrene, diabetes, extension of the arterial occlusion, and poor runoff.

Similarly, the 2-year patency rate is reduced in the above conditions except for rest pain and/or gangrene. Hypertension, smoking, and age did not seem to be influential in the population described. The functional stage was markedly improved in our patients 2 years after PTA, when 70% of the patients examined were asymptomatic.

Summary

Early and long-term patency rates were observed in 254 patients after percutaneous transluminal angioplasty (PTA). PTA of 250 femoropopliteal arteries resulted 199 times in early success. Overall patency rate after 2 years was 71%. In patients with occlusions longer than 3 cm, poor runoff, and diabetes the patency rate was significantly reduced. After 53 PTAs of iliac arteries an early success was observed in 50 cases. Patency rate after 2 years was 89%. Complications (hemorrhage, dissection, embolization) occurred in 8% of the interventions, necessitating surgical interventions in 2%.

References

1. Grüntzig A (1977) Die perkutane transluminale Rekanalisation chronischer Arterienverschlüsse mit einer neuen Dilatationstechnik. Witzstrock, Baden-Baden
2. Spence RK, Freiman DB, Gantenby R, Hobbs CL, Barker CF, Berkowitz HD, Roberts B, McClean G, Oleaga J, Ring EJ (1981) Long-term results of transluminal angioplasty of the iliac and femoral arteries. Arch Surg 116: 1377–1386
3. Zeitler E, Grüntzig A, Schoop W (eds) (1978) Percutaneous vascular recanalization. Springer, Berlin Heidelberg New York

32. Long-Term Results of Iliac and Femoropopliteal Angioplasty

Ronald F. Colapinto

Transluminal angioplasty of the peripheral arteries using the Grüntzig balloon catheter has been performed at the Toronto General Hospital since 1978. The method used is the same as that originally described by Grüntzig except that almost all stenoses, and some obstructions, are initially passed with a curved catheter rather than the guide wire. All patients receive acetylsalicylic acid 600 mg (lately reduced to 300 mg) and dipyridamole 50 mg three times a day beginning 3 days before the procedure and continuing for 2–3 weeks after. An intraarterial injection of 5,000 units heparin is given during the procedure but no long-term anticoagulant therapy is used. However, no heparin has been administered during the last 34 iliac dilatations in an attempt to reduce the incidence of hematoma formation at the puncture site. No increase in the incidence of early reocclusion has been noted in this group of patients. Heparin is still used during femoropopliteal angioplasty to prevent thrombus formation related to the stasis which often occurs during these procedures.

Complications

Hematomas at the puncture site were common. Three were large enough to prolong the patients' hospital stay. On other patient bled from the puncture site and required transfusion. Although distal emboli are not uncommon, most are clinically insignificant. In this series, only one surgical embolectomy was required. Two emboli were removed successfully by catheter during angioplasty. Two patients died in hospital within 1 week of the procedure but from unrelated causes. There were no instances of rupture of the dilated segment. Although several balloon ruptures occurred early in the series, there was never any difficulty in removing the catheter.

Results

Dilatation of 359 iliac and femoropopliteal segments was attempted between July 1978 and December 1981. There were 12 technical failures and 10 immediate failures, giving an immediate success rate of 94%; 337 dilatations

Percutaneous Transluminal Angioplasty
(ed. by C. T. Dotter, A. Grüntzig, W. Schoop, E. Zeitler)

were available for long-term follow-up (Table 1). The long-term results were assessed by:

1. Clinical status
2. Ankle-arm Doppler pressure ratio
3. Doppler flow studies
4. Angiography.

Repeat angiography was carried out only if symptoms recurred or during the performance of unrelated vascular investigations. Angioplasty was considered successful if improvement was demonstrable both clinically and by objective laboratory tests.

Cumulative success rates were determined by life table analysis (Figs. 1–5, Table 2). Angioplasty is now considered the procedure of choice for isolated iliac stenoses at our hospital, with a success rate after 43 months of 77%. In contrast, we found the success rate in combined stenosis of the common and external iliac arteries to be only 49%. This lower rate is likely to be a reflection of the higher incidence of distal disease that often accompanies diffuse disease of the iliac arteries.

Dilatation of complete iliac occlusions was found to have the surprisingly high success rate of 94% (Fig. 6). Only 1 of the 18 recanalized iliac occlusions has failed in a 34-month period. Although these results are gratifying, it must be cautioned that treatment of iliac occlusions is probably the most difficult of angioplastic procedures.

Table 1. Immediate results of iliac and femoropopliteal angioplasty 1978–81

	At-tempted	Technical failure	Early failure	Early success	
Solitary iliac stenosis	195	4	7	184	(94%)
Common and external iliac stenosis	31	1	3	27	(90%)
Iliac obstruction	21	3	0	18	(86%)
Femoropopliteal stenosis	78	2	0	76	(97%)
Femoropopliteal obstruction	34	2	0	32	(94%)
Total	359	12	10	337	(94%)

Table 2. Length of follow-up and cumulative success rate of 337 successful angioplasties calculated by life table analysis

	Average follow-up (mos)	Maximum follow-up (mos)	Cumulative success rate (%)
Solitary iliac stenosis	9.2	43	77
Common and external iliac stenosis	9.6	31	49
Iliac obstruction	15	34	94
Femoropopliteal stenosis	8.6	40	61
Femoropopliteal obstruction	6.5	23	31

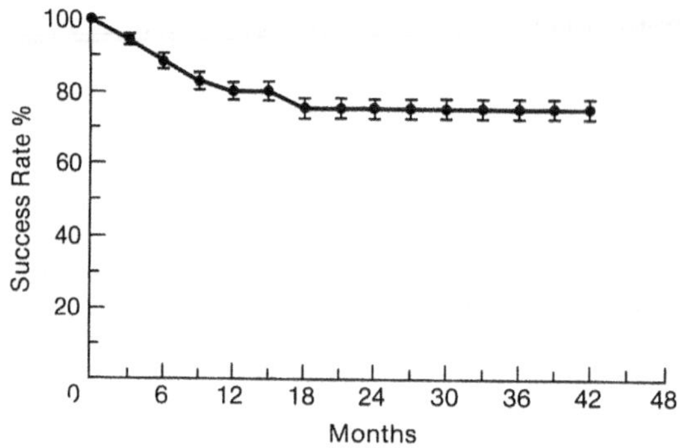

Fig. 1. Cumulative success rate calculated by life table method: solitary iliac stenoses ($n = 184$)

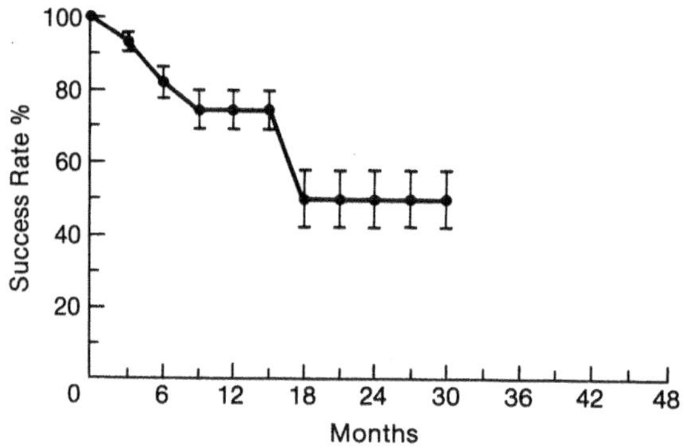

Fig. 2. Cumulative success rate calculated by life table method: common and external iliac stenoses ($n = 18$)

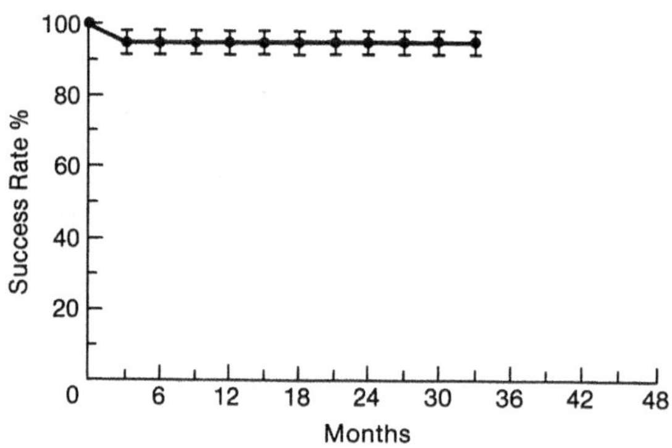

Fig. 3. Cumulative success rate calculated by life table method: iliac obstructions ($n = 18$)

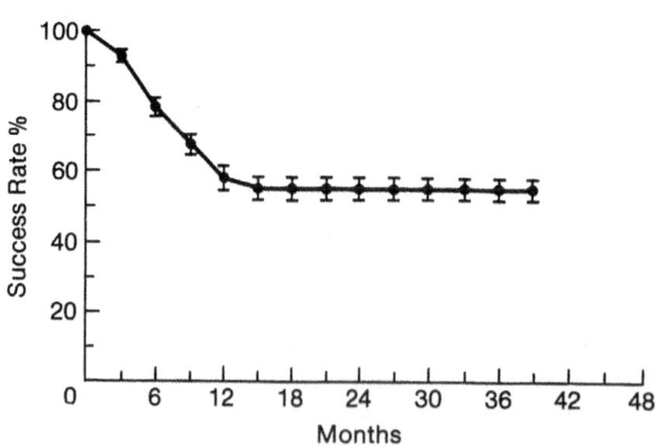

Fig. 4. Cumulative success rate calculated by life table method: femoropopliteal stenoses and obstructions ($n = 108$)

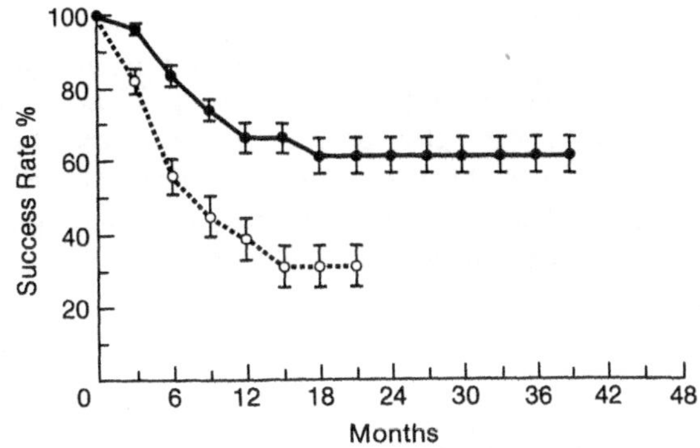

Fig. 5. Comparison of cumulative success rate for femoropopliteal stenoses (●) and femoropopliteal obstructions (○)

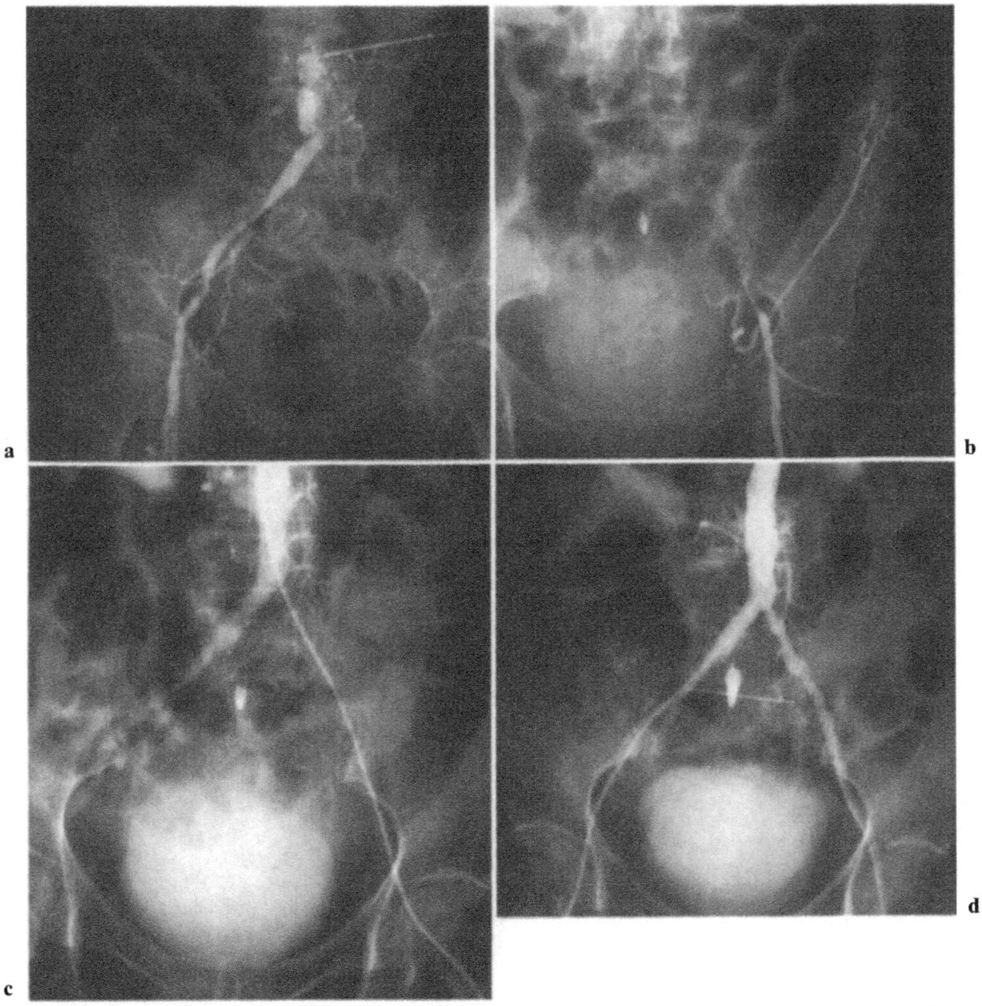

Fig. 6a–d. A 58-year-old woman with severe claudication and ankle-arm pressure ratio of 0.40. **a** Translumbar aortogram shows occlusion of the left common and external iliac arteries. **b** Left femoral arteriogram shows the obstruction to be 13 cm in length. **c** A Kifa catheter has been passed to the aorta through the occlusion. **d** Immediately following dilatation, a patent lumen is demonstrated. This patient is symptom-free with an ankle-arm pressure ratio of 0.95 18 months later

The success rate for femoropopliteal dilatations is lower than that for iliac disease. This is also probably related to the increased incidence of distal vascular disease that accompanies atheroma of the femoral and popliteal arteries. There seems to be little doubt that the results of surgical bypass are better. Nevertheless, both stenoses and obstructions are worth attempting if surgery is contraindicated. If restenosis does occur, dilatation can be repeated and the surgical option is still available.

33. Long-Term Results of Transluminal Angioplasty of the Femoral Arteries

H. D. Berkowitz, R. K. Spence, D. B. Freiman, C. F. Barker,
B. Roberts, G. McLean, and E. Ring

Percutaneous transluminal angioplasty (PTA) as a means of treating occlusive vascular disease of the lower extremities has become widespread. Within the last 3 years, reports of experience in centers across the United States and Europe have been published in both radiological and surgical literature [1–7]. Many of these reports have only dealt with short-term studies and small numbers of patients. Others fail to examine the variables that a vascular surgeon normally uses to evaluate surgical procedures. In this paper, we report the results of femoral artery PTA from the viewpoint of a vascular surgeon by examining those factors that are known to affect the outcome of surgical treatment of lower extremity occlusive arterial disease in order to provide a better way of comparing the results of angioplasty to those of surgery.

Materials and Methods

A total of 282 iliac and femoral artery lesions were dilated in 239 patients between January 1978 and January 1981. This has provided a significant experience at the Hospital of the University of Pennsylvania and the purpose of this report is to focus on the femoral artery lesions alone. The indications for PTA were based on clinical grounds and consisted of claudication of two blocks or 200 yards or less in 74 (67%), rest pain in 13, and the presence of an ischemic ulcer or gangrene in 23 patients. Patients with rest pain and gangrene are regarded as threatened with limb loss and make up the salvage group, which consisted of only 33% of our patients. All patients were evaluated in the noninvasive peripheral vascular laboratory with measurements of segmental Doppler pressures at thigh, calf, and ankle levels, along with pulse volume recordings. Arteriograms were performed on all patients and the lesions were categorized as to location and the length of stenosis or occlusion. After discussion between the vascular surgeon and the radiologist, patients with suitable lesions were subjected to PTA. All patients were given 5,000 units heparin through the arterial catheter after the stenotic lesion had been traversed. Long-term anticoagulation was not routinely used following dilatation. Most patients were placed on a regime of aspirin 600 mg orally twice a day and dipyridamole 50 mg three times a day.

Initial succes or failure was assessed angiographically by the appearance of the dilated vessel or the restoration or improvement of distal pulses in the

Percutaneous Transluminal Angioplasty
(ed. by C. T. Dotter, A. Grüntzig, W. Schoop, E. Zeitler)

angiographic suite. Initial failures were categorized as those lesions which could not be traversed by the dilating catheter or lesions whose angiographic appearance was unchanged following inflation of the balloon catheter. Noninvasive studies were repeated usually within 24–48 h and then at 3–6 month intervals. Initial pressure measurements were usually lower than the pressures that were ultimately obtained 3 months after the initial determination. In order to be considered a success on the basis of noninvasive studies, the segmental pressure index had to be increased by 0.15 at the calf or ankle level. In addition, the height of the plethysmographic pulse volume tracing was also used to assess patency and was sometimes improved even when the pressure indexes were unchanged. At follow-up visits, patients were assessed for degree of symptomatic relief and the status of the peripheral pulses was recorded. Follow-up angiographic examination of a dilated vessel was performed if a significant change had occurred in the symptoms, strength of distal pulses, or vascular laboratory parameters. Patients were not brought back for routine arteriographic follow-up, but examination of the dilated vessel was often possible in conjunction with evaluation of obstruction in vessels at proximal or distal sites.

Late failure was defined as return of symptoms, diminution or loss of pulse, or decrease in pressure index by 0.2 or more, and angiographic evidence of restenosis or occlusion. If a stenotic lesion was successfully redilated, it was considered as continuously patent and not a failure. However, if total occlusion occurred in a successfully dilated area, it was listed as a failure.

Results

Percutaneous transluminal angioplasty was attempted in 110 femoral arteries, consisting of 107 superficial femoral and 3 common femoral vessels. There were 14 initial failures and an initial success rate of 87.3%. Six of these failures occurred in arteries with lesions that were 5–10 cm long or longer, or in cases with diffuse disease and multiple stenotic areas. Eight failures occurred in patients who were being treated with a view to limb salvage: three of these underwent a prompt amputation and four had a femoropopliteal or femorotibial bypass graft. In only one patient did a longer segment occlusion ensue as a result of the failed angioplasty. In this patient, a femoral below-knee popliteal bypass graft was performed successfully and the only significant consequence was that the graft could have been placed above the knee prior to the failed dilatation procedure. Eight patients developed evidence of recurrent stenosis and returned for redilatation. In all, ten redilatations were done, six of these for new lesions that developed in the superficial femoral segment and four for restenosis of previous lesions. All were initially successful and only two eventually failed. There were four deaths in the group, none of which were directly attributable to the dilatation procedure. Most of them occurred within 6 months of treatment. Patency rates for femoral PTA are given in Table 1 and Fig. 1 in a life table format [8]. The results are tabulated with the initial failure rates included and

Table 1. Femoral artery patency: life table analysis

Interval (months)	At risk (*n*)	Failed (*n*)	Dead (*n*)	Not followed up entire interval	Interval failure rate (%)	Interval patency rate (%)	Accumulated patency rate (%) (immed. fail.)	Accumulated patency rate (%) (no immed. fail.)
0	110	14	0	0	12.7	87.3	87.3	
0– 6	96	14	3	3	15.1	84.9	74.6	85.5
6–12	76	11	1	14	16.2	83.8	63.8	73.1
12–18	50	3	0	10	6.7	93.3	60.0	68.7
18–24	37	1	0	17	3.5	96.5	58.4	66.8
24–30	19	1	0	9	6.9	93.1	55.3	63.4
30–36	9	0	0	5	0	100.0	55.3	63.4
36–42	4	0	0	3	0	100.0	55.3	63.4

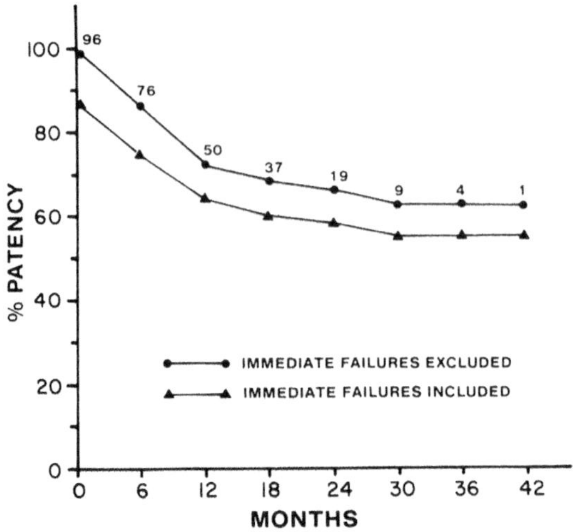

Fig. 1. Femoral artery patency after PTA with and without immediate failures

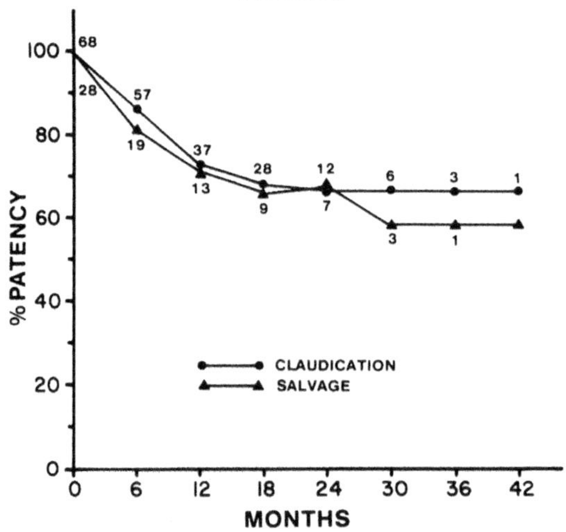

Fig. 2. Femoral artery patency after PTA: treatment for claudication vs. salvage

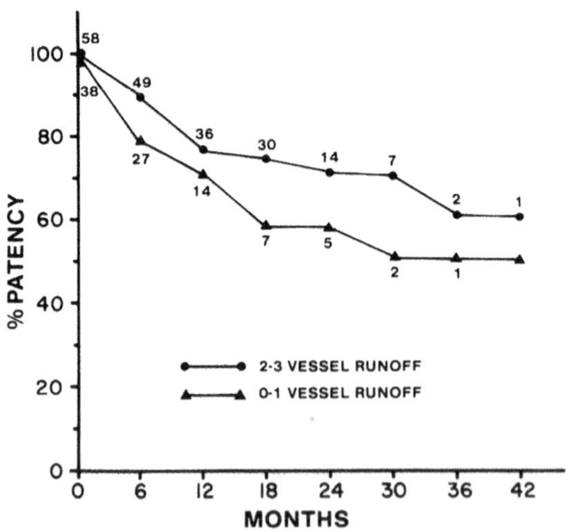

Fig. 3. Femoral artery patency after PTA: good vs. poor runoff

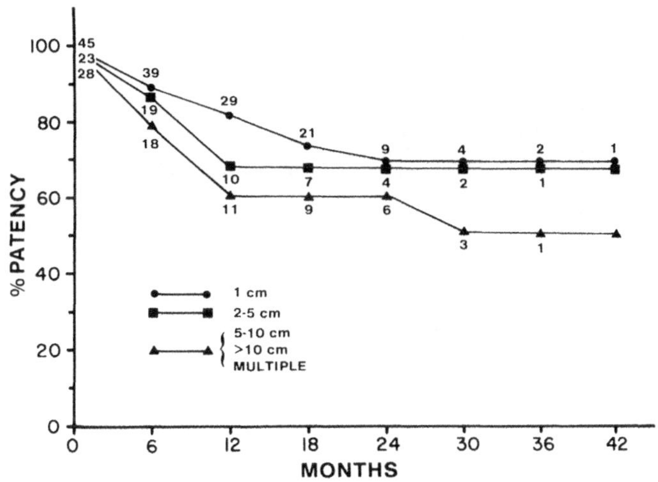

Fig. 4. Femoral artery patency after PTA: influence of length of stenosis

also with the initial failure rates excluded. While it is reasonable to exclude initial failures, since the dilatation was attempted but never accomplished, an appropriate comparison with surgical results must consider initial failures, and we have therefore expressed the results both ways. Redilatations are not included in this analysis, in keeping with our rule that a recurrent stenosis does not constitute a failure, and this is consistent with our policy of reporting surgical results. Patency rate at 1 year was 73.1% with the initial failures excluded and about 10% lower (63.8%) when they were included. At 2 years patency rates were 66.8% and 3 years they were 63.4%, with an approximately 8% lower patency when initial failures were included. Figure 2 shows the patency rates when patients were grouped in to claudication and limb salvage cases. The claudication group tended to show a higher patency at 36 months (67% compared to 58% in the limb salvage group), although this does not represent a significant difference because of the small numbers of patients available for follow-up. Patency rates are also listed according to the number of runoff vessels in continuity with the popliteal, and are expressed as a favorable group with two or three vessels patent and an unfavorable group with only one vessel or none patent (Fig. 3). At 1 year the favorable group showed a 77% patency rate compared to 67.3% in the unfavorable group. This difference was greater at 2 years, with a 72% patency rate in the favorable group and a 57.7% patency rate in the poor runoff group. Patency rates were also calculated on the basis of the length of the lesion dilated (Fig. 4). There was no significant difference seen between the short lesions that measured 1 cm or 2–5 cm, but the longer lesions (lesions of 5–10 cm and > 10 cm and multiple diseased segments) showed some tendency to a poor long-term patency rate at 3 years, 50.9% compared to 70.1% patency in the case of the 1-cm lesions. The majority of lesions dilated were 1 cm long, and this group comprised 43% of the total vessels dilated; the 2–5 cm lesions comprised 26%. Therefore, 69% of our patients had dilatations of short

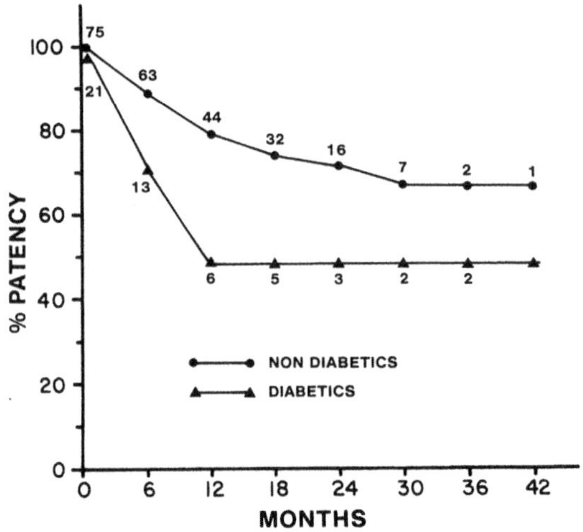

Fig. 5. Femoral artery patency after PTA: influence of diabetes

lesions, while only 31% had dilatations of lesions greater than 5 cm long. Diabetics have poorer long-term patency in reconstructive surgical procedures than nondiabetics, and diabetes also had an adverse effect on long-term patency rates in the present series. At 1 year, only 49.3% of the diabetic patients' vessels were patent, compared to 79.4% in nondiabetic patients (Fig. 5). At 2 and 3 years, the differential patency was approximately 18%.

Comments

Since the beginning of our experience with PTA in 1978, we have attempted to record not only the results of dilatation, but a wide variety of parameters that might influence outcome and allow us to compare the results of PTA with conventional bypass procedures. Two previously published series of long-term follow-up after femoropopliteal bypass performed at our institution [9, 10], as well as numerous reports in the literature, provided a basis for comparison [11]. The results at 1, 2, and 3 years are shown in Table 2, along with data obtained by Metha [11] in his review of saphenous vein bypass grafts performed for claudication and salvage and reported in the literature. The results of PTA for claudication are not as good as those obtained with femoropopliteal bypass grafting, but the results in terms of limb salvage were actually better than those figures reported previously by us and only slightly worse than the figures collected by Metha.

While an important consideration in the comparison of PTA and surgery is success or patency, and even more important point is the penalty for failure. Even though PTA has a lower long-term patency rate than surgery, a failed PTA has entirely different consequences from those of a failed surgical procedure. If morbidity and mortality continue to remain low with PTA, then the worst

Table 2. Femoral PTA vs. femoropopliteal bypass (FPB) – % patency

Years	PTA	FPB	
		Naji [9, 10]	Mehta [11]
Claudication			
1	73.1	86.3	86
2	66.6	81.9	81
3	66.6	79.5	77
Salvage			
1	73.5	66.6	75
2	67.8	57.5	70
3	58.1	54.1	68

consequences of a failed PTA are that the lesion remains unchanged, a stenosis is converted to an occlusion, or there is some distal progression of the lesion. The patient remains a viable surgical candidate and can still have the indicated surgical procedure performed without any significant new complications because of the failed PTA.

The morbidity of a failed bypass procedure has more significant complications. There is a significant period of hospitalization and convalescence, wounds may not heal, and there is a small but significant mortality which averages 4% in the reported literature [11]. Of major importance is that a precious nonrenewable resource, the saphenous vein, is destroyed.

The long-term patency with the short (1-cm and 2- to 5-cm) stenoses in the femoral system is so good that we usually recommend PTA before even considering surgery. The longer lesions (greater than 5 cm) and the multiple lesions have only a 50% 3-year patency compared to the 70% patency with the shorter lesions, and we only recommend PTA in these patients if they are poor operative risks.

There is no question that the length of hospital stay, recuperative period, and ultimately the cost to the patient are much less with PTA, since patients are often discharged within 2 days after successful dilatation. There therefore seems to be little reason to withhold PTA from a patient, even if the patient is an acceptable candidate for surgery. If the PTA is successful, the patient has avoided an operation. If the PTA fails, the patient is still an excellent candidate for surgery and nothing has been lost. If the PTA works for a short period of time and then develops a restenosis, the lesions can be dilated again or the surgeon still has the option of performing surgery. Although diabetic patients have a poorer prognosis following dilatations than nondiabetic patients, we still consider them to be acceptable candidates if they have short lesions or are extremely poor operative candidates. However, since 67% of our patients had symptoms of claudication and 69% of the lesions were 5 cm or less, and 87% of the patients were not diabetic, it appears that PTA has its greatest utility in the most favorable group of patients, who are also excellent surgical candidates.

Summary

One hundred and ten femoral artery lesions were treated using percutaneous transluminal angioplasty (PTA). Patency rates were 73.1%, 66.8%, and 63.4% at 1, 2, and 3 years and were adversely affected by the presence of diabetes, lesions longer than 5 cm, poor runoff, and threatened limb loss. The results of PTA compare favorably with those of bypass surgery.

References

1. Katzen BT, Chang J, Know WG (1979) Percutaneous transluminal angioplasty with the Grüntzig balloon catheter. Arch Surg 114: 1389–1399
2. Kalman PG, Colapinto RF, Harries-Jones EP (1980) Preliminary results of transluminal dilatation in the treatment of peripheral arterial occlusive disease. Surg Gynecol Obstet 150: 865–868
3. Van Andel G (1980) Transluminal iliac angioplasty: long-term results. Radiology 135: 607–611
4. Bachman DM, Casarella WJ, Sos T (1979) Percutaneous transluminal angioplasty via the contralateral femoral artery. Radiology 130: 617–621
5. Motarjeme A, Keifer JW, Zuska AJ (1980) Percutaneous transluminal angioplasty of the iliac arteries: 66 experiences. AJR 135: 937–944
6. Waltman AC (1980) Percutaneous transluminal angioplasty: iliac and deep femoral arteries. AJR 135: 921–925
7. Johnson KW, Colapinto RF, Harries-Jones EP (1980) Transluminal dilatation in the treatment of peripheral arterial occlusive disease. Can J Surg 23: 547–548
8. Cutler SJ, Ederer F (1958) Maximum utilization of the life table method in analyzing survival. J Chronic Diss 8: 699–712
9. Naji A, Chu J, McCombs PR et al. (1978) Results of 100 consecutive femoropopliteal vein grafts for limb salvage. Ann Surg 188: 162–165
10. Naji A, Barker CF, Berkowitz HD et al. (1978) Femoropopliteal vein grafts for claudication: analysis of 100 consecutive cases. Ann Surg 188: 79–82
11. Mehta S (1980) A statistical summary of the results of femoropopliteal bypass surgery. Gore Newark, pp 1–32

34. Late Results After Percutaneous Transluminal Angioplasty of Iliac and Femoropopliteal Obstructive Lesions – A Cooperative Study

H. Gailer, A. Grüntzig, and E. Zeitler

The comparability of long-term results after percutaneous transluminal angioplasty (PTA) depends upon standardized, quantitative methods of follow-up control. In this regard, simple unidirectional Doppler ultrasound examinations [1–3] provide a complement to manual checks of the pulse status and vascular auscultation. Additionally, intravenous digital subtraction angiography (DSA), because of its low complication rate and limited invasiveness, is finding increasing application as a method for following the results of PTA [4–6]. Conventional arteriographic studies can then be limited to those cases in which there is good reason to suspect recurrent obstruction and in which PTA may need to be repeated immediately.

The problematics of follow-up control in a large patient series, as well as the statistical evaluation, have already been addressed by Rieger et al. (see Chap. 30 in this volume). Series at different institutions should be compared with caution, since there may be differences in patient selection, PTA technique, adjunct medical therapy, and methods of follow-up (e.g., prospective, retrospective, cohort selection) and differing numbers of patients lost to follow-up. However, even if these differences are not taken into account, the late results of the various institutions represented in this symposium agree surprisingly well (Tables 1 and 2).

Table 1. Summary of long-term results after PTA for iliac artery stenoses[a]

n	Working group	Cure rate (3 years)
200	Zurich	79%
306	Aggertal Klinik	70%
63	New York	86%
145	Säckingen	64%
195	Toronto	72%
120	Chicago	72%
53	Bern	85%
1082		

[a] Cure rate (%) = $\frac{\text{primary success (\%)} \times \text{patency rate (\%)}}{100}$

Table 2. Summary of long-term results after PTA for femoropopliteal obliterations

n	Working group	Cure rate (3 years)
682	Zurich	60%
441	Freiburg	66%
108	Toronto	53%
250	Bern	60%
110	Philadelphia	58%
197	Säckingen	71%
316	Vienna	58%
2104		

Percutaneous Transluminal Angioplasty
(ed. by C. T. Dotter, A. Grüntzig, W. Schoop, E. Zeitler)

Table 3. Working group of the collective statistics

Berkowitz	Philadelphia (USA)	Roth, Schoop, Schmidtke, Rieger	Engelskirchen (FRG)
Colapinto	Toronto (Can)		
Schwarten	Indianapolis (USA)		
Le Goff	Limoges (F)	Schneider, Grüntzig, Bollinger	Zurich (CH)
Levade	Toulouse (F)		
Mahler	Bern (CH)		
Mathias	Freiburg (FRG)		
Motarjeme	Chicago (USA)	Sos	New York (USA)
Olbert	Vienna (A)		
Ostheim	Bad Säckingen (FRG)		

Table 4. Success rate following PTA for 2337 femoral artery obliterations

Primary success rate	87% (2031)				
Follow-up period	6 mos	1 year	2 years	3 years	5 years
Patency rate	84%	79%	74%	67%	64%
Cure rate	≈ 70%			≈ 60%	

Table 5. Success rate following PTA for 518 femoral artery occlusions

Primary success rate	86% (445)		
Follow-up period	6 mos	2 years	3 years
Patency rate	82%	72%	68%
Cure rate	≈ 71%		≈ 58%

Table 6. Success rate following PTA for 751 femoral artery stenoses

Primary success rate	96% (721)				
Follow-up period	6 mos	1 year	2 years	3 years	5 years
Patency rate	86%	82%	76%	75%	72%
Cure rate	≈ 83%			≈ 72%	

Table 7. Complications following PTA

	Puncture site	General (occur. within 10 days)	Requiring surg. interv.
Iliac artery stenoses ($n = 1915$)	33 (1.7%)	6 (0.3%)	15 (0.8%)
Femoropopliteal obliterations ($n = 1963$)	62 (3.2%)	49 (2.4%)	39 (2.0%)

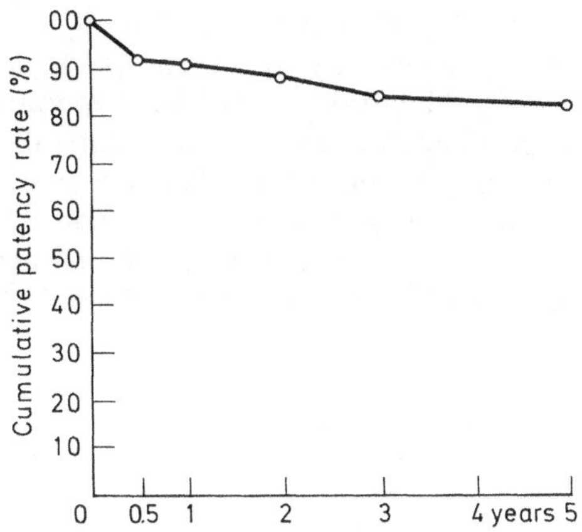

Fig. 1. Patency rate following PTA for 1725 iliac artery stenoses in 1,600 patients: primary success rate 93%

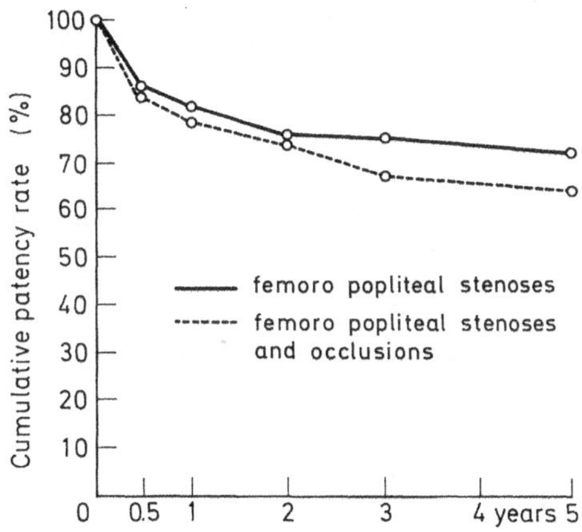

Fig. 2. Patency rate following PTA for 751 femoropopliteal stenoses (*solid line;* primary success rate 96%) and for 2,337 femoropopliteal stenoses and occlusions (*broken line;* primary success rate 87%)

Encouraged by the good agreement of the treatment results, we feel it is justified to combine and summarize the results of all those groups with long-term observations reaching 5 years (Table 3). Since some of the series did not differentiate between obstructive lesions and occlusions (e.g., short occlusions were sometimes combined with stenoses for purposes of evaluation), Tables 4–6 show success rates of PTA for obstructions, occlusions, and stenoses. Table 7 illustrates the complication rates associated with PTA. These were divided into:

1. Complications at the site of arterial puncture.
2. Systemic complications within 10 days after PTA. These included pulmonary emboli, myocardial infarct, congestive heart failure, and stroke with or without mortality.
3. Complications requiring surgical intervention.

The data regarding complications include the results of those groups that are not yet able to provide long-term results. The combined results show that PTA in a patient with an isolated iliac stenosis has a 93% chance of being primarily successful. Complications leading to surgical intervention occur only in 0.8%. The patency rate at 2 years is 88%, and at 3 years 84% (Fig. 1).

Of dilatations in the femoropopliteal region, 87% are primarily successful. Approximately 2% of these patients have to undergo surgery as a result of bleeding or occlusion. Patency rates for dilated femoropopliteal obstructive lesions are 84% at 6 months and 67% at 3 years (Fig. 2).

These are average values which vary from series to series as a function of the extent of the lesion being dilated, the severity of atherosclerotic occlusive disease (as classified by Fontaine), and the presence of further disease in distal vessels. The results are further influenced by the experience of the various groups, modifications in dilatation technique, and the use of anticoagulants and other medications. Thus the Zurich group, who treated 70% of their patients with warfarin show the best long-term results. There have so far been no randomized studies providing information about the value of warfarin versus platelet aggregation inhibitors in achieving good long-term results.

The influence of the various factors listed above can only be analyzed in future studies designed for that purpose.

References

1. Bollinger A (1979) Funktionelle Angiologie. Lehrbuch und Atlas. Thieme, Stuttgart
2. Kaufman SL, Barth KH, Kadir S et al. (1982) Hemodynamic measurements in the evaluation and follow-up transluminal angioplasty of the iliac and femoral arteries. Radiology 142: 329–336
3. Kriessmann A (1982) Diagnostik peripherer arterieller und venöser Stenosen und Verschlüsse mit Hilfe der Doppler-Sonographie. Internist (Berlin) 23: 393–395
4. Starck E, Harth P, Kollath J, Walter M, Riemann H (1982) Die digitale Subtraktionsangiographie – eine wertvolle Hilfe bei der Diagnose von Gefäßkrankheiten. Internist (Berlin) 23: 338–392
5. Seyferth W, Dilbat G, Marhoff P, Zeitler E (1982) Digitale Subtraktionsangiographie – diagnostische Bereicherung oder technische Spielerei? – Standortbestimmung und Ausblick. Herz/Gefäße 2: 742–757
6. Baert AL, Marchal G, Wilms G, et al. (1981) Computerangiographie – intravenöse Arteriographie. Electromedica 2: 122

35. Late Results After Percutaneous Transluminal Angioplasty for Iliac Artery Stenosis

W. Ostheim-Dzerowycz

Between June 1978 and December 1980 percutaneous transluminal angioplasty was performed for iliac artery stenosis in 145 (90.5% men, 9.5% women) patients. The treatment was successful in 133 cases. The mean age was 56 ± 10 years range (21–81). Sixty-four percent had a bad runoff with additional occlusions in the thigh and in the calf; 31.7% suffered from rest pain and necrosis.

The results of PTA in iliac artery stenosis are shown in Fig. 1. The patency rate after 1 year in the surviving 123 patients was 85.4%. The amputation rate was 1:117 (0.85%) after 6 months. The amputated leg was 1 out of 21 with necrosis, so that for stage IV the 6-month amputation rate was 4.7%. In 76.7%

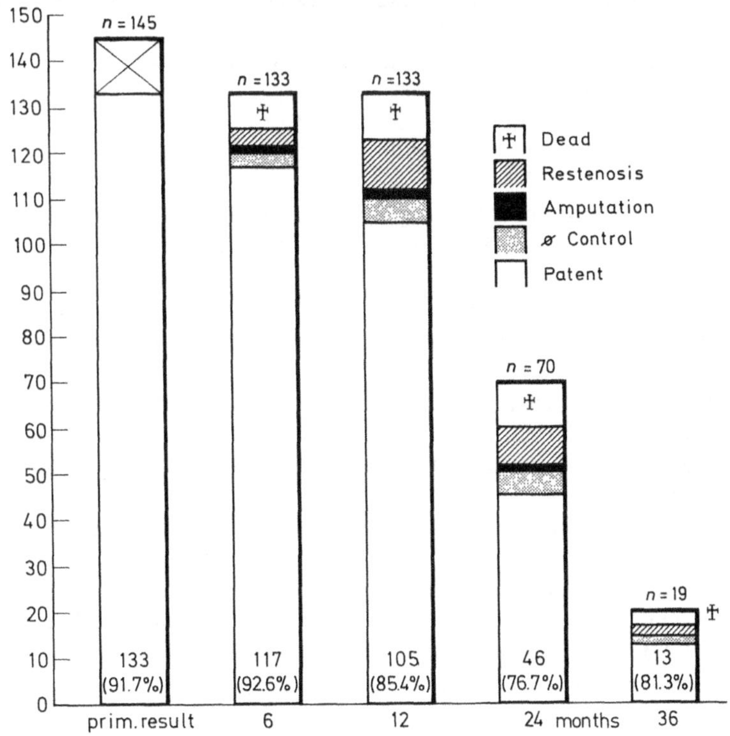

Fig. 1. Results of PTA for iliac artery stenosis

Percutaneous Transluminal Angioplasty
(ed. by C. T. Dotter, A. Grüntzig, W. Schoop, E. Zeitler)

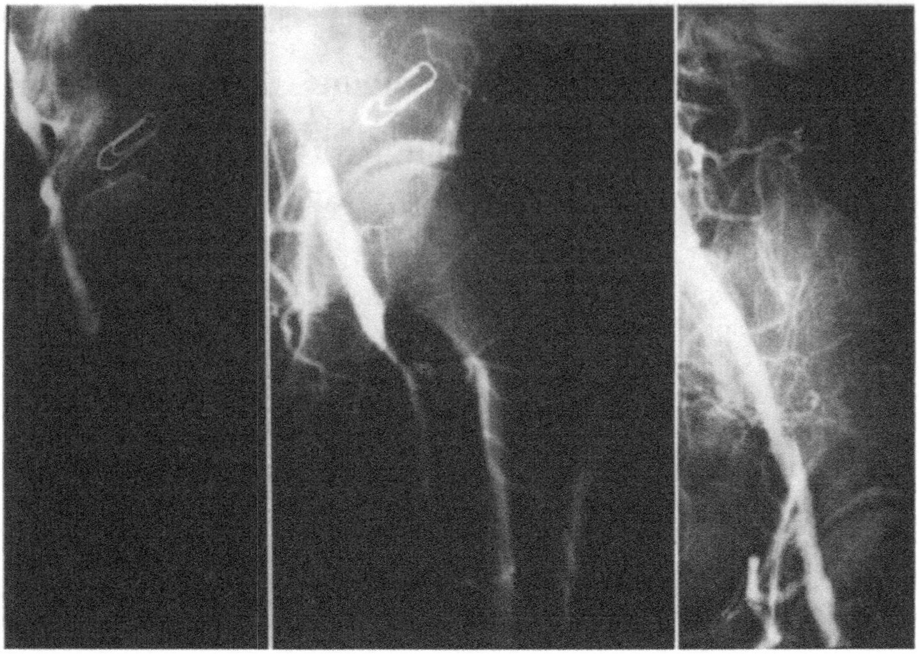

a b c

Fig. 2a–c. A 73-year-old man with a long femorocrural occlusion and additional pelvic stenosis, which was dilated from the contralateral side. **a** predilatation angiogram; **b** postdilatation angiogram; **c** 3-year follow-up angiogram

of the 60 patients surviving after 2 years, the treated arteries were patent. The 3-year result (81.3% patency in the 16 survivors) shows the positive trend but is not representative.

We gave special attention to the group of patients who suffered rest pain and necrosis and had additional occlusions in the femorocrural axis. Dilatation of the pelvic artery stenosis, followed by conservative therapy, treatment of risk factors, and care of necrosis, brought good results even without surgical reconstruction of distal occlusions, which was important especially in elder people. Of 41 patients who had rest pain and necrosis only 1 still had rest pain after 1 year.

Figure 2 shows the pre- and postdilatation angiograms and 3-year follow-up angiogram taken in a 73-year-old man with long femorocrural occlusion and additional pelvic stenosis, which was dilated from the contralateral side. Figure 3 shows the necrotic fifth toe before and 3 years after PTA. In high-risk patients, PTA ist the method of choice in proximal stenosis, not only for immediate but also for long-term amelioration.

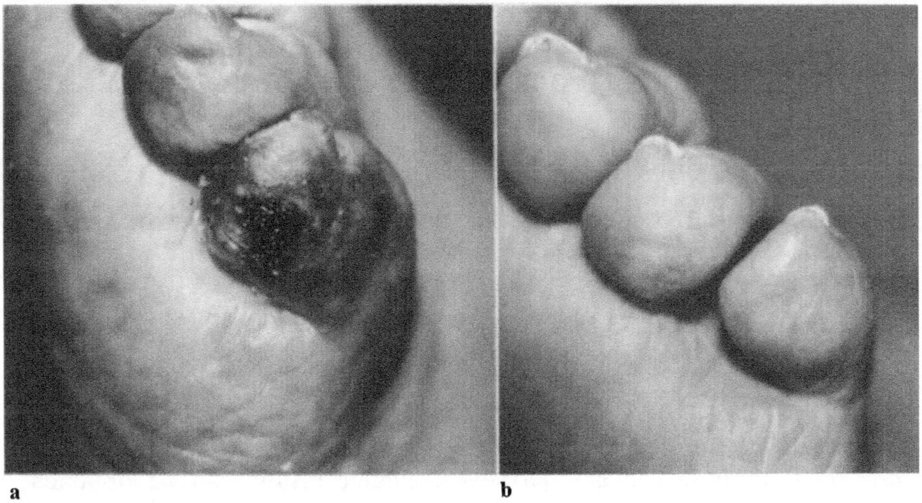

Fig. 3. **a** Necrotic fifth toe before dilatation and **b** the good results still to be seen 3 years after dilatation in the same patient as in Fig. 2

36. Percutaneous Transluminal Angioplasty for Limb Salvage – Progress in Therapy for Severe Leg Ischemia With Rest Pain and Gangrene

E. Schneider, A. Grüntzig, and A. Bollinger

For patients with ischemic rest pain (Fontaine stage III) and gangrene (Fontaine stage IV), revascularization therapy is urgently required to save the limb threatened with imminent amputation. Reconstructive surgery [2, 7, 10, 13] is best suited to limb salvage. However, similar results can be obtained by percutaneous transluminal angioplasty (PTA) in selected cases [5], provided the stenoses and occlusions are suited for this kind of therapy. The advantages of the procedure are low costs and a low complication rate that allows the use of PTA in high-risk patients who are not candidates for vascular surgery [3, 14, 15, 16] [see Chap. 54 in this volume and 12–14].

As far as we know, no studies on PTA for threatened limb based on a large, strictly selected patients series have been published. The following study reports the results for 173 patients in whom PTA was used as a new approach to limb salvage, out of a total of 980 patients treated between 1974 and 1981.

Patients and Method

The patients with severely ischemic limbs threatened with amputation were selected by means of strict clinical, apparative, and angiographic criteria to exclude not only acute ischemic syndromes, acral necroses originating from arterioarterial emboli, and diabetic microangiopathy with patent major arteries, but also patients with peripheral arterial occlusive disease in stage II complicated by nonhealing wounds after local traumata.

The criteria for selection were as follows:

1. Nocturnal acral rest pain depending on reclining position (Fontaine stage III) or acreal necroses (Fontaine stage IV) in patients with a long history of peripheral vascular disease
2. Missing or severely pathological pulse tracings from the big toe on measurement using electronic oscillograms, even after induction of hyperemia (nitroglycerin, warm water bath)
3. Systemic ankle (Doppler) pressures measured from the posterior tibial and dorsalis pedis artery below 60 mm Hg
4. Angiographically proved multilevel arterial occlusive disease with an obligate involvement of at least two calf arteries

In 7 years (1974–1981), 173 out of 980 patients (18%) fulfilled the required criteria. Table 1 shows ages, sexes, and incidence of diabetes mellitus. PTA was

Percutaneous Transluminal Angioplasty
(ed. by C. T. Dotter, A. Grüntzig, W. Schoop, E. Zeitler)

Table 1. Patients with rest pain or gangrene

	n	Age	Diabetes
Men	61	73	31
Woman	112	76	57
Total	173	75 (55–97)	88 (51%)

performed according to the technique described by Grüntzig [5] using double-lumen balloon catheters (Schneider Medintag, Zurich).

The criterion for successful treatment was the preservation of the threatened limb for 6 months after PTA. This interval is usually decisive. At a later date, the progression of the atherosclerotic disease in other, untreated segments plays an important role. For 146 (52 males, 94 females) of the 173 patients the follow-up period was 6 months or more.

All patients were examined immediately prior to and after PTA and 3 and 6 months later. Besides a careful evaluation of clinical and angiologic status, pulse volume recordings and digital pulse tracing (electronic oscillogram) and systolic ankle pressure measurements (Doppler) were made. Primary success was the patency of at least one hemodynamically important segment, resulting in a clinical improvement (relief of rest pain) and improvement in the arm-ankle pressure gradient by at least 20 mm Hg. However, pressure measurements could not be taken into account in a high percentage of patients because of diffuse and extensive calcification of the limb arteries.

Results

Table 2 summarizes the primary success rate in the 173 patients with threatened limbs treated. The multilevel atherosclerotic occlusive disease involved an average of 2.5 segments. In patients treated primarily successfully, a mean of 1.6 segments were dilated by PTA. In 112 patients of 146 followed up for 6 months, the transluminal recanalization was primarily successful (Table 3).

In 16 of the 34 patients in whom PTA failed, surgical revascularization was possible. However, in the remaining 18 patients below- or above-knee amputation had to be performed. In addition, 16 amputations were necessary, 15 (13%) despite primarily successful PTA and 1 after successful vascular surgery. Thirteen amputations were carried out above knee level and 21 below the knee. Seven deaths were probably directly related to amputation. In the remaining patients the acral necroses healed spontaneously or minor amputations had to be performed.

During the 6-month follow-up period 22 of the 146 patients (15%) died. Of those remaining, the limbs of 99 (80%) had been preserved and 25 (20%) had suffered amputation (Table 4).

The only severe complication due to PTA was a popliteal embolus which was treated successfully by the vascular surgeon. In three cases a hematoma at the

Table 2. Primary results of PTA in patients with rest pain or gangrene ($n = 173$)

Success	137 (79%)
Failure	36 (21%)
Lesion not passed	22
Early reocclusion	9
PTA of deep femoral art. without improvement	4
Popliteal embolization	1

Table 3. Revascularization, amputation and mortality 6 months after PTA for rest pain or gangrene

		Surgical revascul.		Amputated legs	Patient dead
Primary success	112	3		15 (13%)	17 (15%)
Failure	34	16		19 (68%)	5 (15%)
Total	146	19		34 (23%)	22 (15%)
			Thigh	13 (3[a])	
			Calf	21 (4[a])	

[a] Deaths after major amputations

Table 4. Results 6 months after PTA for rest pain or gangrene

		Saved legs	Amputations
Patients alive	124	99	25
Patients dead	22	13	9
Total	146	112	34

puncture site had to be removed under local anesthesia. The total complication rate was 3%, with a preponderance of inguinal spontaneously resorbed hematoma. There were no deaths directly related to the PTA.

Discussion

For the evaluation of the therapeutic effect of PTA in patients with severely ischemic limbs threatened with amputation, the efficiency of the procedure should be compared with established surgical revascularization methods. However, a direct comparison is only possible if both procedures can be performed in a comparable series of patients. In the present study a direct comparison cannot be made, as many patients were unsuitable for surgical revascularization because of severe debilitation due to generalized atherosclerosis, involving coronary and cerebral arteries. This is reflected in the mean age of the patients (75 years) and the high percentage of diabetics (51%). In two series of patients with threatened limbs treated with surgical revascularization [7, 10] the mean age was 70 and 62.6 years, and so markedly lower than in the present study. Also, the frequency of diabetes in those series was lower (30% and 41.6% respectively).

The primary success rate of 79% in the present study on patients suffering from rest pain and gangrenous feet is markedly lower than the primary success rate of 88% of a total of 682 consecutive angioplasties of the femoropopliteal segment [11]. The highest primary success rate (96.2%) was achieved in patients with a pain-free walking distance of more than 200 m (stage IIa), provided they had ideal morphological patterns for a PTA in the femoropopliteal segment [6]. However, a primary success rate of 79% is still relatively high, since there was a preponderance of inoperable patients. The lower success rate of the present series cannot be explained by a failure of the technique per se. It mainly results from the occlusive pattern (multilevel occlusion), the age, and the organizational stage of the thrombotic material. As there was a threat of amputation, maximum occlusion length of 10 cm for PTA was not adhered too strictly.

The low complication rate (3%) and the almost complete absence of fatalities [see Chap. 31 in this volume and 4, 8, 11, 15, 16] speak in favor of PTA. In case of PTA failure surgical revascularization can still be attempted, see Chap. 54 in this volume provided the patient is in an operable condition [1, 3]. This applies to 16 of 34 patients of the present series in whom transluminal recanalization failed.

As already stated, the criterion for success and efficiency of PTA in the present study was the preservation of the endangered limb for a 6-month period. It must be mentioned that all limbs where PTA was not successful and reconstructive surgery was not applicable had to be amputated in this follow-up period. This speaks in favor of the adequacy of the criterion and shows clearly that all selected patients really did have endangered limbs.

At the end of the follow-up period of 6 months, 124 of 146 patients were alive, 99 (80%) with good limb function and restored arterial circulation. These results are due only to PTA in 82 patients, in the other cases due to surgical revascularization or combined procedures. In patients treated exclusively with vascular surgery a femoropopliteal venous bypass graft preserved the threatened limbs primarily in 82.8% [10] and 97% [7] respectively. In cases where femorocrural reconstructions were necessary, the success rate was 67.9% [10]. The perioperative mortality after bypass implantation during the 1st month was 1.7% and 2.9% respectively.

On the basis of the results of the present study on 173 patients and of other series with smaller groups [5, 9, 14], it may be concluded that PTA represents an advancement among the types of therapy available for severe lower limb ischemia where legs are endangered. PTA should therefore be considered for all patients for whom amputation seems inevitable and for those for whom extensive vascular surgery represents a high risk.

Summary

Primary and 6-month results after PTA for the purpose of limb salvage are evaluated in 173 patients (61 men and 112 women, mean age 75 years, 51%

diabetics) with rest pain and/or gangrene. The patients were selected on the basis of clinical examination, noninvasive techniques, and angiographic pattern. The main parameter for successful therapy was the primary limb salvage and the preservation of the threatened extremities over 6 months. Of 173 patients, 146 were followed up for 6 months and more. PTA was primarily successful in 79% of the whole group (137/173) and in 77% (112/146) of those in whom follow-up was completed. In 16 of 34 primary failures surgical revascularization was possible; in the remaining 18 primary amputation could not be avoided. Six months later 17 successfully treated legs also had to be amputated. During the 6-months follow-up 22 patients died; 124 were still alive at the end, 99 with preserved and 25 with amputated limbs. PTA alone saved 82 legs, PTA combined with surgery 2 more, and surgery alone 15 after primary failure of PTA. Thus PTA is an efficient, less invasive therapeutic procedure, which should be considered whenever an amputation of in ischemic leg seems inevitable, especially in patients for whom extensive vascular surgery involves high risk.

References

1. Abbott WM (1980) Percutaneous transluminal angioplasty: surgeon's view. AJR 135:917
2. Bollinger A (1979) Funktionelle Angiologie. Thieme, Stuttgart
3. Brunner U, Schneider E, Gygax P (1982) Kombination der PTA mit chirurgischen Eingriffen im femoro poplitealen Bereich. VASA 11:278
4. Gallino A, Mahler F, Probst P, Nachbur B (1982) Früh- und Spätergebnisse bei 250 perkutanen transluminalen Dilatationen (PTA) an der unteren Extremität. VASA 11:319
5. Grüntzig A (1977) Die perkutane transluminale Rekanalisation chronischer Arterienverschlüsse mit einer neuen Dilatationstechnik. Witzstrock, Baden-Baden
6. Jäger K, Schneider E, Grüntzig A, Bollinger A (1982) Perkutane transluminale Angioplastie (PTA) im frühen Stadium II der peripheren arteriellen Verschlußkrankheit. VASA11:332
7. LoGerfo FW, Corson JD, Mannick JA (1977) Improved results with femoropopliteal vein grafts for limb salvage. Arch Surg 112:567
8. Neiman HL, Brandt TD, Greenberg M (1981) Percutaneous transluminal angioplasty: an angiographer's viewpoint. Arch Surg 116:821
9. O'Mara CS, Neiman HL, Flinn WR, Herman RJ, Yao JS, Bergan JJ (1981) Hemodynamic assessment of transluminal angioplasty for lower extremity ischemia. Surgery 89:106
10. Reichle FA, Raskin KP, Tyson RR, Finestone AJ, Shuman C (1979) Long-term results of 474 arterial reconstructions for severely ischemic limbs: a fourteen-year follow-up. Surgery 85:93
11. Schneider E, Grüntzig A, Bollinger A (1982) Langzeitergebnisse nach transluminaler Angioplastie iliakaler und femoro-poplitealer Obstruktionen. VASA 11:322
12. Veith FJ, Gupta SK, Samson RH, Scher LA, Fell SC, Weiss P, Janko G, Flores SW, Rifkin H, Bernstein G, Heimovici H, Gliedman ML, Sprayregen S (1981) Progress in limb salvage by reconstructive arterial surgery combined with a new or improved adjunctive procedures. Ann Surg 194:386
13. Vollmar J (1975) Rekonstruktive Chirurgie der Arterien. Thieme, Stuttgart
14. Zarins CK, McDonnell AE, Whitehouse WM jr (1980) Limb salvage by percutaneous transluminal recanalization of the occluded superficial femoral artery. Surgery 87:701
15. Zeitler E, Grüntzig A, Shoop W (1978) Percutaneous vascular recanalization. Springer, Berlin Heidelberg New York Tokyo
16. Zeitler E (1982) Komplikationen nach PTA femoraler und iliacaler Obstruktionen. VASA 11:270

IX. Percutaneous Transluminal Angioplasty of Coronary Arteries

37. Percutaneous Coronary Angioplasty – a Critical Review of its Clinical Application

A. R. Grüntzig, J. W. Hurst, and C. R. Hatcher

Atherosclerosis is a progressive disease which occurs focally and usually in a staggering course and cannot be cured. Progression of the disease may be favorably influenced by reducing the risk factors, and a sense of well-being may be enhanced with physical exercises. Often we are unable to control the symptoms and are, therefore, compelled to consider surgical treatment even though this treatment is known to be merely palliative. Besides the operative bypass techniques, percutaneous transluminal angioplasty of coronary arteries is now available with a reasonable primary success and patency rate [1].

Coronary dilatation is done with a guiding catheter and a double-lumen balloon catheter, which are introduced under local anesthesia at the groin with the aid of an introducer sheath and advanced into the right or left coronary artery. The balloon is filled with a contrast medium mixture and inflated in a stepwise fashion to 4–10 atm. The new Geon-PVC allows even higher pressures. By means of this overpressure, the atherosclerotic material is compressed and dislodged into the vessel wall, thereby partly disrupting and dissecting the intima and overstretching the media. The so-called "controlled injury" is repaired and the inner surface of the vessel wall is smoothed in the follow-up period. The factors influencing the repair of the vessel wall after dilatation are still not known. The induction of a foreign body reaction may contribute to this.

General Prerequisites for Percutaneous Transluminal Coronary Angioplasty

The results of previous invasive and noninvasive examination of the candidate for the procedure should be discussed with the cardiac surgeon. This is not only important for goodwill and cooperation within the hospital, but also in case complications arise. If the surgeon is informed about the case, any necessary operative treatment can be carried out immediately. After the method has been established and agreement on the indications has been reached within the group, discussion of individual cases may not be necessary.

The possible benefits and the risks of the procedure, and alternative treatments available, should be explained to the patient and informed consent obtained. The procedure should be performed at a time when surgical facilities are available. Physicians now beginning to use percutaneous transluminal

Percutaneous Transluminal Angioplasty
(ed. by C. T. Dotter, A. Grüntzig, W. Schoop, E. Zeitler)

coronary angioplasty (PTCA) should be trained in centers which have already gained experience with the technique.

There are no general contraindications to the application of the technique. A short history of angina pectoris seems to be important. If the onset of pain goes back for more than 1 or 2 years, the stenosis is very likely to be hardened or calcified, and passage of the coronary dilatation catheter may become difficult. The introduction of a smaller version of the dilatation catheter with an outer diameter of less than 1 mm has been of great help in some of these cases.

Indications for and Results of PTCA

The ideal candidate should have a proximal discrete stenosis, not more than 15 mm long, located in the left anterior descending (LAD), left circumflex, or right coronary artery. According to our results, and results of other groups, the passage of the LAD stenosis seems to be the easiest one. The right coronary artery and circumflex stenosis still represent technical difficulties. The introduction of the "steerable" catheters will be of great help.

The patient should have clinical symptoms that compromise his quality of life. Disabling angina pectoris necessitates consideration of blood flow augmentation procedure. These patients are, therefore, candidates for coronary bypass surgery. If the circumstances and anatomic conditions are appropriate, the dilatation should be done first. These rules apply because, should serious complications arise, surgery would have been indicated in any case. At the present time we do not feel justified in recommending the procedure in mild asymptomatic coronary stenosis.

Since September 1977 we have attempted PTCA 875 times in 789 patients. We were able to pass the lesion and achieved angiographic, hemodynamic, and clinical success in 743 (85%). In 5.5% of the cases, emergency aortocoronary bypass operations were required due to reclosure of the stenosis or unresolvable spasm. Myocardial infarction (Q wave) occurred in 2.5%. Other complications were pericardial tamponade (0.2%), ventricular fibrillation (1.4%), and false aneurysm at the puncture site (groin) (0.7%).

Long-term follow-up results from Switzerland are now available. Of the 134 primary successes, 34 had recurrences (25%). The 25 patients in whom the 34 recurrences of the Swiss series occurred were available for a second dilatation. Of these patients, 16 demonstrated continuing success during a mean follow-up period of 7 months (3–4 months), and 8 had recurrences necessitating aortocoronary bypass grafting. One patient had partial recurrences and is on medical therapy only.

As in all technically oriented therapies, a learning curve exits. We had a primary success rate of 65% with our first 50 cases [2]; the primary success rate in the last 104 consecutive cases (between February and March 1982) has risen to 92%. Three emergency operations and one myocardial infarction occurred. Of the vessels dilated, the LAD was the most successful one, with a 95% success rate, whereas in the right coronary artery this was only 85%. The lower success rate reflects the specific problems of this vessel, which are similar to the ones in the left circumflex artery:

1. These vessels are tortuous.
2. Usually the onset and duration of chest pain are underestimated, and it is therefore difficult to predict the hardness of the stenosis. In contrast, hemodynamically significant LAD stenosis reveals itself very early by chest pain.
3. Anatomic difficulties are the shepherd's crook form of the proximal vessel, right ventricular branches right in or immediately after the stenosis, a long left main stem with a sharp angulation of the circumflex, etc.

The general improvement in our results reflects not only improved skill and better case selection, but also the improvement of the catheter system. The improvements introduced since 1979 have been: (a) a flexible guiding catheter; (b) the use of G-and J-type dilatation catheters, instead of DG- and DJ-type; (c) step-by-step increase of balloon pressure, making it possible to avoid abrupt opening of stenosis; (d) and intracoronary injection of nitroglycerin through the dilatation catheter in front of the stenosis. The introduction of the "over the guide wire" dilatation catheter with torque control of the wire tip represents a major step forward. The primary success rate of 92% in the last 2 months is partially due to the availability of this system. By means of an additional tightly fitted Y-connector it enables distal ejection of contrast medium as well as pressure measurement.

In summary, it can be foreseen that with properly selected cases, PTCA will achieve the same primary and long-term success rates as bypass surgery in this subset of patients. The socioeconomic and psychological advantages of the procedure, as compared to heart surgery, are obvious. The classic candidate for the procedure is the patient with single-vessel disease. At the present level of experience and case selection, approximately 10% of the surgical candidates could undergo dilatation. If patients with double-vessel disease suffering from discrete proximal stenosis are included, the number is slightly higher. Future developments in technique as well as increased experience will broaden the spectrum of this promising treatment alternative.

References

1. Grüntzig A, Fischer M, Goebel N, Schlumpf M (1981) Percutaneous transluminal coronary angioplasty (PTCA). Ann Radiol 24: 377
2. Grüntzig A, Senning A, Siegenthaler W (1979) Non-operative dilatation of coronary artery stenosis: percutaenous transluminal coronary angioplasty (PTC). N Engl J Med 301: 61
3. Cowley M, Block P (1981) Percutaneous transluminal coronary angioplasty. Mod Concepts Cardiovasc Dis 50: 25

38. Transbrachial Coronary Dilatation: Technique, Indications, Results, and Complications

G. Kober, N. D. Scherer, S. Dowinsky, R. Hopf, and M. Kaltenbach

Since 1977, transluminal coronary angioplasty (TCA) has evolved into a technique which is currently performed throughout the world at a limited number of centers. Between October 1977 and May 1982, 284 TCA procedures were performed in Frankfurt*. With increasing experience as well as the cooperation of more angiographers from other hospitals, the number of procedures rose from 10 in 1978 to 114 in 1981. Figure 1 shows the rapidly increasing numbers of procedures being performed between 1977 and 1982. During 1981 alone, 61 patients from 25 different hospitals were accepted for TCA. Among those patients undergoing diagnostic catheterization for coronary heart disease at our institution, 5.9% were found to be suitable for TCA. This figure corresponds to 11% of all patients requiring coronary revascularization.

With the exception of one patient, TCA was invariably carried out during a second catheterization. Criteria required for the indication included angina pectoris, electrocardiographic or radionuclide evidence of myocardial ischemia, and the presence of a discrete stenosis requiring treatment in the context of single- or multivessel disease. Only in exceptional situations were two stenoses treated at one or two sessions. A surgical indication as well as fundamental operability had been established for each patient.

Of the 284 procedures, 7 (2%) were performed using a transfemoral approach; 277 (98%) were carried out transbrachially employing our own preformed, thin-walled 8-F Teflon guiding catheters (external diameter 2.7 mm, internal diameter 1.83 mm), which are introduced into the ascending aorta via a guide wire after the brachial artery has been cut. Three different catheters are currently available for probing the right and five for the left coronary artery. They differ primarily in terms of their varying tip lengths (Fig. 2).

After the guiding catheter has been firmly positioned in the ostium of the coronary artery, the Grüntzig angioplasty catheter is entroduced into the coronary vascular system while pressure is monitored and small amounts of contrast material are injected. From this point on the technique applied is almost the same as for the transfemoral approach.

Starting the day before angioplasty, the patient receives acetylsalicylic acid at a daily dose of 1.5 g. This treatment is maintained for at least 3 months. Following arteriotomy, 100 units heparin per kilogram body wt. is given

* The number of TCA-interventions has increased to 635 until September 1983

Percutaneous Transluminal Angioplasty
(ed. by C. T. Dotter, A. Grüntzig, W. Schoop, E. Zeitler)

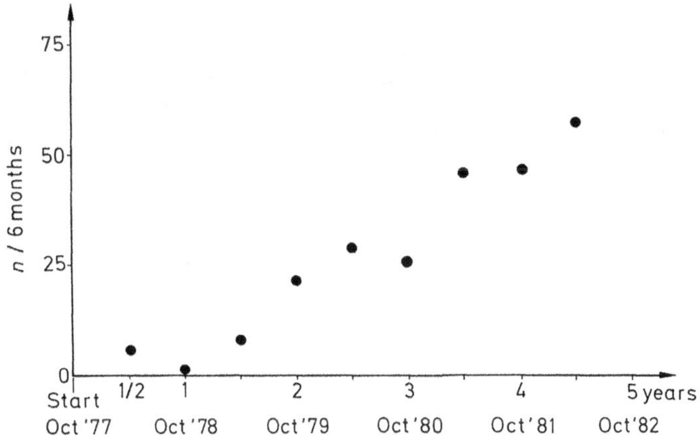

Fig. 1. Increase in the number of TCA procedures performed between October 1977 and May 1982

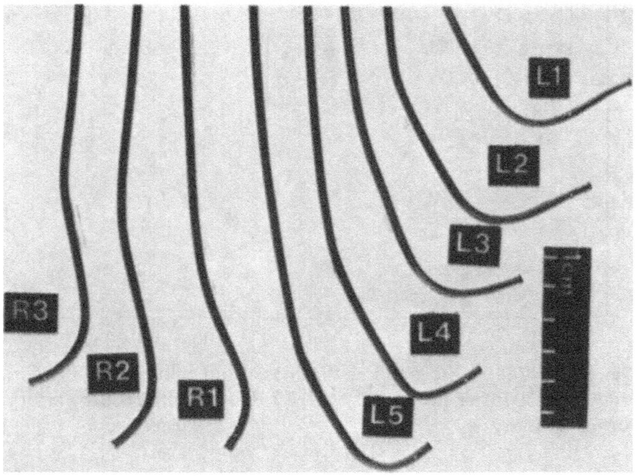

Fig. 2. Different preshaped guiding catheters for probing the left (L1–L5) and right (R1–R3) coronary artery

intraarterially, and half this dose injected after each subsequent 1-h period. At the end of the procedure, the arteriotomy is sutured. Anticoagulation is not reversed. To identify coronary spasm, prior to TCA angiograms before and after nitroglycerin (generally 0.5 mg intracoronarily) and nifedipine (10 mg sublingually) are recorded in all patients.

Results

Among the first 250 TCA-treated stenoses, left anterior descending branch (LAD) stenoses were attempted most often (69%), followed with a wide margin by those in the right coronary artery (20%). Circumflex, left main, and

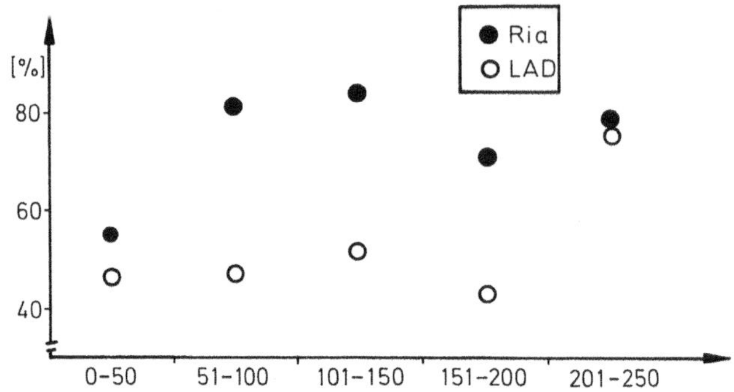

Fig. 3. TCA success rate per 50 consecutive procedures ($\Delta D \leqslant 20\%$) *RCA,* right coronary artery; LAD; left anterior descending coronary artery

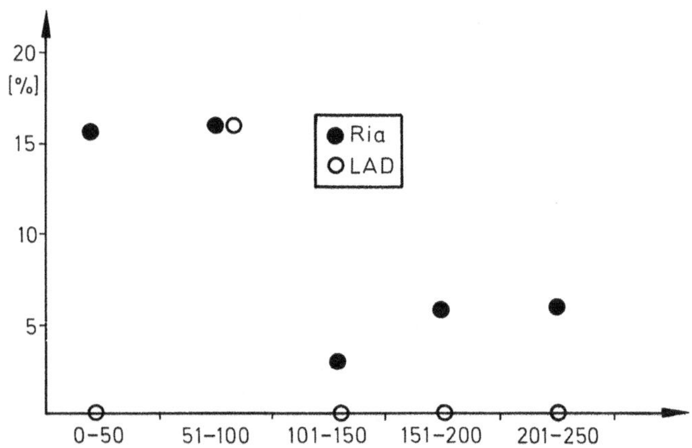

Fig. 4. Decline in the number of crossed but undilatable stenoses between the first 100 and the following 150 procedures ($\Delta D \leqslant 20\%$) *RCA,* right coronary artery; *LAD,* left anterior descending coronary artery

aortocoronary bypass graft stenoses represented rather uncommon indications (4% each). Seventy-five percent of the patients had single-vessel disease, 33% double- and triple-vessel disease.

The mean success rate per 50 consecutive procedures increased from an initial 52% to 74%. The success rate referred to treated stenoses is greater because of second attempts following initially unsuccessful TCA.

Until very recently, the success rate for LAD stenoses exceeded that for right coronary artery stenoses. This is primarily attributable to the course of the vessels, which permits LAD stenoses to be reached and crossed with greater ease (Fig. 3).

The progressive improvement in the success rate during the early part of our TCA experience was achieved by more accurate placement of the guiding catheter. Whereas the guiding catheter could not be positioned properly in 14% of the first 100 procedures, poor placement currently accounts for only 2% of TCA failures – a negligible figure.

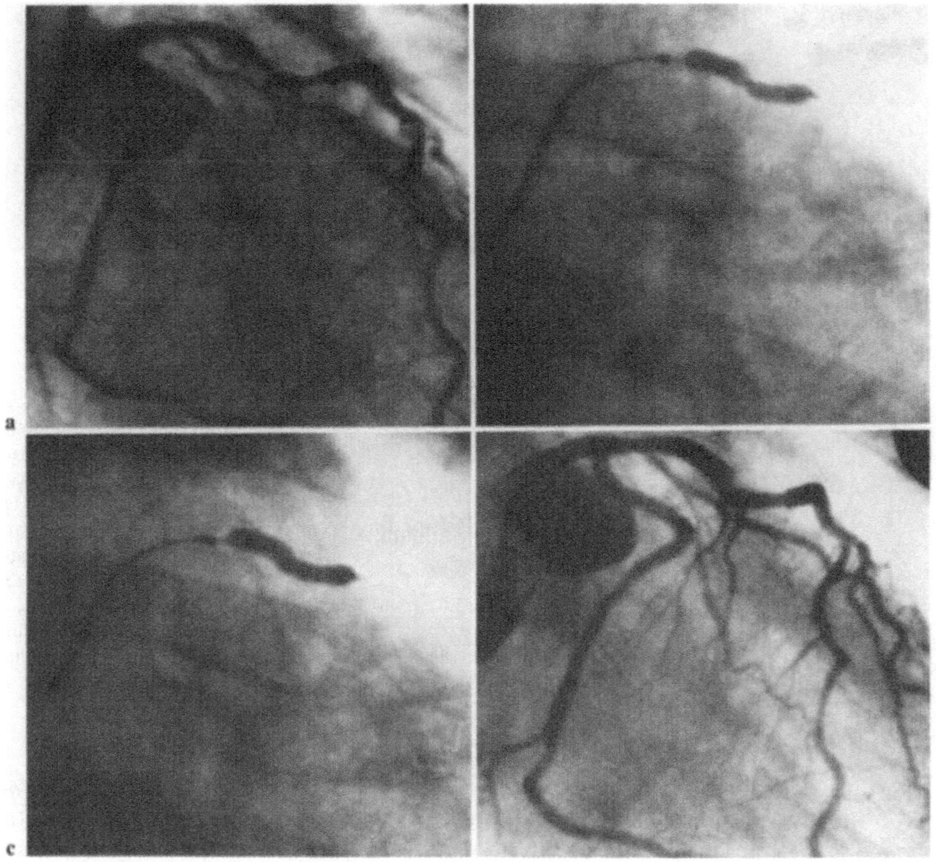

Fig. 5. a 80% LAD stenoses proximal to the first septal branch. **b** Compression of the balloon within the stenosis during the first dilatation. **c** Totally distented balloon during the fourth consecutive dilatation. **d** Angiogram immediately following TCA with successful reduction in stenoses

Failure to reach the stenosis after the guiding catheter had been positioned also declined considerably (from 10% to 4%). By contrast, the incidence of tight stenoses which could not be crossed remained relatively constant at 12%. Although several tight stenoses have been crossed and successfully dilated recently using the newly available 2-mm balloon catheter, these successes have not yet had an impact on the overall picture.

The percentage of stenoses crossed but unsuccesfully dilated, however, has declined considerably – from 17% in the first 100 procedures to 6% in the most recent 150 procedures (Fig. 4). This improvement may be attributed to more frequent (up to ten times) and longer (up to 90 s) balloon inflations. Not infrequently, gradually increasing inflation and reduction in external compression of the balloon is observed, which parallels a progressive increase in poststenotic pressure (Figs. 5 and 6).

If the success rate is evaluated in terms of case history, no clear differences can be found with regard to the nature of the symptoms, for example the

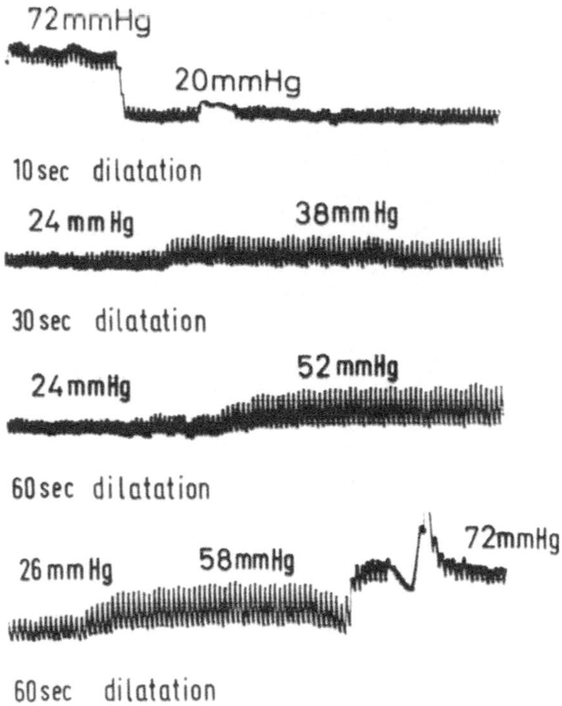

Fig. 6. Recording of intracoronary pressure during TCA in the same patient as in Fig. 5. Pressure drop from 72 to 20 mm Hg during passage of the stenoses (gradient 52 mm Hg) *(1st panel)*. No pressure change after 10 s dilatation. Gradually increasing poststenotic pressure to reach 58 mm Hg after the second (30 s, 2nd panel), third (60 s, 3rd panel), and fourth (60 s, 4th panel) dilatations. Remaining gradient 14 mm Hg

presence of stable or unstable angina pectoris. Sex- and age-related differences were also not apparent. There did seem to be a trend toward slightly better primary success in patients with a recent history of complaints but better long-term results when the patient had a long history of angina.

This observation suggests that stenoses in patients with a brief history of complaints tend to progress more rapidly. When the history has been longer, however, atheroma development may have already reached maturity. The failure of such stenoses to progress further could account for the disappointing primary results in some of these patients but on the other hand also for the low rate of recurrence.

There was no clear correlation between the angiographically proven morphology of the lesion (eccentric, concentric) and its ability to be dilated. With a success rate of 38% calcified stenoses were markedly less amenable to TCA than noncalcified ones, for which the success rate was 85%.

In 101 successfully treated patients, the mean rate of recurrence after 3 months at the time of the routine reangiogram was 13%. During the following 12 months, after which a second follow-up angiogram was made in 34 patients, no further recurrence was observed.

The complications can be broken down into serious and minor events. Emergency bypass surgery was performed in 12 cases or 4.8% of all procedures. Four cases involved vascular occlusion, six dissection with obstructed flow, and two severe unstable angina pectoris which had also been present before the procedure. There was never any evidence of thrombotic occlusion; in every instance the problem was due to vascular dissection with impaired blood flow. One female patient with double-vessel disease and evidence of previous inferior wall infarction due to occlusion of the right coronary artery died of intractable pump failure, despite successful emergency bypass surgery after a dissection had occluded the LAD during angioplasty.

Minor complications were encountered in 28 patients, often those with successfully treated significant stenoses. These involved depots of contrast material within the vessel wall which did not inhibit flow and were generally no longer visible in follow-up angiograms. In two patients, small hemodynamically insignificant myocardial infarctions occurred after branches originating in the region on the stenosis became occluded. All these cases were treated conservatively.

Conclusions and Summary

Between October 1977 and May 1982, 284 TCA procedures were performed using both the brachial (98%) and the femoral (2%) techniques. For the preferred brachial approach, special guiding catheters were developed which have been made available commercially. The mean rate of success for all procedures increased from 52% to 74%. This improved success rate is attributable to a reduction in the number of failed attempts due to difficulty in positioning the guiding catheter and reaching the prestenotic vessel segment. The percentage of stenoses which could not be crossed, however, did not decline. It became possible to dilate a greater percentage of crossed stenoses by using longer and more frequent balloon dilatation. Prediction of success or failure on the basis of history or angiographic findings was not possible.

Severe complications requiring emergency bypass surgery occurred in 12 of 250 procedures (4.8%). Of these, one patient died due to irreversible pump failure despite successful aortocoronary bypass surgery. Restenosis was observed in 13 out of 101 patients who underwent follow-up angiography after a period of 3 months. No further recurrence was seen subsequently.

As with the transfemoral approach, firm placement of the guiding catheter at the coronary ostium can also be achieved in almost every case using the transbrachial approach. An advantage of the transbrachial technique is precise control of hemostasis under direct vision, which enables TCA to be carried out using effective anticoagulation and eliminates the need to reverse heparinization following completion of the procedure. The absence of thrombotic complications is attributable to use of this approach.

39. Transbrachial Transluminal Dilatation of Abdominal and Peripheral Arteries

K. Bachmann and G. Raab

Everything has two sides and, in the case of angiography, two approaches. This is also the case with the Dotter technique [3]. The intravascular routing via the femoral artery primarily used by Dotter for intraluminal dilatation has been generally accepted and followed not only for dilatation of peripheral and abdominal arteries but also for coronary angioplasty [5]. In 1974 Grüntzig introduced a new dilatation catheter, and in 1977 he made the first attempt at dilatation of coronary artery stenosis in man, an attempt that met with success [5, 6].

The transfemoral routing has always been the preferred approach in both diagnostic and therapeutic procedures, especially in angiology [3, 4, 6–8, 10]. In 1972 we started to extend coronary angiography to "total angiography", using the Sones method [1]. This procedure includes left ventricular angiography, coronary angiography, and opacification of peripheral, abdominal and supraaortic arteries, and in patients with arterial hypertension it also includes selective renal angiography (Fig. 1). Thus more information is gained by this method than by selective coronary angiography, with no increase in risks and complications. The task of this diagnostic procedure was primarily to exclude severe peripheral arterial occlusive disease in patients who were considered to be candidates for coronary bypass surgery. Up to now the method has been applied to more than 4,000 subjects without a single serious complication [2]. Of course, there is an increase in fluoroscopic time from 2.8 to 8.6 min, in radiation from 6,200 to 15,300 R cm^2, and in the total amount of contrast material injected from 0.3 to 3.2 ml/kg body wt. (mean values from 100 consecutive examinations).

It turned out from these diagnostic investigations that the Sones catheter could easily be advanced from the brachial artery as far as the popliteal artery. This led us to attempt intraluminal dilatation of abdominal and peripheral arteries with Grüntzig catheters 140–160 cm long, using the same transbrachial approach. At present we use a 9-F 40/80 catheter 140 cm in length for dilatation of iliac arteries and a 7-F 40/60 catheter 160 cm in length for the femoral or popliteal artery.

After completion of the diagnostic procedure with identification and location of the peripheral or abdominal vascular lesion, a guide wire 250 cm or 300 cm in length is introduced into the Sones catheter and the tip advanced distal to the arterial stenosis. Then, with the guide wire in place, the Sones catheter is withdrawn and replaced by the Grüntzig catheter. We start by filling the balloon

Percutaneous Transluminal Angioplasty
(ed. by C. T. Dotter, A. Grüntzig, W. Schoop, E. Zeitler)

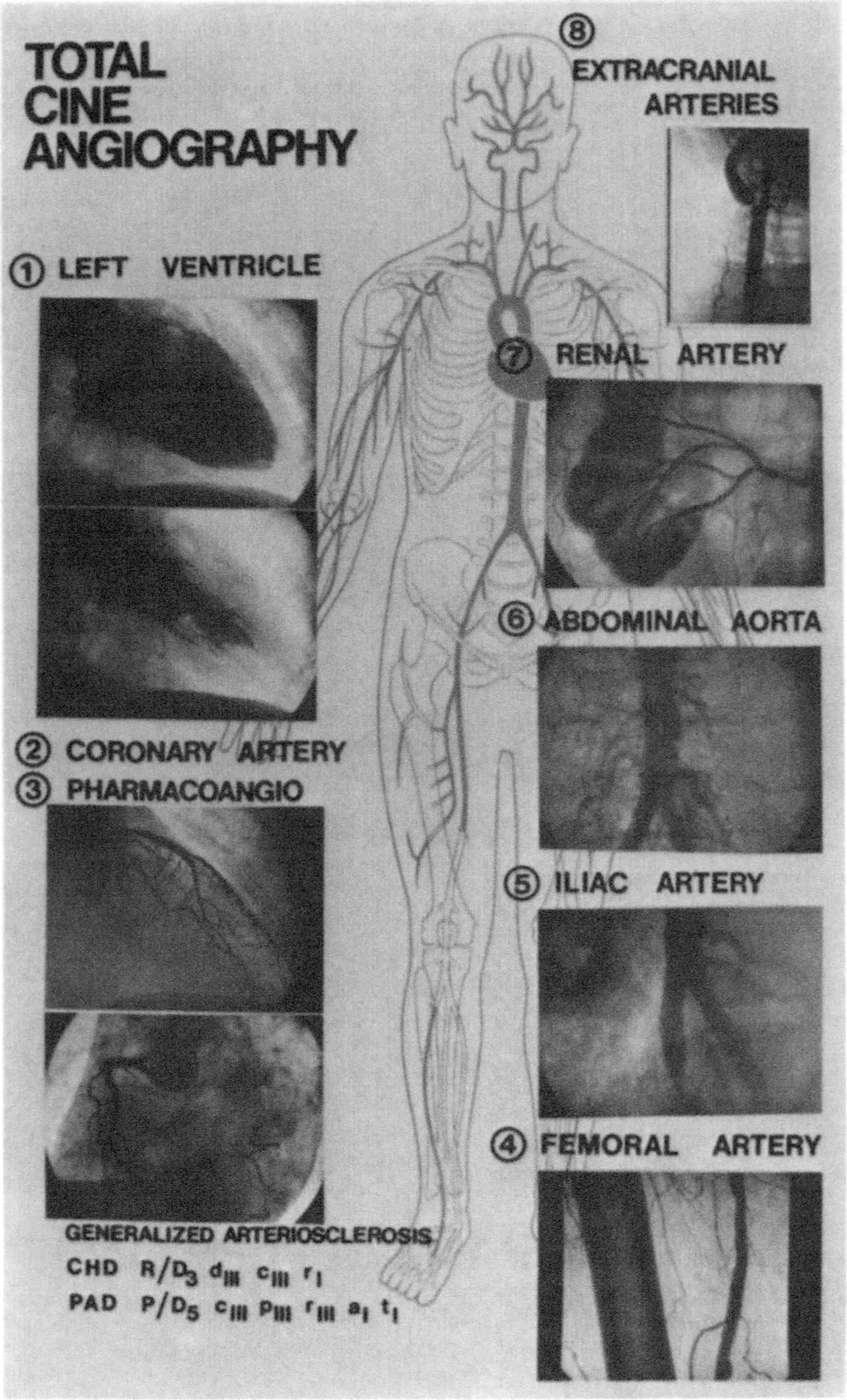

Fig. 1. Total cineangiography in a 59-year-old patient suffering from arterial hypertension and generalized arteriosclerosis with severe segmental obstruction of the LAD and circumflex arteries and severe segmental luminal narrowing of the right internal carotid artery, right renal artery, and right common iliac artery

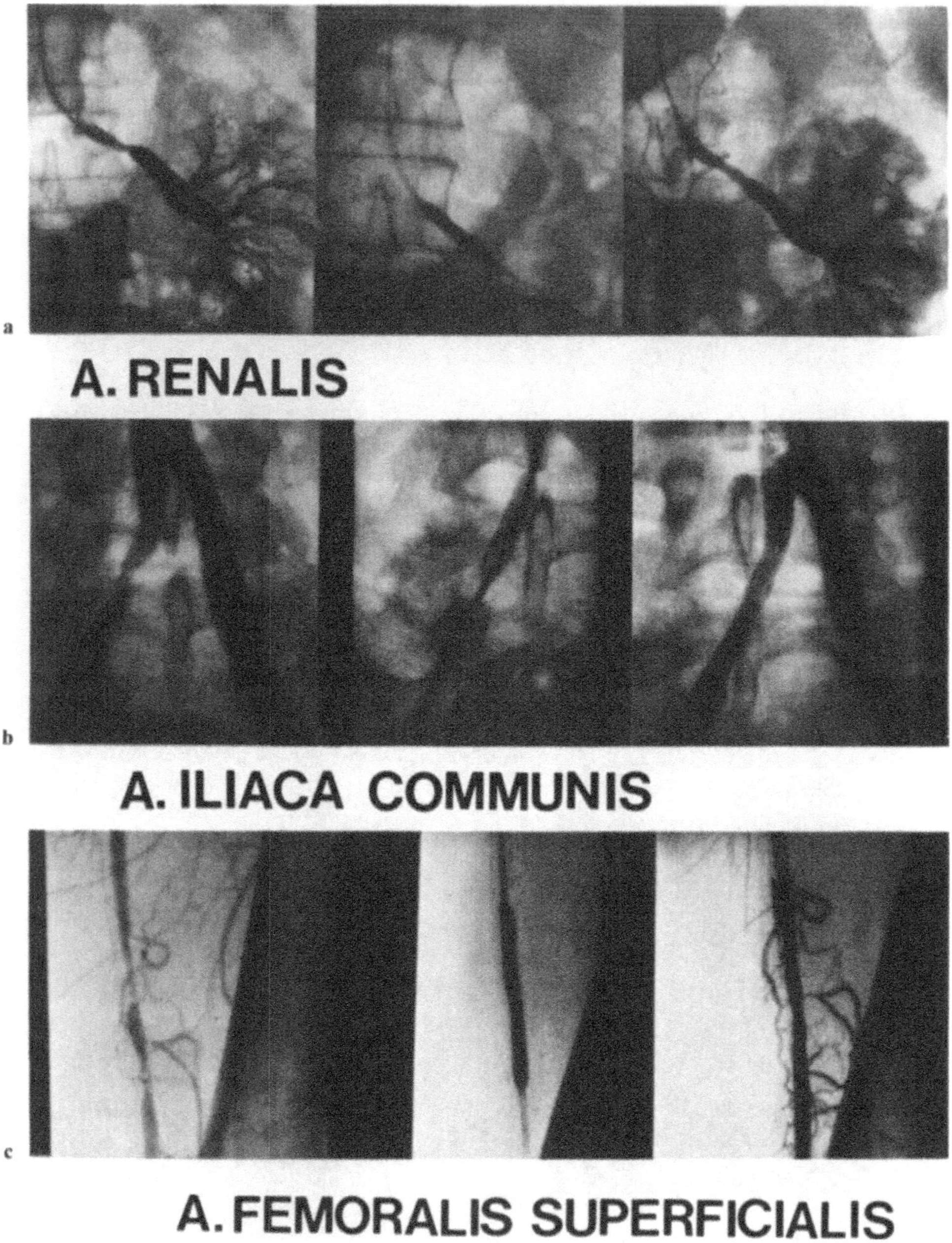

Fig. 2a–c. Examples of transbrachial transluminal dilatation in cases of severe segmental stenosis of **a** the left renal artery, **b** the right common iliac artery, and **c** the left superficial femoral artery

manually and then we proceed with dilatation under fluoroscopic control by adding stepwise 1 ml of contrast material with the same automatic injector that we use for angiography (Contrac).

The method was first used in December 1978 in a 40-year-old patient with severe stenosis of the left common iliac artery. Up to now we have performed transbrachial transluminal dilatation (BTD) immediately following total angiography in 25 patients with 26 stenotic lesions. The overall primary success rate was 84.6%: eight out of nine stenoses in the femoral artery, seven out of ten in the iliac artery, two in the subclavian artery, and all five renal artery stenoses were successfully dilated (Fig. 2). We experienced one complication due to dissection of a tortuous right renal artery in which we achieved primary dilatation with a 7-F 40/60 dilatation catheter.

Transbrachial transluminal dilatation is far from being a substitute for PTD, but in our limited experience it has some advantages over the percutaneous transfemoral technique [9] in some special situations:

1. In coronary patients with suspected or previously diagnosed peripheral arterial occlusive disease, coronary angiography and opacification of peripheral arteries can be performed using the same catheter.
2. After identification of a high-grade peripheral arterial lesion, arterial dilatation can be performed immediately by the same transbrachial approach. This technique avoids puncture of the femoral artery and thereby most of the local complications encountered with the percutaneous transfemoral approach.
3. Neither coumarin therapy, nor heparin therapy initiated immediately before the procedure, need be discontinued. Anticoagulation may be continued throughout BTD and afterward.

In our series the results of the disadvantages were:

1. Recanalization was not attempted because of the long distance between the site of catheter insertion and site of the occlusion.
2. There was one complication: dissection in a very tortuous renal artery. This may just as easily occur when the transfemoral route is employed. In this patient we used a 7-F 40/60 femoral-type dilatation catheter for the renal artery.

In summing up one should critically state that transbrachial dilatation (BTD) has limited indications. It is an alternative in patients who need combined angiography of coronary and peripheral arteries and who, during arteriography, demonstrate severe segmental stenosis in peripheral, abdominal, or subclavian arteries.

Furthermore, BTD may be an alternative in peripheral arterial disease in patients with anatomic difficulties, such as stenotic lesions of both femoral arteries close to the puncture site; in patients in whom retrograde catheterization of the iliac arteries is not possible; and, for example, in patients whose lower legs have been amputated. BTD is a safe, reliable, highly successful, and in combination with total angiography a nontraumatic method. BTD serves to widen the application potentials of the Dotter technique.

References

1. Bachmann K (1976) Total cineangiography. In: Lichtlen PR (ed) Coronary Angiography and angina pectoris. Symp. Europ. Soc. Cardiol., Hannover 1975. Thieme, Stuttgart
2. Bachmann K, Raab G, Niederer W (to be published) Coronary angiography in combination with opacification of the peripheral vessels and transbrachial transluminal dilatation of peripheral stenoses. Symp Eur Soc Cardiol, Titisee, 1982
3. Dotter CT, Judkins MP (1964) Transluminal treatment of arteriosclerotic obstruction. Description of a technique and a preliminary report of its application. Circulation 30: 654
4. Dotter CT, Rösch J, Judkins MP (1968) Transluminal dilatation of atherosclerotic stenosis. Surg Gynecol Obstet 121: 194
5. Grüntzig A (1978) Transluminal dilatation of coronary artery stenosis. Lancet I: 263
6. Grüntzig A (1978) Percutaneous transluminal recanalisation (PTR) with the double lumen dilatation catheter. In: Zeitler E, Grüntzig A, Schoop W (eds) Percutaneous vascular recanalisation. Springer, Berlin Heidelberg New York
7. Grüntzig A, Hopff H (1974) Perkutane Rekanalisation chronischer arterieller Verschlüsse mit einem neuen Dilatationskatheter. Modifikation der Dotter-Technik. Dtsch Med Wochenschr 99: 2502
8. Porstmann W (1973) Ein neuer Korsett-Ballonkatheter zur transluminalen Rekanalisation nach Dotter unter Berücksichtigung von Obliterationen an den Beckenarterien. Radiol Diagn (Berl) 14: 239
9. Zeitler E (1978) Complications in and after PTR. In: Zeitler E, Grüntzig A, Schoop W (eds) Percutaneous vascular recanalisation. Springer, Berlin Heidelberg New York
10. Zeitler E, Schoop W, Zahnow W (1971) The treatment of occlusive arterial disease by transluminal catheter angioplasty. Radiology 99: 19

X. Percutaneous Transluminal Angioplasty for Supraaortic Stenoses

40. Percutaneous Transluminal Angioplasty of the Vertebral Arteries

A. Motarjeme, J. W. Keifer, A. J. Zuska, and P. Nabavi

Introduction

Since the introduction of the balloon dilatation catheter by Grüntzig and Hopff [1] in 1974, transluminal angioplasty, originally described by Dotter and Judkins [2], has been widely used to treat atherosclerotic occlusive disease of the coronary, renal, iliac, and femoral arteries [3–9]. However, due to fear of cerebral emboli, transluminal angioplasty of vertebral arteries has only rarely been performed. We have reported successful dilatation of four vertebral arteries [10], and here we describe our experience in dilatation of 16 vertebral arteries during a 3-year period.

Subjects and Methods

Dilatation of 16 vertebral arteries was attempted in 14 patients (both vertebral arteries in two patients) complaining of the typical symptoms of vertebral basilar insufficiency: dizziness, blurred vision, ataxia, and drop attack. A complete angiographic assessment of the cerebral circulation, including both carotid arteries and vertebral basilar system, was made in all patients. Five patients had isolated vertebral artery disease, while the others had had carotid artery stenosis treated by arterectomy without relief of symptoms. Both vertebral arteries were successfully dilated in one patient. Transluminal angioplasty was performed only when stenoses were at the origin of the vertebral artery and only when there was no additional occlusion of the vertebral basilar system. Patients with both vertebral and carotid artery stenosis were first treated with carotid endarterectomy, and vertebral artery dilatation was only considered if the symptoms were not relieved. Furthermore, transluminal dilatation was performed when reconstructive vascular surgery was warranted and, in some, already planned.

After selective catheterization of the vertebral artery, via the femoral artery, an exchange guide wire, usually straight, was advanced well beyond the point of stenosis. With the guide wire in place, the angiographic catheter was exchanged for a 7-F Grüntzig balloon catheter, having a balloon 1 cm long and 4 mm in diameter. The balloon was inflated by hand using dilute contrast medium for about 5 s, and this was repeated two or three times. The balloon catheter was

Percutaneous Transluminal Angioplasty
(ed. by C. T. Dotter, A. Grüntzig, W. Schoop, E. Zeitler)

then withdrawn back to the subclavian artery and a postangioplasty subclavian arteriogram was routinely obtained. No intraarterial pressures were measured, since the catheter occludes the lumen of the vertebral artery. Dilatation was considered successful when the postangioplasty arteriogram showed a normal-appearing artery or considerably increased lumen of the artery (at least 50%) and when the vertebral basilar insufficiency symptoms were relieved.

Results

Thirteen vertebral arteries, nine on the left and four on the right, were successfully dilated in 16 attempts. The procedure failed in three arteries due to tortuosity of the vertebral artery in two and of the the right subclavian artery in one. Both vertebral arteries were successfully dilated in one patient. Carotid endarterectomy was ineffective in relieving symptoms in four patients with both vertebral and carotid stenoses, but the symptoms were relieved by dilatation of the vertebral artery. Arteriotomy and venous patch of the left vertebral artery in a patient with bilateral vertebral artery stenosis diminished his dizziness, but it was only entirely relieved after successful dilatation of the right vertebral artery.

Case Presentation

A 72-year-old man had dizziness. A four-vessel cerebral arteriogram revealed no carotid artery disease, but there was severe stenosis of the origin of both vertebral arteries (Fig. 1a). Percutaneous transluminal angioplasty of both

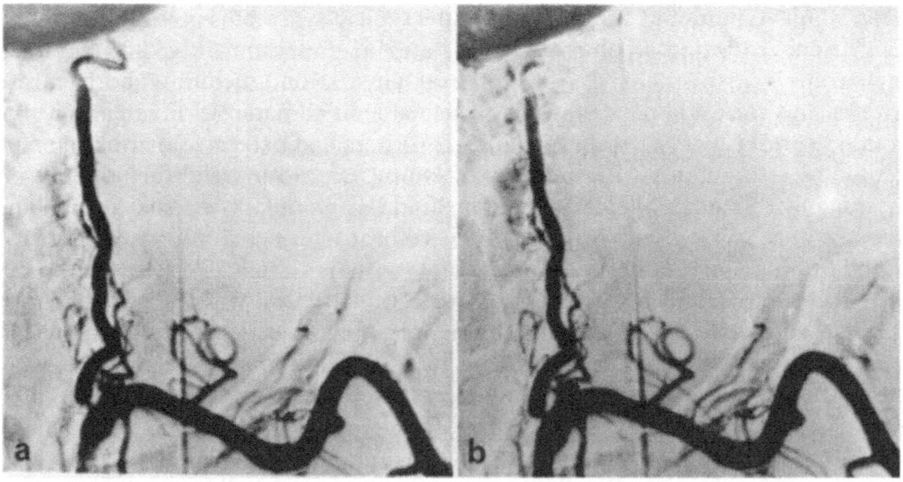

Fig. 1. a Left subclavian arteriogram shows severe stenosis of the origin of the left vertebral artery. **b** Post-angioplasty left subclavian arteriogram shows satisfactory dilatation of the origin of the vertebral artery

vertebral arteries was attempted, but only the left one was successfully dilated (Fig. 1b). Dilatation of the right vertebral artery was technically unsuccessful due to tortuosity of the right subclavian artery. The dizziness was alleviated and the patient was still asymptomatic 18 months after the procedure.

Discussion

Endarterectomy of the carotid artery bifurcation is a rather simple and generally effective procedure, but surgical treatment of subclavian vertebral artery disease is more complex. We believe transluminal angioplasty, on the other hand, to be an effective nonsurgical treatment with few complications when it is applied in selected cases. Our series, although small in number, shows favorable results. This is mainly due to careful selection of cases and exclusion of potentially high-risk patients. Dilatation of a vertebral artery stenosis was never attempted if the diseased vertebral artery was the only contributor to the basilar system circulation; neither was an isolated vertebral artery dilated if it was feeding an isolated posterior inferior cerebellar artery.

Substantial experience in arterial dilatation is a prerequisite for any angiographer attempting to dilate a vertebral artery stenosis. If catheterization of the vertebral artery or insertion and advancement of the guide wire within the vertebral artery are technically difficult, the procedure should be terminated. Dilatation of carotid stenoses bears a high risk of cerebral emboli from an ulcerated plaque; however, ulcerated plaques are rarely seen in the vertebral artery. Stenotic lesions of the vertebral artery occur mainly at the origin of the artery and are nonulcerated. We consider vertebral artery angioplasty only when the stenotic lesion is at the origin of the artery and when there is no additional atherosclerotic disease in the vertebral basilar system or carotid arteries. Vertebral artery dilatation should only be attempted if surgery is warranted and can be scheduled as a back up measure.

Summary

Percutaneous transluminal angioplasty was used to treat atherosclerotic lesions of 16 vertebral arteries in 14 patients during a 3-year period. Thirteen arteries were successfully dilated, but dilatation of three vertebral arteries failed. The first patient was still asymptomatic at 36 months and no symptoms recurred in any of the successfully treated patients. No complications were encountered during these procedures.

References

1. Grüntzig A, Hopff H (1974) Perkutane Rekanalisation chronischer arterieller Verschlüsse mit einem neuen Dilatationskather – Modifikation der Dotter-Technik. Dtsch Med Wochenschr 99: 2502–2505

2. Dotter CT, Judkins MP (1964) Transluminal treatment of arteriosclerotic obstruction. Description of a new technic and a preliminary report of its application. Circulation 30: 654–670
3. Grüntzig A, Myler R, Stertzer S, Kaltenback M, Turina M (1978) Coronary percutaneous transluminal angioplasty: preliminary results. Circulation 56–211
4. Grüntzig A, Vetter W, Meier B, Kuhlmann U, Lütolf U, Siegenthaler W (1978) Treatment of renovascular hypertension with percutaneous transluminal dilatation of a renal-artery stenosis. Lancet 1: 801–820
5. Tegtmeyer CJ, Dyer R, Teates C, et al. (1980) Percutaneous transluminal dilatation of the renal arteries. Radiology 135: 589–599
6. Schwarten DE, Yune HY, Klatte EC, Grim CE, Weinberger MH (1980) Clinical experience with percutaneous transluminal angioplasty (PTA) of the stenotic renal arteries. Radiology 135: 601–604
7. Katzen BT, Chang J (1979) Percutaneous transluminal angioplasty with the Grüntzig balloon catheter. Radiology 130: 623–626
8. Motarjeme A, Keifer JW, Zuska AJ (1980) Percutaneous transluminal angioplasty of the deep femoral artery. Radiology 135: 613–617
9. Motarjeme A, Keifer JN, Zuska AJ (1980) Percutaneous transluminal angioplasty of the iliac arteries: 66 experiences. AJR 135: 937–944
10. Motarjeme A, Keifer JW, Zuska AJ Percutaneous transluminal angioplasty of the vertebral artery

40a. Percutaneous Transluminal Angioplasty of the Supra-aortic Arteries

E. Zeitler, G. Berger, and R. Schmitt-Rüth

Introduction

Dilatation of arterial stenoses by means of percutaneous transluminal angioplasty (PTA), introduced by Dotter and Judkins [4] with coaxial Teflon catheters in 1964, has achieved increasing application in special clinics and medical centers for the treatment of arterial obstructions in the pelvis and lower extremities, particularly after the development of balloon catheter systems [12]. It did not take long before experimental studies were initiated to determine the efficacy of this simple therapeutic procedure free of the hazards of a general anesthesia in treating lesions of the coronary, carotid, and vertebral arteries. In 1976 and 1978 [46] the first reports appeared on experimental results in the dilatation of coronary artery stenoses [9, 10] and of carotid artery stenoses in dogs [17, 21]. As this book goes into print, the first results of clinical studies in the percutaneous treatment of coronary artery stenoses [10, 11] have become available. Cardiologists have embraced the technique, and it is now being tried in several clinics. On the other hand, the first experimental results in the internal carotid arteries are being greeted with criticism and scepticism by vascular surgeons. This criticism is summarized by a statement made by the vascular surgeon van Dongen [40]: "The performance of percutaneous transluminal angioplasty in the carotid can bring an otherwise generally recognized therapeutic principle in disrepute." Such criticism is apparently unjustifiable, however, if one assumes that the frequency of embolization (1%–3%) caused by PTA is the same in arteries supplying the brain as it is in the femoral and popliteal arteries [46].

Operative Risks

The results of surgical management of carotid stenoses in the region of the carotid bifurcation have been excellent in experienced hands. Operative mortality can be expected to be 1% in stage I disease, 1%–3% in stage II, and 2%–8% in stage IV [5, 8, 28, 35, 43]. The stern warnings of the surgeons should naturally be taken seriously by cardiovascular radiologists before an arteriosclerotic carotid lesion is approached by PTA. The danger of embolization must be seriously considered. However, one should also realize that besides the operative mortality in stage II, an operative morbidity of 1%–4% has been

Percutaneous Transluminal Angioplasty
(ed. by C. T. Dotter, A. Grüntzig, W. Schoop, E. Zeitler)

reported [34, 43], usually from emboli causing a postoperative neurologic deficit. From the available results, one can assume that 85% of stage II patients whose carotid stenosis is operatively treated will be asymptomatic after the procedure [5, 7, 8, 28, 34, 35, 42, 43].

Preclinical Studies

Animal experiments performed in dogs [18, 21, 22] showed that it was possible to pass and successfully dilate 23 of 31 experimentally induced carotid stenoses (lumen narrowing between 50% and 90%) using PTA. In the remaining eight cases, the stenosis could not be passed by the balloon catheter and no dilatation was attempted. Histologic investigations have shown that besides intimal changes, there is clear damage to the elastic fibers of the media. No emboli were seen angiographically and no complications occurred in the dog experiments. As a result of this study, Mathias [24] has formulated prospective indications for PTA:

1. Stenoses of the origin of major aortic branches (branchiocephalic, common carotid, and subclavian arteries)
2. Stenoses in the midportion of the common carotid artery
3. Stenoses of the external carotid artery in the presence of internal carotid occlusions, where one hopes to improve the collateral circulation
4. Fibromuscular stenoses of the internal carotid artery

Clinical Results

The results of PTA in the supra-aortic arteries are reported in Table 1 for 134 patients treated before April 1983, of whom 127 were treated successfully.

Table 1. Results of PTA in supra-aortic arteries before April 1983

Artery	Patients	Authors
Left subclavian	85	Athanasoulis 3; Castaneda 2; Galachia 6; Mathias 32; Olbert 11; Roth 10; Seurot 3; Zeitler 13
Right subclavian		Galachia 1; Olbert 2; Zeitler 2
Left common carotid	2	Kerber 1; Zeitler 1
Internal carotid (AS)	6	Mathias
Internal carotid (FMD)	10	Belan 1; Hasso 3; Mathias 1; Mullan 1 (Disc. 4)
External carotid	5	Vitek 3; Zeitler 2
Vertebral	17	Motarjeme 16; Schulz 1
Basilar	2	Sundt
Innominate	7	Kobinia 1; Roth 2; Seurot 2; Zeitler 2
	134	

Unsuccessful cases, 7; complications, 1 (embolization of the hand).
AS, atherosclerotic; FMD, fibromuscular dysplasia

Table 2. Results of PTA of the supra-aortic arteries at the Radiological Center of the Nuremberg Clinic from 1976 to May 1983

Lesion	Patients	Results
Left subclavian stenosis	13	11 + follow-up 2–52 months 2 + recurrent stenosis
Left subclavian occlusion	2	2 – unpassable
Right innominate stenosis	2	2 + follow-up 2+ 9 months
Right subclavian stenosis	2	2 + follow-up 26+28 months
Left common carotid stenosis	1	1 + follow-up 7 months
External carotid stenosis	2	2 + follow-up 2+34 months
Total	22	24 dilatations, 22 successful

In the course of 5 years, a group from Freiburg, working with the cooperation of neurologists and vascular surgeons, has successfully performed dilatation in 39 patients with disease of supra-aortic arteries without a single complication. The most commonly dilated vessel was the subclavian artery.

The indications for and results of PTA in the supra-aortic branches must be analyzed with respect to the risks involved, the degree of disease, and the operative alternatives in the following groups:

1. Obstructions of the left subclavian artery
2. Obstructions of the brachiocephalic or right subclavian arteries
3. Stenoses of the right and left common carotid arteries
4. Stenoses of the internal carotid arteries near the carotid bifurcation (predominantly atherosclerotic)
5. Stenoses of the internal carotid artery near the base of the skull (predominantly caused by fibromuscular dysplasia)
6. Stenoses of the external carotid artery in the presence of internal carotid occlusion
7. Stenoses of the vertebral artery
8. Stenoses of the basilar artery

The results of therapy of supra-aortic arteries in the Department of Radiology in the Klinikum Nürnberg are given in Table 2.

Obstructive Lesions of the Left Subclavian Artery

Lesions in the prevertebral segment of the left subclavian artery are very common, constituting 10.2%–17% of the obstructions in the extracranial vessels supplying the brain; after carotid obstructions, they are the most common pathologic finding in this region [45].

The only clinical indication for recanalization or dilatation of this segment is the subclavian steal syndrome. Studies comparing conservative and operative forms of treatment have failed to show any considerable difference in the long-term neurologic symptoms [3]. A surgical procedure frequently employed to avoid the need for thoracotomy is carotid subclavian bypass [32, 33, 42, 43].

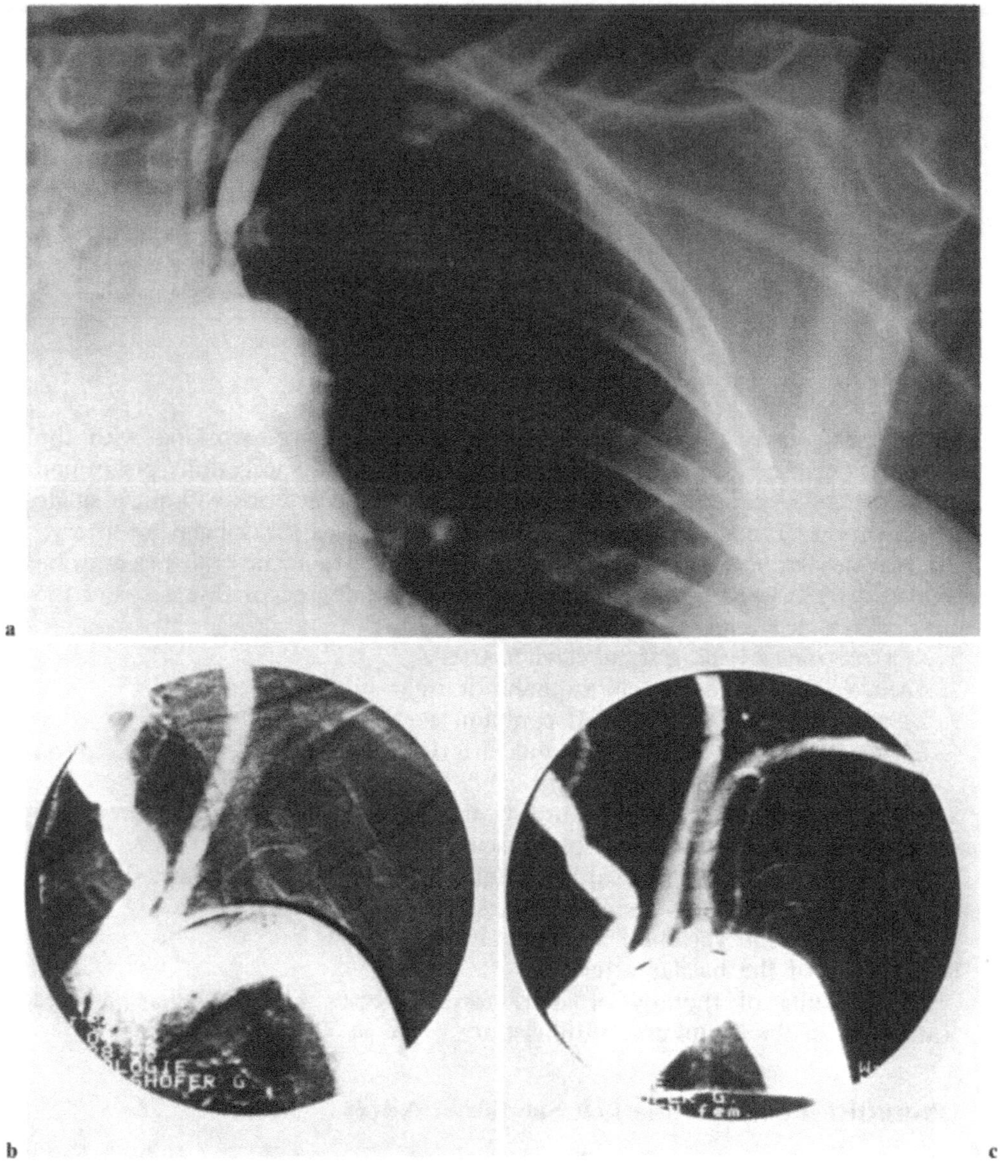

Fig. 1a–c. Left subclavian stenosis. **a** Left subclavian artery stenosis with no orthograde filling of the left vertebral artery. **b** Intra-arterial digital subtraction angiography before dilatation. **c** Digital subtraction angiography after dilatation. No signs of a hemodynamically significant residual stenosis

There have been many reports on the treatment of subclavian stenoses with PTA [1, 6, 16, 19, 20, 23, 26, 27, 29, 30, 31, 36, 44]. Combining the results of the Freiburg group and the Aggertal Clinic with our own experience and that of the literature, positive hemodynamic and angiographic results have been seen in 81 of 85 dilatations of left subclavian stenoses. To date, only one complication has been reported, that being embolization with signs of ischemia in the left hand. Attempts at recanalization of a subclavian occlusion have only occasionally been successful. The observations at present seem to indicate that the chances for recanalization of such an occlusion without complication are better if a retrograde technique from the axillary artery is employed [20, 24].

We have had primary success in all 13 patients with 11 left subclavian stenoses that we have treated. The indications were in 11 a subclavian steal syndrome (Fig. 1), as confirmed either clinically or by Doppler ultrasound. Two of our patients suffered small peripheral digital artery emboli. In two patients there continued to be a significant blood pressure difference between the arms, and repeat PTA was performed and achieved the desired result. No peripheral or central emboli were observed after the procedure. In two of our patients, the left vertebral artery originated from the aortic arch; thus there was no real risk of cerebral embolization.

The dilatation of subclavian stenoses as well as the recanalization of a subclavian occlusion appear to be associated with only slight risk, which is even lower if the vertebral artery arises directly from the aortic arch.

The long-term results that are presently available from individual articles indicate that results have remained satisfactory in 85% of those who have been followed up for 6–24 months. In these patients, hemodynamic follow-up is very simple. In our own series, only the two patients with previous digital artery emboli have been placed on long-term anticoagulation with coumadin. All others receive aggregation inhibitors.

Obstructive Lesions of the Brachiocephalic Artery and the Right Subclavian Artery

Hemodynamically significant right subclavian and innominate artery stenoses are considerably less common than lesions on the left-hand side [45]. The frequency of the stenotic changes in both segments which can be angiographically demonstrated approaches the frequency of those in the left subclavian artery; however, most of these do not prove to be hemodynamically significant. Stenoses of the brachiocephalic artery have rarely been treated by PTA because of the increased possibility of cerebral emboli [14, 20, 36].

In the example reported by Kobinia [15], a 40-year-old man suffered aortic arch syndrome, with a left carotid occlusion and stenosis of the brachiocephalic artery. Peripheral venous bypass had been placed on both the left and the right. The bypass on the right became occluded, that on the left developed a stenosis. Under these exceptional circumstances, a dilatation of the brachiocephalic artery was performed and led to clinical and hemodynamic improvement.

Two patients were successfully treated by Seurot [36] for brachiocephalic artery stenoses and right subclavian steal syndrome.

We have dilated the brachiocephalic artery in one patient. This was a 55-year-old man with decreased blood pressure in the right arm, proven by oscillography and blood pressure control before and after PTA, and with a subclavian steal syndrome on the right (Fig. 2). He had had successful PTA

a
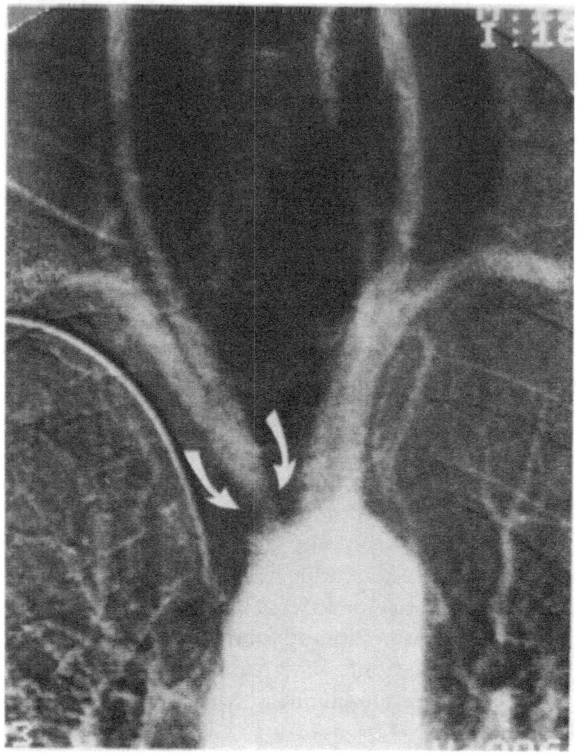

Fig. 2. a DSA of a brachio-cephalic artery stenosis prior to treatment. b Blood-pressure control before and after angioplasty of the stenosis

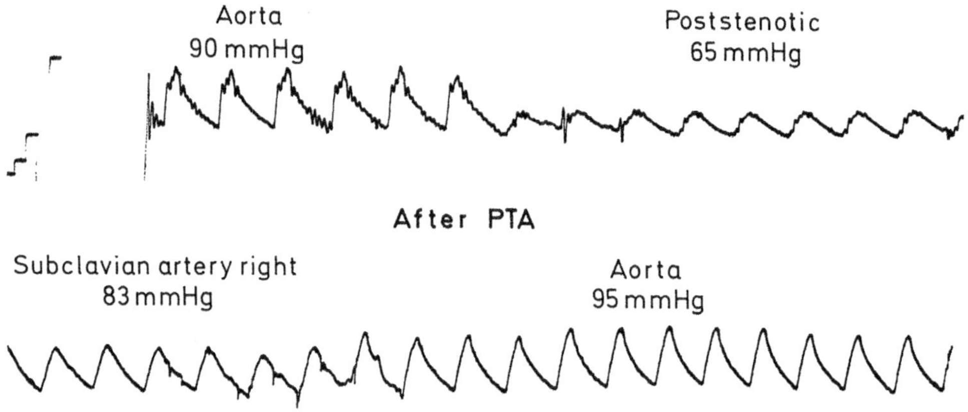

b

treatment of a femoropopliteal lesion 2 years before. The hemodynamic findings of Doppler sonography before and after dilatation are portrayed in Fig. 3. Pretherapeutically, the lesion was imaged by means of intravenous digital subtraction angiography (DSA). This minimally invasive procedure has also proven to be a very good method of post-therapeutic follow-up [37].

With regard to dilatating a lesion of the right subclavian artery, it is necessary to consider the possible compression of the origin of the common carotid artery.

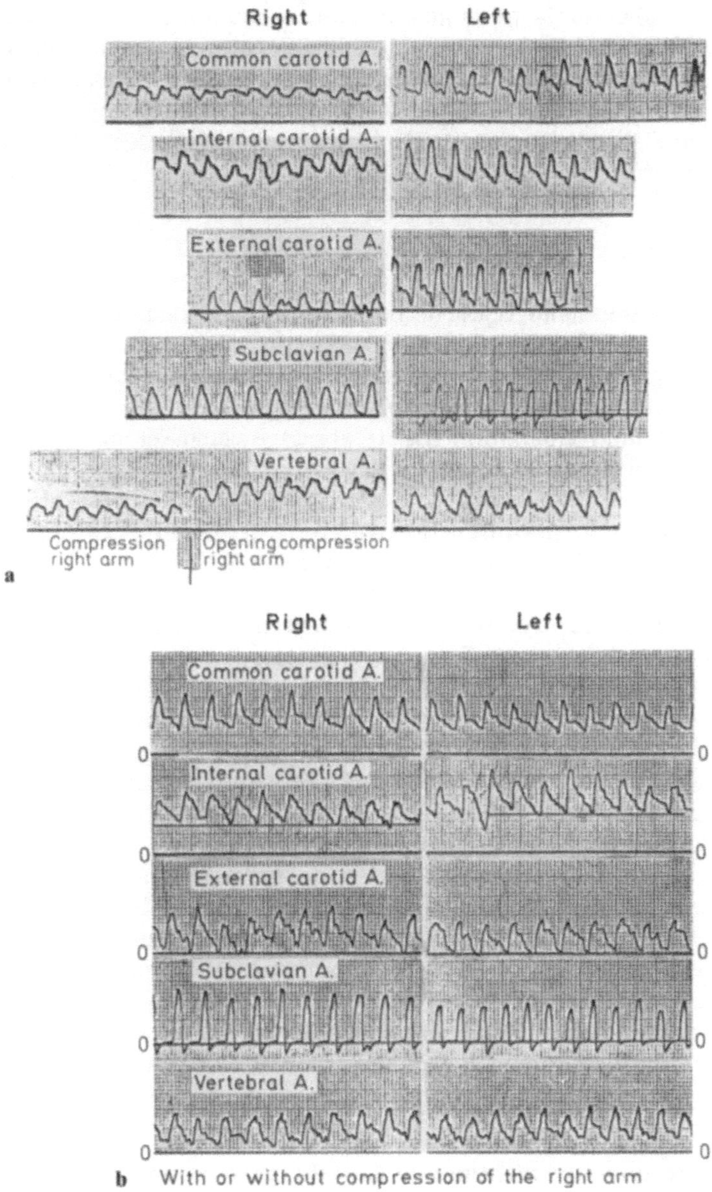

Fig. 3a, b. Confirmation of the hemodynamic effects of the innominate stenosis by Doppler sonography **a** before angioplasty, **b** after angioplasty

In order to prevent cerebral emboli, Mathias [19, 23] prefers the transaxillary approach. In our own series, we have dilated two right subclavian arteries in the portion proximal to the origin of the vertebral artery. Both of these cases showed good hemodynamic results despite an initial residual gradient.

Due to the possibility of cerebral embolization, the indications for dilatating obstructive lesions of the brachiocephalic and right subclavian arteries are most stringently defined. However, if the subclavian stenosis is distal to the origin of the vertebral artery, there is less risk. We have seen one patient with proximal and distal stenoses. PTA was successful, and the clinical results were postive.

Stenoses of the Common Carotid Artery

Stenoses in the region of the common carotid artery are found at the origin of the left common carotid artery and in the midsections of the common carotid artery bilaterally. As a rule, an isolated stenosis of the left common carotid presents no indication for recanalization, as long as the remaining arteries provide adequate collateral circulation. The treatment of such a stenosis is only meaningful if there are lesions in multiple arteries. Kerber [14] has reported the intraoperative balloon dilatation of a common carotid artery stenosis at the artery's origin at the aortic arch in conjunction with the treatment of a carotid bifurcation stenosis on the left. The procedure was successful.

At the expressed wish of the referring vascular surgeon, we treated a common carotid stenosis with dilatation in a 68-year-old patient prior to further surgical therapy. Thromboendarterectomies were planned for both internal carotid arteries, and the left internal carotid lesion was high grade (Fig. 4). The angiogram shows the high-grade common carotid stenosis in addition to the bifurcation lesion. The dilatation was performed after selective catheterization with a Sidewinder II catheter. The systolic pressure gradient was considerably reduced. The subsequent surgical treatment of the left carotid bifurcation stenosis was also successful.

In another patient with a high-grade stenosis of the left common carotid artery shown by DSA, dilatation was felt to be clinically warranted since this patient also had an occlusion of the right common carotid artery with collateral circulation through the vertebral basilar system. In preparation for PTA, our routine transcatheter pressure measurements failed to show a gradient, despite the angiographic appearance of a high-grade stenosis. In this case we refrained from performing PTA, and this underlines the importance of hemodynamic measurements in confirming the significance of an angiographic finding.

Stenoses of the Internal Carotid Artery and the Carotid Bifurcation

If there are no contraindications to surgery, only highly unusual situations can be imagined in which percutaneous dilatation might be preferred to operative vascular reconstruction at present. Dilatation of atherosclerotic stenoses in the region of the bifurcation have only rarely been performed. We ourselves have had no experience in this area. Mathias [19, 20, 22] reports six atherosclerotic stenoses of the internal carotid artery that were approached percutaneously with a balloon catheter. In five cases the stenosis was successfully dilated, but in one case the balloon could not be properly placed. No clinically apparent neurologic

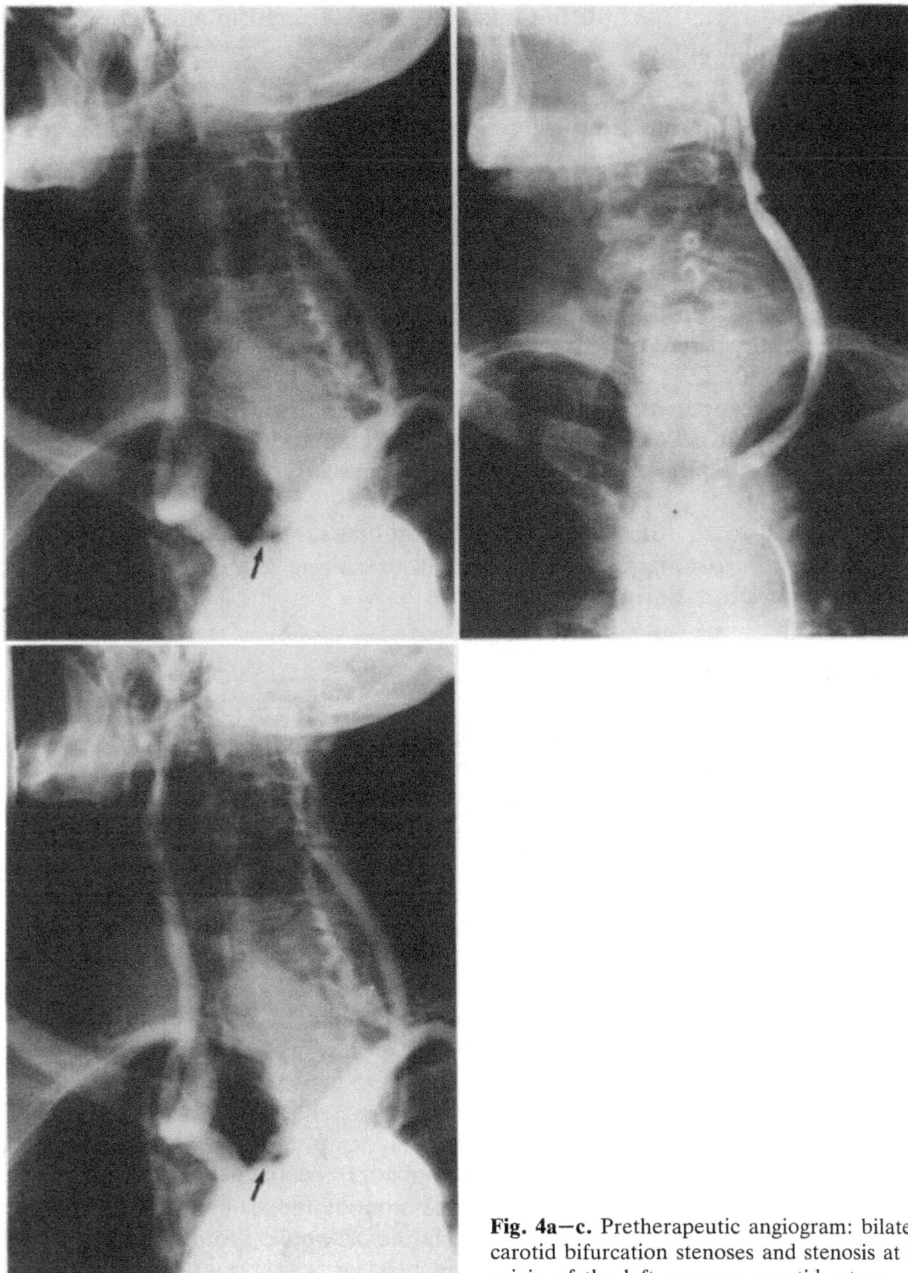

Fig. 4a–c. Pretherapeutic angiogram: bilateral carotid bifurcation stenoses and stenosis at the origin of the left common carotid artery

complications arose. Each of these patients was selected in close cooperation with the vascular surgeon.

Stenoses of the Internal Carotid Artery near the Skull and Fibromuscular Dysplasia

Balloon dilatation of fibromuscular stenoses of the internal carotid has been used as an intraoperative procedure. However, due to the easy passage of stenoses more than 4 cm from the carotid bifurcation, the percutaneous treatment of these lesions is also possible. Hasso [13] has reported positive results in treating three patients, and single successful cases have been reported by Mathias [20, 22], Belan [2], and Mullan [27]. Discussions at various congresses have concentrated on the positive use of Grüntzig balloon catheters in fibromuscular dysplasia both in intraoperative and percutaneous procedures. Which of these approaches will prove to be more effective remains to be decided.

In contrast to atherosclerotic stenoses, fibromuscular lesions do not present the danger of dislodging mural thrombi or cholesterol crystals from an atheromatous ulcer during dilatation.

External Carotid Stenoses

The risk of producing intracerebral emboli in dilatation of an external carotid lesion is considerably lower when an internal carotid occlusion is present. Vitek and Morawetz [41] have reported successful treatment of three patients with an external carotid stenosis in association with a homolateral internal carotid occlusion, in order to provide adequate flow to a planned bypass from the superficial temporal artery to the middle cerebral artery. This concept could be successfully extended to patients with transient ischemic attacks (TIAs), particularly if an internal carotid occlusion is present on the opposite side. We ourselves have treated one patient with external carotid stenosis in 1980 and another in 1983. A 78-year-old woman presented with transient ischemic attacks and acute onset of muscle weakness in the left arm, aphasia, and numbness in the oral region. A bruit was present over the right carotid. Clinical examination revealed a central facial paresis on the left, a persistent aphasia, brisk reflexes on the left, and gross weakness of the left arm compared to the right. Sensory changes were not detected. The right medial supratrochlear artery could not be found using Doppler ultrasonography. The hemodynamics in its counterpart on the left were unremarkable (Fig. 5). Direct Doppler sonography of both bifurcations revealed a turbulent flow, which was more marked on the right than on the left and present in both the internal and external carotids. On echoflow examination a high-grade acceleration of flow was found in the right carotid bifurcation as well as in the internal carotid, while on the left there was a moderate high-grade increase in flow rate at the carotid bifurcation. These examinations led to the diagnosis of high-grade carotid bifuration stenosis on the right and a moderate carotid bifurcation stenosis on the left.

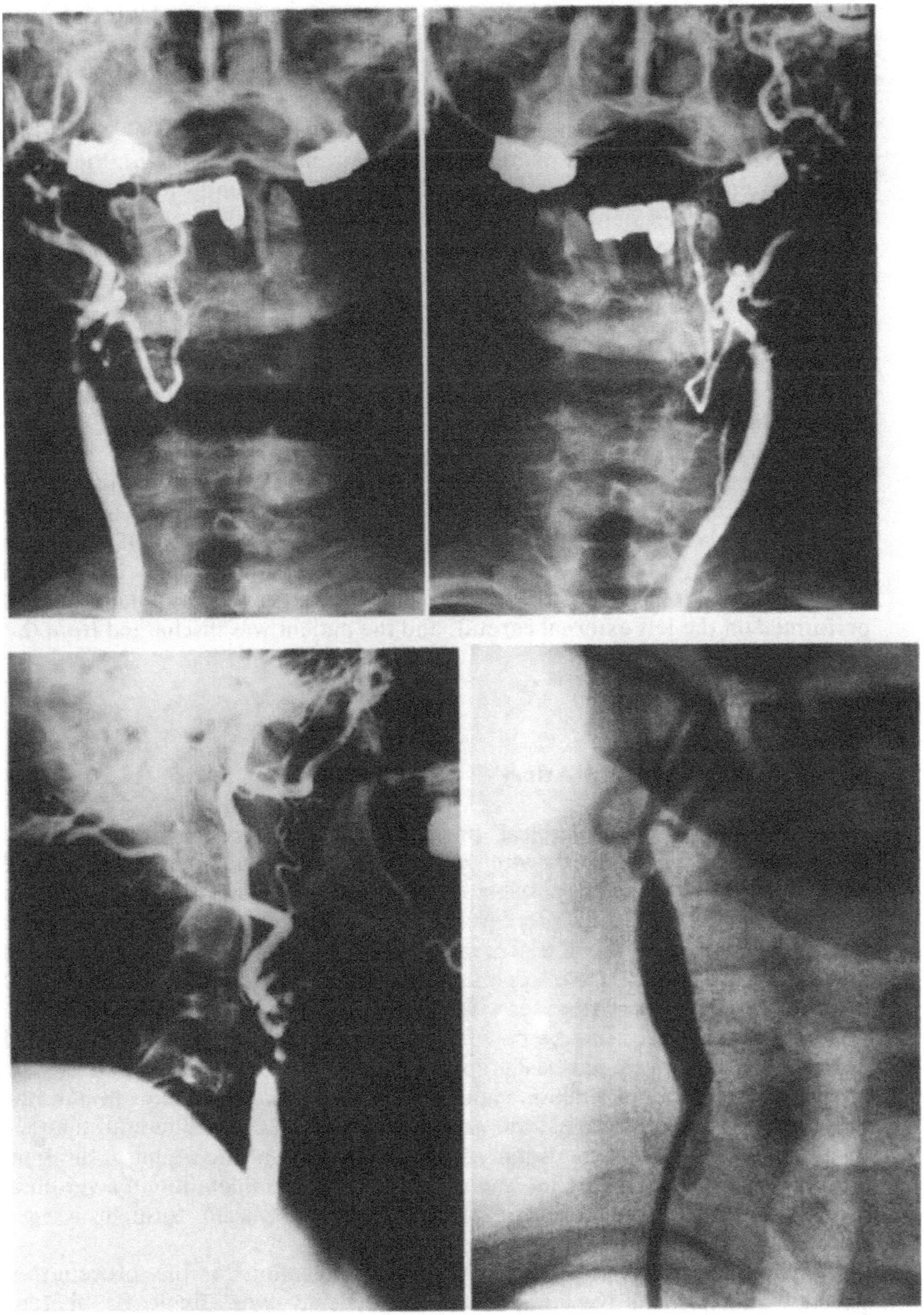

a

b c

Fig. 5a–c. Bilateral external carotid stenoses and internal carotid occlusion. **a, b** Before therapy; **c** after dilatation of the external carotid stenosis

Carotid angiography revealed a high-grade external carotid stenosis on the right, a moderate external carotid stenosis on the left, and occlusion of both internal carotid arteries. Collateral flow was provided over the ophthalmic artery bilaterally.

After a period of conservative treatment with dextran 40 injections (Rheomacrodex, piracetam; pentoxifylline; cortisone, and digitoxin), there was no improvement of the patient's clinical status; consequently the patient was submitted to a transfemoral percutaneous procedure. Advancement of a 5 F catheter through the right external carotid stenosis showed occlusive pressures beyond the lesion. Dilatation proceeded with a balloon catheter of 6-mm diameter, with the inflating pressure limited to 4 atm. Final pressure measurements showed that the catheter no longer occluded the vessel; however, there was a persistent systolic gradient of 20 mm Hg.

Angiography performed immediately after dilatation showed a considerable reduction in the right external carotid stenosis and no change with respect to the carotid occlusion. After this intervention, the left arm paresis resolved completely, as did the residual aphasia. The patient no longer complained of paresthesia in the region of the mouth. A repeat Doppler ultrasound examination showed good filling of the ophthalmic artery through the right external carotid, as well as a marked retrograde flow through the medial supratrochlear artery. Since the clinical situation improved, no dilatation was performed on the left external carotid, and the patient was discharged from the hospital.

Stenosis of the Vertebral Artery

Reconstructive vascular surgical procedures in the vertebral arteries are understandably undertaken with great reluctance and narrowly defined indications. PTA makes it possible to approach and dilate these lesions in a relatively simple way. The prerequisite is that appropriate clinical symptoms justify the procedure. To the present, experience with such lesions has been limited. Motarjeme [25] has reported the successful treatment of single and bilateral vertebral artery stenoses with balloon catheters of 3–5 mm in diameter. The 11 patients treated had a total of 16 vertebral artery stenoses and presented a clinical picture of vertebrobasilar insufficiency. Three of the 16 stenoses could not be dilated since the balloon could not be appropriately placed, despite the initial good selective passage of the stenosis. Five patients had bilateral stenoses, and five had stenoses at the origin of the left and one at the origin of the right vertebral artery. Schutz [39] has reported the successful dilatation of a vertebral artery stenosis with a Grüntzig balloon catheter placed through a right subclavian arteriotomy.

We have no experience in this area. An indication for this procedure is probably unequivocal vertebrobasilar insufficiency with single or bilateral vertebral artery stenosis in the presence of occlusive lesions in other arteries supplying the brain.

Stenoses of the Basilar Artery

The only published results of basilar artery balloon dilatation have come from the Mayo Clinic [38]. The two patients involved were gravely ill with frequent and severe TIAs and vertebrobasilar insufficiency. Both had had multiple previous operative procedures, and the prognosis was very poor. In these cases the catheter was introduced directly into the vertebral artery intraoperatively after resection of the arch of the atlas. The balloon used had a diameter of 3.7 mm. This procedure is only justified in patients with brain stem and cerebellar ischemia if no extra- to intracranial bypass procedure can be performed and the only alternative is no therapy at all.

We have not performed a basilar artery stenosis dilatation. However, we have had the opportunity of examining a patient with acute and severe basilar insufficiency where the question of such a possible therapeutic measure arose. Selective vertebral angiography showed a complete occlusion of the basilar artery. The only possible intervention in this situation was intra-arterial clot lysis therapy with streptokinase. Using a total of 150,000 IU of streptokinase, we were successful in lysing the thrombus in the basilar artery. We could find no stenosis after the clot was lysed, so dilatation did not come into question. Despite performing the clot lysis within 2 h of diagnosis of acute quadriplegia, there was no improvement in the clinical picture. The patient died on the 3rd post-therapeutic day.

Discussion

Since 1978, on the basis of animal experimental data from Mathias [18, 21, 22] and the increasing experience with PTA in other vasuclar areas, in particular in the coronary and renal arteries, the percutaneous treatment of obstructive lesions in the supra-aortic arteries has achieved increasing success. The results available at present, however, are certainly not adequate to allow a definitive judgement on the use of a balloon dilatation in this area (Fig. 6).

With the prerequisite that all patients and indications be considered in close cooperation with the neurologist and the vascular surgeon, and taking into account the individual clinical situation and age of the patient, the following indications can be proposed:

1. Transfemoral dilatation of left subclavian stenoses in circulatory disturbances of the left arm and in the subclavian steal syndrome
2. Dilatation of external carotid stenoses in the presence of internal carotid occlusions for treating clinically symptomatic patients, and also in preparation for a possible bypass from the external carotid branch to the middle cerebral artery
3. Dilatation of symptomatic stenoses of the internal carotid artery (from fibromuscular dysplasia or other causes) if these are located close to the base of the skull in an area inaccessible to the vascular surgeon

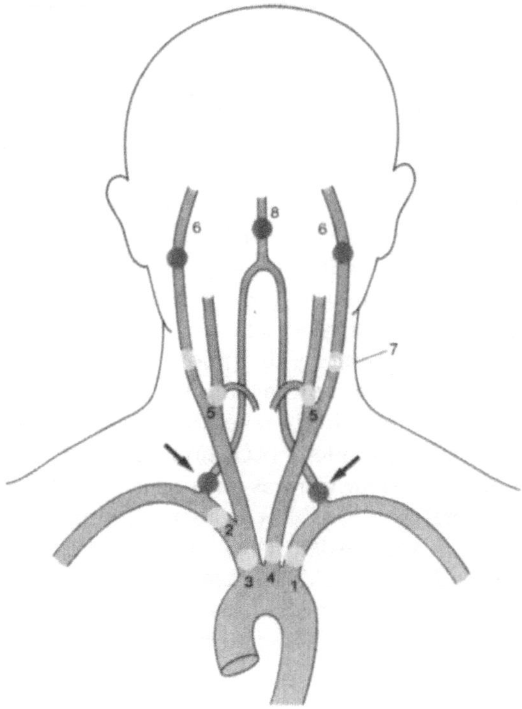

Fig. 6. Possible locations for application of PTA in the extracranial arterial branches supplying the brain. *1* left subclavian artery, *2* right subclavian artery, *3* brachiocephalic trunc, *4* left common carotid artery, *5* external carotid artery, *6* internal carotid artery (FMD and below the base of skull), *7* internal carotid artery (AS), *8* basilar artery, *9* vertebral artery

Table 3. Obstructive lesions in arteries of the neck

Carotid bifurcation stenoses	→ operation
International carotid stenoses of typical location	→ operation
International carotid stenoses	
close to the skull base	→ PTA
fibromuscular dysplasia	↗ operation ↘ PTA
prior to other operative procedures	↗ operation ↘ ? PTA
External carotid stenoses with internal carotid occlusion	↗ PTA ↘ operation
a) alone	
b) prior to temporal artery – middle cerebral artery bypass	

4. In selective clinical situations where the operative risk is high, balloon dilatation can be employed in treating stenoses of the brachiocephalic artery, the right subclavian artery, and the left common carotid artery. The choices between pre- or intraoperative access and retrograde or orthograde dilatation must be made in close cooperation of all members of the vascular team
5. Dilatation of ostial stenoses of the vertebral artery when bilateral disease is present or in combination with obstructive lesions in other arteries supplying the brain and severe symptomatic vertebrobasilar insufficiency

6. In all other cases (Table 3), dilatation is to be used only as a last resort in exceptional situations, where all other therapeutic possibilities have been exhausted. Possible dilatation or clot lysis of the basilar artery is one of these rare indications.

No area requires such close cooperation among the various specialists involved as the dilatation or recanalization of supra-aortic arteries. It is very important to follow up all patients closely in order to be able to assess the results of these therapeutic measures since a randomized study is certainly not feasible.

Summary

Results of percutaneous dilatation of supra-aortic arteries are reported in a series of 24 patients with a review of 134 cases in the literature. PTA of left subclavian artery stenosis can be considered an alternative to surgical therapy, but should be reserved for selected patients presenting a considerable operative risk.

References

1. Bachmann DM, Kim RM (1980) Transluminal dilatation for subclavian steal syndrome. AJR 135: 995–996
2. Belan A, Vesela M, Vanek I, Weiss K, Peregrin JH (1980) Percutaneous Transluminal Angioplasty of fibromuscular dysplasia of the internal carotid artery. Cardiovasc Intervent Radiol 5: 79–81
3. Buchwalsky R, Genswein R, Schlosser V, Blümchen G (1977) Subclavian Steal Syndrom: Postoperativer und spontaner Verlauf bei 27 Patienten über 3 Jahre. Thoraxchirurgie 25: 288–290
4. Dotter CT, Judkins MP (1964) Transluminal treatment of arteriosclerotic obstruction: Description of a new technic and a preliminary report of its application. Circulation 30: 654–670
5. Fields WS, Maslenikov V, Meyer JS, Hass WK, Remington RD, MacDonald MC (1970) Joint study of extracranial arterial occlusion. V. Progress report of prognosis following surgery or nonsurgical treatment for transient cerebral ischemic attacks and cervical carotid artery lesion. JAMA 211: 1993
6. Galichia JP, Bajaj AK, Vine DL, Roberts RW (to be published) Subclavian artery stenosis treated by transluminal angioplasty: Six cases. Cardiovasc Intervent Radiol
7. Giessler R, Gehl H, Heberer G (1969) Die chirurgische Behandlung der cerebrovaskulären Insuffizienz. Chirurg 40: 433
8. Giessler R, Schoop W, Zeitler E (1973) Indikationen zur operativen Therapie bei koronaren und zerebralen Durchblutungsstörungen. Huber, Bern
9. Grüntzig A (1976) Perkutane Dilatation von Coronarstenosen – Beschreibung eines neuen Kathetersystems. Klin Wochenschr 54: 543–545
10. Grüntzig A (1978) Transluminal dilatation of coronary artery stenosis – Experimental report. In: Zeitler E, Grüntzig A, Schoop W (eds) Percutanous vascular recanalisation. Springer, Berlin Heidelberg New York, pp 57–65
11. Grüntzig A (1978) Transluminal dilatation of coronary artery stenoses. Lancet I: 263
12. Grüntzig A, Hopff H (1976) Perkutane Rekanalisation chronischer arterieller Verschlüsse mit einem neuen Dilatationskatheter (Dotter-Prinzip). Fortschr Röntgenstr 124: 80

13. Hasso AN, Bird CR, Zinke DE, Thompson JR (1981) Fibromuscular dysplasia of the internal carotid artery: percutaneous transluminal angioplasty. AJNR 2: 175–180
14. Kerber CW, Cromwell LD, Loehden OL (1980) Catheter dilatation of proximal carotid stenosis during distal bifurcation endarterectomy. AJNR 1: 348–349
15. Kobinia GS, Bergmann H Jr (to be published) Angioplasty in stenosis of the innominate artery. Cardiovasc Intervent Radiol
16. Martin EC, Diamond NG, Casarella WJ (1980) Percutaneous transluminal angioplasty in non-atherosclerotic disease. Radiology 135: 27–33
17. Mathias K (1976) Technik und Erfolgsrate der transfemoralen zerebralen Angiographie. Fortschr Röntgenstr 124: 511–515
18. Mathias K (1977) Ein neuartiges Katheter-System zur perkutanen transluminalen Angioplastie von Karotisstenosen. Fortschr Med 95: 1007–1011
19. Mathias K (1981) Perkutane transluminale Katheterbehandlung supraaortaler Arterienobstruktionen. Angiology 3 (1): 47–50
20. Mathias K (1983) Dilatationsbehandlung hirnversorgender Arterien. Ed. Trübestein, Thieme, Stuttgart (im Druck)
21. Mathias K, Rohrbach R, Neff W, Ensinger H (1978) Percutaneous transluminal dilatation (PTD) of carotid artery stenosis. In: Zeitler E, Grüntzig A, Schoop W (eds) Percutaneous vascular recanalization. Springer, Berlin Heidelberg New York, pp 66–72
22. Mathias K, Mittermeyer C, Ensinger H, Neff W (1980) Perkutane Katheterdilatation von Karotisstenosen. Fortschr Röntgenstr 133: 258–261
23. Mathias K, Staiger J, Thron A, Spillner G, Heiss HW, Konrad-Graf S (1980) Perkutane Katheterangioplastik der Arteria subclavia. Dtsch Med Wochenschr 105: 16–18
24. Mathias K, Bockenheimer S, Von Reutern G, Heiss HW, Ostheim-Dzerowycz W (1983) Katheterdilatation hirnversorgender Arterien. Radiologie 23: 208–214
25. Motarjeme A, Keifer JW, Zuska AJ (1981) Percutaneous transluminal angioplasty of the vertebral artery. Radiology 139: 715–717
26. Motarjeme A, Keifer JW, Zuska AJ (1982) Percutaneous transluminal angioplasty of the brachiocephalic arteries. AJR 138: 457–462
27. Mullan S, Duda EE, Patronas NJ (1980) Some examples of balloon technology in neurosurgery. J Neurosurg 52: 321–329
28. Neugebauer J (1975) Die cerebrovaskuläre Insuffizienz infolge extrakranieller Arterienveränderungen. VEB-Verlag, Berlin
29. Novelline RA (1980) Percutaneous transluminal angioplasty. Newer applications. AJR 135: 983–988
30. Novelline RA (1982) Other applications of percutaneous transluminal angioplasty. In: Athanasoulis CA, Pfister RC, Greene RE, Robertson GH (eds) Interventional radiology. Saunders, Philadelphia, pp 326–333
31. Olbert F, Schidrich W, Kasprzak P, Schlegl A (1981) Ein neuer Dilatationskatheter. Röntgen-Bericht 10: 297–308
32. Raithel D (1974) Gefäßchirurgische Maßnahmen bei zerebralen Durchblutungsstörungen. In: Wieck HH (ed) Zerebrale und periphere Durchblutungsstörungen. Aesopus, München
33. Raithel D, Bürger L (1973) Das Subclavian Steal Syndrom. Med Welt 24: 1478
34. Raithel D (1977) Komplikationen operativer Maßnahmen – Indikation zur Reintervention. In: Raithel D (ed) Zerebrale Insuffizienz durch extrakranielle Gefäßverschlüsse. Perimed, Erlangen, pp 215–221
35. Raithel D (1977) Zerebrale Insuffizienz durch extrakranielle Gefäßverschlüsse. Perimed, Erlangen
36. Seurot M, Pernesse JM, Angel C, Gaux JC (1983) Angioplastie percutané transluminale des artères des membres. Ed. Trübestein, Thieme, Stuttgart (im Druck)
37. Seyferth W, Marhoff P, Zeitler E (1982) Transvenöse und arterielle digitale Video-Subtraktionsangiographie (DVSA). Fortschr Röntgenstr 136 (3): 301–309
38. Sundt TM Jr, Smith HC, Campbell JK, Vlietstra RE, Cucehiara RF, Stanson AW (1980) Transluminal angioplasty for basilar artery stenoses. Mayo Clin Proc 55: 673–680
39. Schutz H, Yeung HP, Chiu MC, Terbrugge K, Ginsberg R (1981) Dilatation of vertebral artery stenosis. N Engl J Med 304: 732

40. Van Dongen RJAM (1981) Perkutane transluminale Katheterbehandlung supraaortaler Arterienobstruktionen. Angiology 3 (2): 111–112
41. Vitek JJ, Morawetz RB (1982) Percutaneous transluminal angioplasty of the external carotid artery (preliminary report). AJNR 3: 541–546
42. Vollmar J (1974) Chirurgische Behandlungsmöglichkeiten bei zerebrovaskulärer Insuffizienz. Dtsch Med Wochenschr 99: 465
43. Vollmar J (1975) Rekonstruktive Chirurgie der Arterien. Thieme, Stuttgart
44. Zeitler E (1980) Percutaneous dilatation and recanalization of iliac and femoral arteries. Cardiovasc Intervent Radiol 3: 207–212
45. Zeitler E, Holik B (1977) Angiographische Diagnostik. In: Raithel D (ed) Zerebrale Insuffizienz durch extrakranielle Gefäßverschlüsse. Perimed, Erlangen
46. Zeitler E, Grüntzig A, Schoop W (1978) Percutaneous vascular recanalization. Springer, Berlin Heidelberg New York

XI. Percutaneous Transluminal Angioplasty of Renal Arteries

41. Long-Term Results of Percutaneous Transluminal Angioplasty for Renovascular Hypertension Using the Coaxial Catheter Technique in Patients With Atherosclerosis and Fibromuscular Dysplasia

F. Mahler, Z. Glück, P. Probst, P. Weidmann, and B. Nachbur

During the last few years percutaneous transluminal angioplasty (PTA) has been established as alternative therapy for renovascular hypertension in patients who would otherwise be treated medically or surgically [3–10]. Our group has gathered experience by using almost exclusively the coaxial catheter system [2, 6, 7]. The mean follow-up time of 2 years in our study and the inclusion of patients with different diagnoses allows us to draw some tentative conclusions regarding prognostically significant features [8].

Technique

The choice of technical approach depends not only on the vascular conditions but also on the local school and experience of the team. Our group prefers the modified coaxial technique introduced by Grüntzig for the coronary arteries [2]. It consists of a guiding catheter (F-8) inserted in the femoral artery and a dilatation catheter with a balloon at its tip and a diameter of 3.7 mm or 5 mm. This set has the advantage of working for almost all types of stenoses in the renal arteries except for those in vessels branching at very acute angles from the aorta. The system is specially suited in very tight or distally located stenoses, even those located in polar branch arteries, such as frequently occur in fibromuscular dysplasia (FMD) or in children [1]. With a special, modified right coronary guiding catheter (type FR-S, Schneider), it was easily possible to reach the arteries of three transplanted kidneys from the contralateral femoral artery as shown in Fig. 1. We needed to use the transaxillary approach in only one case (2%).

Patients

Percutaneous transluminal angioplasty of renal arteries was performed in 40 patients. The total number of 59 PTAs encompasses 47 primary unilateral or bilateral interventions (i.e., the first PTA per artery) and 12 secondary

Percutaneous Transluminal Angioplasty
(ed. by C. T. Dotter, A. Grüntzig, W. Schoop, E. Zeitler)

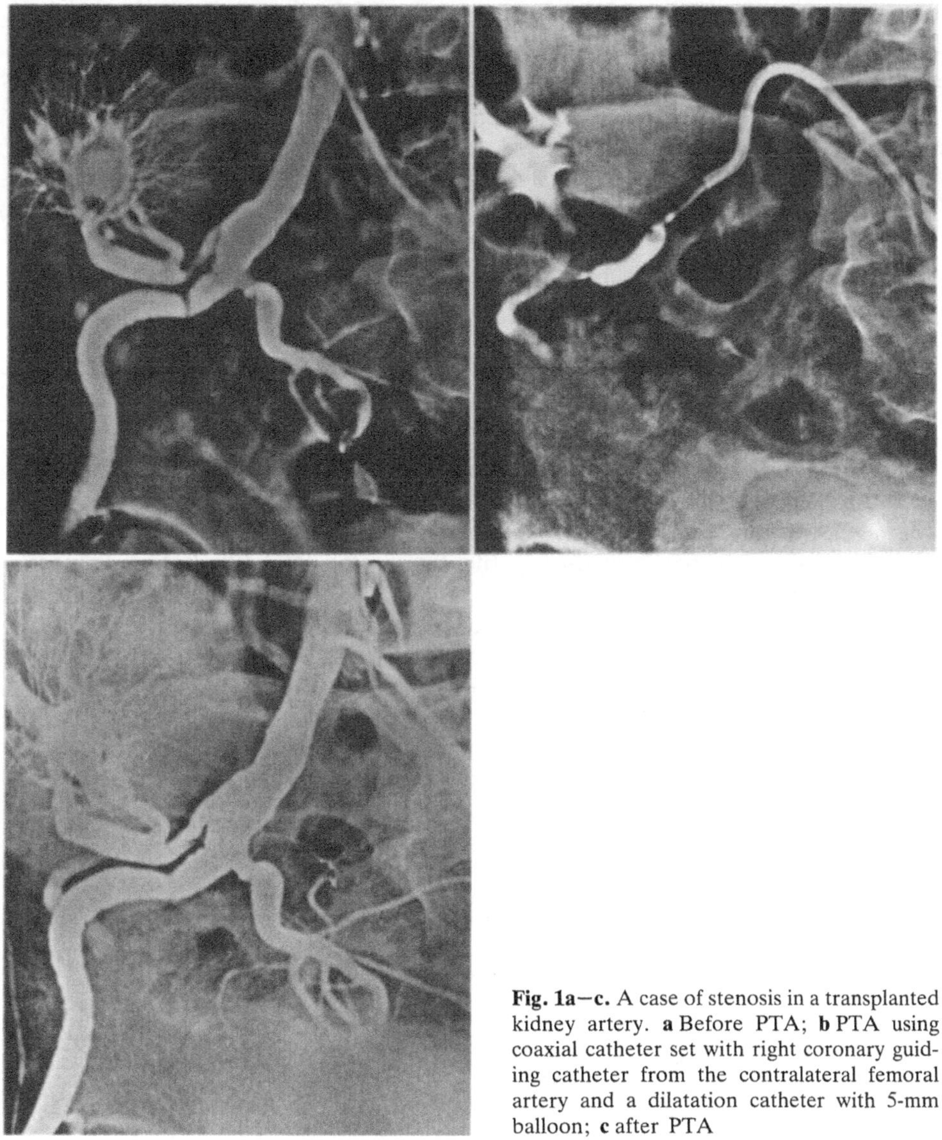

Fig. 1a–c. A case of stenosis in a transplanted kidney artery. **a** Before PTA; **b** PTA using coaxial catheter set with right coronary guiding catheter from the contralateral femoral artery and a dilatation catheter with 5-mm balloon; **c** after PTA

dilatations (i.e., repeated PTA). The patients were divided into groups as follows: atherosclerosis (AS; $n = 15$, 3 bilateral, mean age 53 years); fibromuscular dysplasia ($n = 11$, 2 bilateral, mean age 31 years); miscellaneous (vasculitis and/or renal insufficiency; $n = 6$, 2 bilateral, mean age 58 years); and transplanted kidneys ($n = 3$). Follow-up ranged from 3 to 54 months and included clinical examination (blood pressure, renal function) in all cases, late angiograms in 20, and postdilatational renal vein renin determination in 24 patients.

Complications

The complications occurring in 12% of our interventions included intimal dissections at the dilatation site and hemorrhages at the puncture site. Only one dissection caused restenosis, treated successfully by repeated PTA, and one hemorrhage needed surgical revision of the puncture site. Complications such as renal artery perforation, acute renal artery thrombosis, and renal infarction were not observed. However, PTA of renal arteries should not be performed where no emergency vascular surgery is available.

Overall Results

For the presentation of long-term results only 32 adult patients are included, with a mean follow-up time of 23 months (range 3–54). In all these cases PTA was indicated for renovascular hypertension. Figure 2 shows the mean blood pressure values before and during the time after PTA, including values in relapsing and repeatedly dilated cases, related to the concomitant antihypertensive treatment. On average, blood pressure was reduced by PTA from 187/108 ± 26/10 mm Hg before PTA to 150/91 ± 29/13 mm Hg initially ($p < 0.001$). Blood pressure values remained statistically unchanged despite a consistent reduction in the use of antihypertensive agents from an average number of 2.3 to 1.2 ($p < 0.001$).

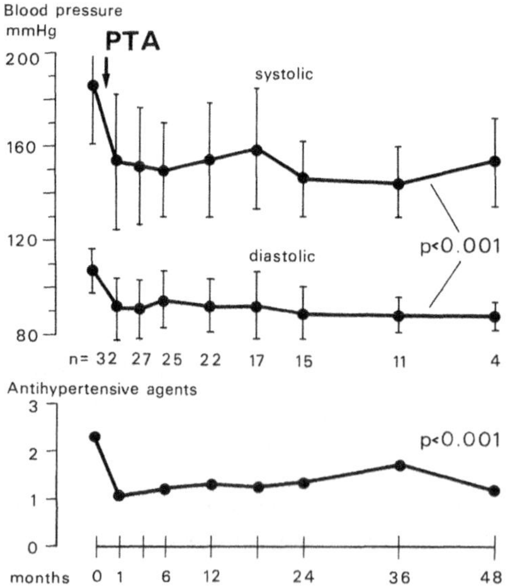

Fig. 2. Mean blood pressure values and number of antihypertensive agents before and 1–48 months after PTA for renovascular hypertension in 32 patients. The decrease in blood pressure is statistically significant and consistent despite reduced treatment. Relapsing and redilated patients are included

Predictive Factors

When the patients are grouped according to the presumed cause underlying the hypertension, the following differences in the results are seen. Figure 3 shows the blood pressure values before and at the end of the follow-up period in relation to the number of antihypertensive agents needed for three subgroups of patients. In the AS and FMD groups blood pressure as well as antihypertensive treatment was significantly reduced, while in the miscellaneous group no significance was observed. The results in patients with FMD are superior to those in patients with AS not only in terms of average values, as shown in Fig. 3, but also in terms of the rate of "cure" and improvement of hypertension among the individual patients, as indicated in Fig. 4. Of 15 patients with AS, 2 reached normal blood pressure levels without the use of antihypertensive drugs (cured hypertension), and 8 experienced an improvement in blood pressure (values reduced by more than 15% of initial pressure with unchanged or reduced antihypertensive treatment). By contrast, out of the 11 patients with FMD 7 cases were cured and 3 cases improved, while in the miscellaneous group only two out of six cases clearly improved. The results in the rest of the patients remained uncertain (changed antihypertensive regimen, treatment of vasculitis, etc.) or unimproved. These differences are statistically significant ($p < 0.05$). It is remarkable that the cured patients in both the AS and FMD groups include only unilaterally affected cases. The only one unimproved patient to date with FMD suffers bilateral reoccurrence.

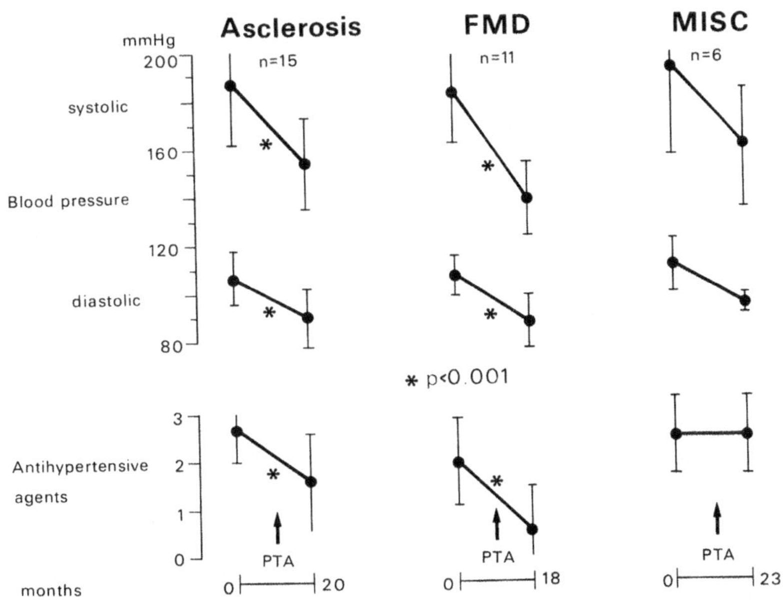

Fig. 3. Influence of PTA on blood pressure and antihypertensive therapy in three subgroups of patients. Reduction in blood pressure and therapy in patients with atherosclerosis *(Asclerosis)* and fibromuscular dysplasia *(FMD)* are statistically significant; the group with miscellaneous disease (*MISC:* vasculitis, renal insufficiency) is less responsive

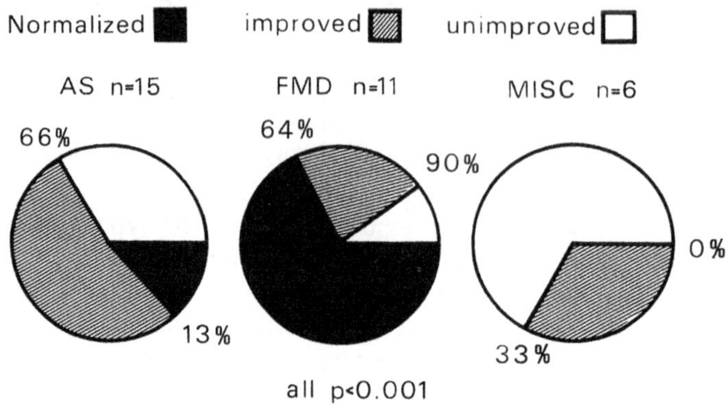

Fig. 4. Proportions of patients with normalized (i.e., not requiring therapy), improved (unchanged or reduced therapy), and uncertain/unimproved blood pressure an average of 21 months after PTA in patients with atherosclerosis *(AS)*, fibromuscular dysplasia *(FMD)*, and miscellaneous diagnoses *(MISC)*

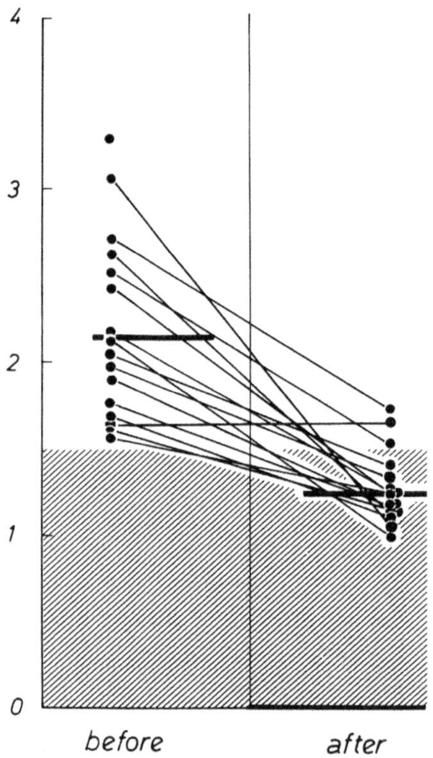

Fig. 5. Renal vein renin ratio before and after PTA in 16 consecutive patients. While each of the patients had an elevated ratio before, only the three cases with clinical relapse showed an elevation (> 1.5, *cross-hatched area*) after PTA

In this context the value of the renal vein renin ratio may be of interest. Figure 5 shows the ratio of affected to unaffected sides in our first 16 consecutive cases. All values exceeded the normal range [11] before PTA and were normalized in the patients who responded well to PTA. The three patients with elevated renin ratio during the follow-up period exhibited clinical relapses of the hypertension. We are aware of the fact that the systemically circulating renin is indicative of the renovascular nature of the hypertension rather than the selective renin ratio. However, for practical reasons (premedication, etc.) a basal renin value is not always easy to obtain in these patients, while the ratio proved reliable after sufficient stimulation with diuretics [11]. It is obvious that renal vein renin ratio is most likely to be elevated in cases with unilaterally stenosed renal arteries and intact contralateral kidney. Elevated renin ratio is therefore indicative of a constellation corresponding closely to those in the candidates described above who were found angiographically and clinically to have the best prognosis [8].

Conclusions

1. Long-term results of PTA for renovascular hypertension are satisfactory and, taken overall, are comparable to surgical results as reported in the literature.
2. The best results are observed in patients with FMD. Factors contributing to this may be absence of renal insufficiency, young age, and unilateral stenosis. Also the elevated renal vein renin ratio belongs to the pattern of the prognostically favorable patient.
3. PTA involves little discomfort, a short hospital stay, low costs, and few complications. It should be regarded as the first step in the therapy program, with surgical repair as a last resort, in patients with renovascular hypertension.

Summary

In nearly all of 59 percutaneous transluminal dilatations the coaxial double-catheter system was used. Only in 1 case was the axillary approach necessary. Clinically relevant complications were one dissection of the dilated renal artery (redilated successfully) and two hemorrhages at the femoral puncture site (one surgical revision). In 32 patients (follow-up 2–54 months, mean 23) blood pressure was lowered from 187/108 to 150/91 mm Hg despite reduction in antihypertensive therapy ($p < 0.001$). Out of 15 patients with atherosclerotic stenoses (unilateral), blood pressure was normalized by PTA in 2 and improved in another 8. Out of 11 patients with fibromuscular dysplasia, blood pressure was normalized in 7 (all unilateral), improved in 3, and unchanged in 1 (bilateral). Of six patients with miscellaneous disease (vasculitis, renal insufficency) only two were improve. Thus PTA of renal arteries is a useful alternative in the management of renovascular hypertension, mainly in patients with fibromuscular dysplasia, unilateral stenosis, and elevated renal vein renin ratio. Long-term results are comparable to surgical results. However, since no surgical dissection is necessary, morbidity is low and long and costly hospital stays can be avoided. The procedure can be repeated in relapsing cases. In case of rare complications a vascular surgical team should be available.

References

1. Ghisla R, Mahler F, Haertel M, Oetliker O, Rossi E (1981) Transluminale Nierendilatation bei einem 5jährigen Knaben. VASA [Suppl] 8:90
2. Grüntzig A, Senning A, Siegenthaler WE (1979) Non-operative dilatation of coronary-artery stenosis. N Engl J Med 301:61
3. Katzen BT, Chang J, Lukowsky GH, Abramson EG (1979) Percutaneous transluminal angioplasty for treatment of renovascular hypertension. Radiology 131:53
4. Kuhlmann U, Vetter W, Furrer J, Lütolf U, Siegenthaler W, Grüntzig A (1980) Renovascular hypertension: treatment by percutaneous transluminal dilatation. Ann Intern Med 92:1
5. Madias NE, Ball JT, Millan VG (1981) Percutaneous transluminal renal angioplasty in the treatment of unilateral atherosclerotic renovascular hypertension. Am J Med 70:1078
6. Mahler F, Probst P, Haertel M, Weidmann P, Krneta A (1982) Lasting improvement of renovascular hypertension by transluminal dilatation of atherosclerotic and non-atherosclerotic renal artery stenoses. Circulation 65:611
7. Mahler F, Krneta A, Haertel M (1979) Treatment of renovascular hypertension by transluminal renal artery dilatation. Ann Intern Med 90:56
8. Martin EC, Mattern RF, Baer L, Fankuchen EI, Caserella WJ (1981) Renal angioplasty for hypertension: predictive factors for long-term success. AJR 137:921
9. Schwarten DE, Yune HY, Klatte EC, Grim CE, Weinberger MH (1980) Clinical experience with percutaneous transluminal angioplasty of stenotic renal arteries. Radiology 135:601
10. Tegtmayer CJ, Dyer R, Teates CD, Ayers CR, Carey RM, Wellon HA, Stanton LW (1980) Percutaneous transluminal dilatation of the renal arteries. Radiology 135:589
11. Weidmann P, De Châtel R, Schiffmann A, Bachmann E, Beretta-Piccoli C, Reubi FC, Ziegler WH, Vetter W (1977) Interrelations between age and plasma renin, aldosterone and cortisol, urinary catecholamines, and body sodium/volume state in normal man. Klin Wochenschr 55:725

42. Treatment of Renovascular Hypertension by Percutaneous Transluminal Angioplasty of Two Renal Arteries in a 5-Year-Old Boy

F. Mahler, R. Ghisla, M. Haertel, O. Oetliker, A. Krneta, and E. Rossi

Case Description

In a 4.5-year-old boy (17.5 kg, 105.5 cm) with dizzy spells, headache, and epileptic attacks a blood pressure of 180/130 mm Hg was observed. Stenoses in the left renal artery and in a right renal polar branch were shown angiographically (Fig. 1a, arrows), and renovascular hypertension was diagnosed after exclusion of other causes. Systemic renin was elevated (40 ng/ml per hour). The boy underwent bilateral percutaneous transluminal angioplasty (PTA) under general anesthesia on 23 October 1980. A F-8 guiding catheter (custom-made prototype by Schneider and Co., Zurich) was introduced through the femoral artery, and a Grüntzig coronary dilatation catheter (balloon width 3.7 mm) was applied. After dilatation both stenoses were widely patent (Fig. 1b). Blood pressure dropped to normal values within 4 h (110/80). During the follow-up of 1.5 years the blood pressure remained normal without any antihypertensive therapy except atenolol for the initial 2 months following PTA. Systemic renin was normal (9.4 ng/ml per hour) 6 months after PTA. Angiography performed 1.5 years after PTA revealed patent renal arteries at the two dilated sites (Fig. 1c, arrows).

Comment

Renovascular hypertension in children is a rare but pertinacious disease [1] requiring careful medical or surgical therapy. The underlying cause is usually fibromuscular dysplasia, and the angiograms suggest that the boy described probably belongs to this group of pediatric patients. Our positive experience with PTA for fibromuscular dysplasia in adult patients [3, 4] and the availability of the coronary dilatation catheter set [2], suitable for small arteries, encouraged us to try PTA for treatment of renovascular hypertension in this small child.

This case demonstrates that PTA of renal arteries in children with renovascular hypertension may result in normalizing blood pressure as observed in follow-up studies in adults [4]. Even though results of renovascular surgery in such patients are excellent [5], PTA compares favorably in terms of morbidity and expense. However, this is an example of an experimental application of PTA that should be performed only with the backing of experienced vascular surgeons in case of failure or complications.

Percutaneous Transluminal Angioplasty
(ed. by C. T. Dotter, A. Grüntzig, W. Schoop, E. Zeitler)

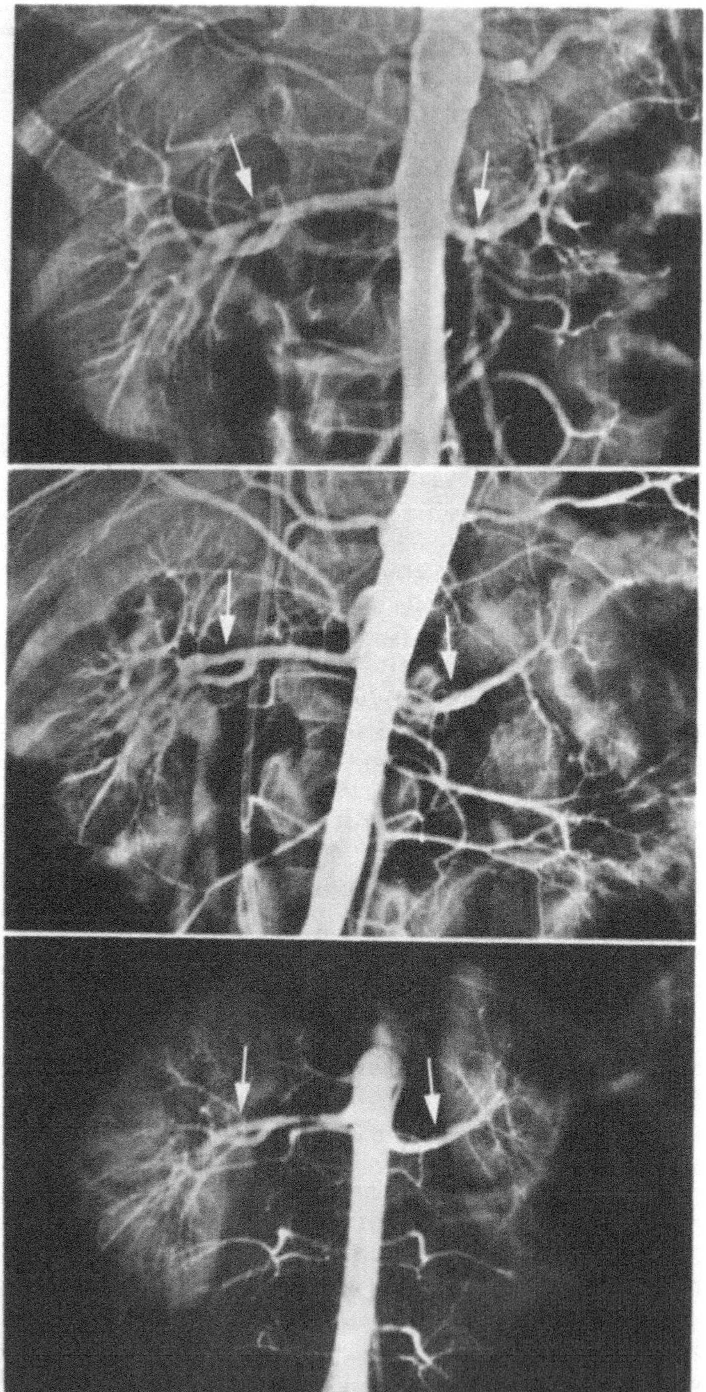

a

b

c

Fig. 1. a Renal angiogram in a 4.5-year-old hypertensive boy before PTA of the upper right polar branch artery and the left main artery *(arrow)*. **b** Angiogram immediately after dilatation of the two stenoses on the left and right sides *(arrows)*. **c** Angiogram 18 months after PTA showing patent renal arteries bilaterally *(arrows)*.

References

1. Foster JH, Pettinger WA, Oates JA, Rhamy RK, Klatte EC, Burko HC, Bolasny BL, Gordon R, Puyau FA, Younger RK (1966) Malignant hypertension secondary to renal artery stenosis in children. Ann Surg 164: 700–713
2. Grüntzig AR, Senning A, Siegenthaler WE (1979) Nonoperative dilatation of coronary-artery stenosis. N Engl J Med 301: 61–68
3. Mahler F, Krneta A, Haertel M (1979) Treatment of renovascular hypertension by transluminal renal artery dilatation. Ann Intern Med 90: 56–67
4. Mahler F, Probst P, Haertel M, Weidmann P, Krneta A (1982) Lasting: improvement of renovascular hypertension by transluminal dilatation of atherosclerotic and non-atherosclerotic renal artery stenosis: a follow-up study. Circulation 65: 611–617
5. Stanley JC, Fry WJ (1977) Surgical treatment of renovascular hypertension. Arch Surg 112: 1291–1297

43. Follow-up in Patients Undergoing Percutaneous Transluminal Angioplasty for Renal Artery Stenosis and Occlusion

W.-D. Bussmann, P. Grützmacher, R. Ruminsky, W. Faßbinder, S. Dowinsky, D. Rummel, M. Kaltenbach, and W. Schoeppe

Since February 1980 we have performed transluminal renal angioplasty [5, 6, 9] in 21 patients, including two with transplanted kidneys. The follow-up time ranged between 2 and 27 months. As a technical modification we used our own 8-F guiding catheters instead of the original 9-F catheters (Angiomed, Esslingen) [1, 2]. Except in one case no attempt was made to cross the stenosis with a guide wire. Angiography was performed using the standard equipment available in the heart catheterization laboratory: 35-mm cinefilm and 6-in amplifier.

Except in a few cases the renin mechanism seems to reflect the hypertension. During the administration of nitroprusside and a decrease in blood pressure, renal vein renin activity increased markedly. Following dilatation, baseline values were reduced and there was no increase attending pharmacologic reduction of blood pressure. One patient developed restenosis, so that renin activity remained high (Fig. 1).

The degree of stenosis declined from 83% to 32% immediately after dilatation and to 20% during the follow-up time of up to 1 year (Fig. 2).

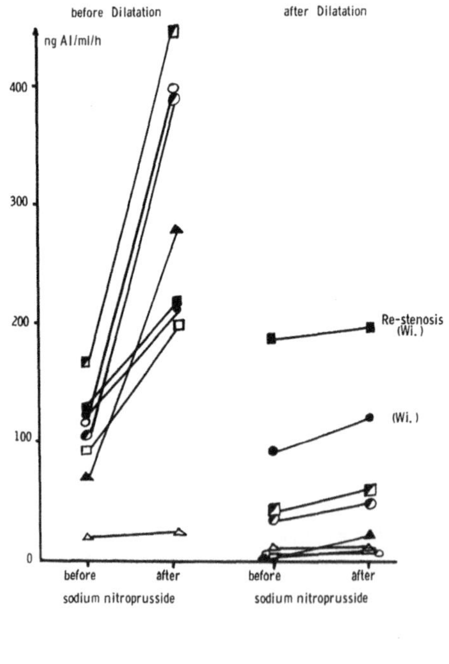

Fig. 1. Selective renin sampling. The pre-angioplasty stimulation of renin activity achieved by lowering blood pressure was no longer observable after successful dilatation *AI*, angiotensin I

Percutaneous Transluminal Angioplasty
(ed. by C. T. Dotter, A. Grüntzig, W. Schoop, E. Zeitler)

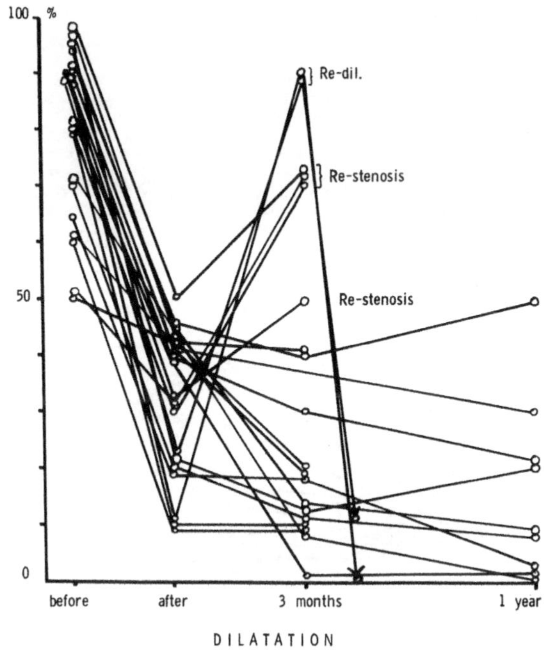

Fig. 2. The degree of stenosis declined from 83% to 32% immediately after the dilatation and further during the follow-up time up to 1 year. $n = 17$ (20)

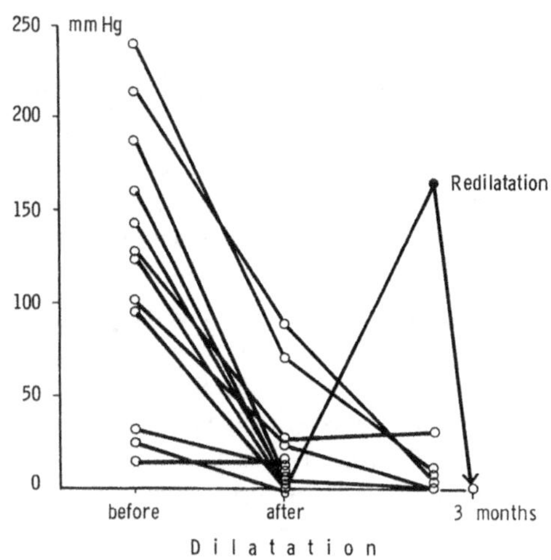

Fig. 3. Pressure gradient across renal artery stenosis before percutaneous transluminal renal angioplasty (PTRA) (123 mm Hg), immediately after PTRA (22 mm Hg), and 3 months after PTRA (7 mm Hg), including the patient who successfully underwent redilatation. $n = 10$ (12)

Significant restenosis was present at 3 months in five cases. Three of them were attempted successfully a second time. The pressure gradient across renal artery stenosis decreased from a mean of 123 mm Hg to 22 mm Hg immediately after transluminal angioplasty. There was a further decrease in most of the cases but restenosis occurred in five cases (Fig. 3). Plasma renin activity [3] declined from 32 to 12 ng immediately and to 10 ng AI ml/h after 3 months, and remained unchanged at 1 year. Restenosis was present in one case (Fig. 4) and could not be explained in a second patient (Fig. 4).

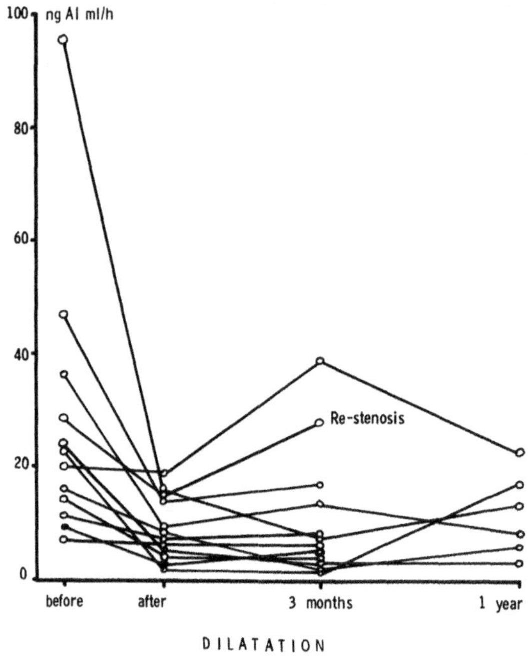

Fig. 4. Plasma renin activity before, immediately after, and 3 months after percutaneous transluminal renal angioplasty. $n = 12$. Values declined from 32 to 13 ng angiotensin I/ml per hour following dilatation and had risen only slightly at 3 months

Figure 5 shows on the left the highest systolic blood pressure – measured before treatment. After successful transluminal angioplasty there is a decrease in average systolic blood pressure, acutely and during the follow-up period. Simultaneously with the decrease in blood pressure, the mean number of antihypertensive drugs was immediately reduced from 3.5 to 2.5 and after 3 months to 2.0; it remained at that level after 1 year.

The dose of antihypertensive agents before and immediately after PTA, at 3 months, and after 1 year is shown in Fig. 6. There was a marked decrease in intake of all antihypertensive agents, diuretics, beta-blockers, antisympathicotonics, and vasodilators. In a few patients the dose of diuretics had to be increased after 1 year.

Renal function improved, especially in those patients with impairment of kidney function prior to angioplasty. This is demonstrated by a decline in serum creatinine immediately after PTA, at 3 months, and at 1 year (Fig. 7). Restenosis was associated with an increase in creatinine in three patients. In one case transient depression of renal function was present due to contrast medium. The increase in creatinine concentration in another case was not explained, and seems to be unrelated to the procedure. The time to the maximum in the radioisotope nephrogram was considerably reduced in most cases. Further improvement was present after 3 months and 1 year (Fig. 8).

The primary success rate was particularly high: all the narrowed arteries except one could be reached. The degree of stenosis was reduced by at least 20%. By 3 months later restenosis had occurred in 5 of the 19 patients. This is a

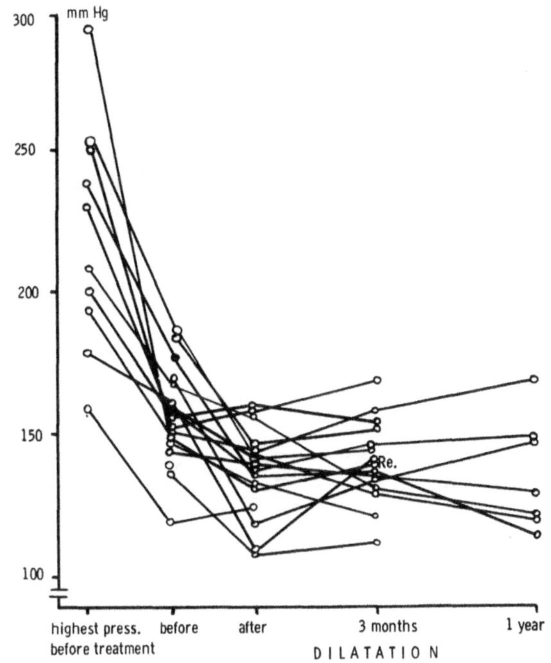

Fig. 5. The maximum systolic arterial blood pressure measured without treatment is shown on the *left side*. $n = 16$. Successful percutaneous transluminal renal angioplasty decreased systolic arterial blood pressure during the follow-up period. The number of antihypertensive drugs fell from 3.5 to 2.0 and less after 1 year. *Re.*, restenosis

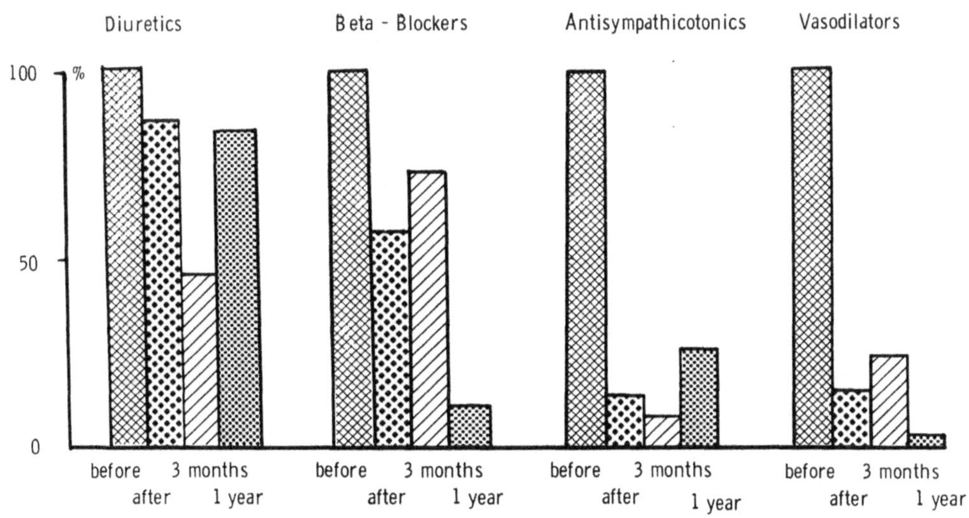

Fig. 6. Dose of antihypertensive agents before, immediately after, 3 months after, and 1 year after percutaneous transluminal renal angioplasty. Note the large decrease in the doses of these agents, except for diuretics

reoccurrence rate of about 25%, which is comparable to the rate in coronary arteries.

Redilatation was necessary in three patients and was successfully attempted. None of the seven patients seen after 1 year had developed restenosis. It is

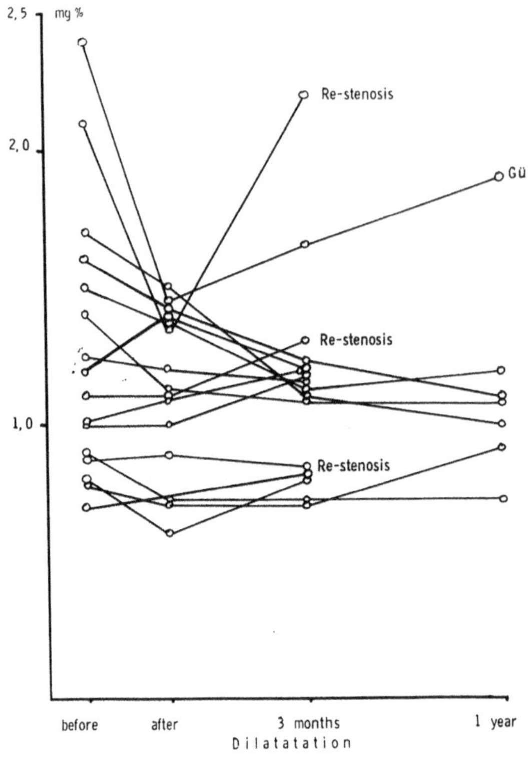

Fig. 7. Decline in serum creatinine immediately after and 3 months and 1 year after percutaneous transluminal renal angioplasty. $n = 16$. *Gü,*

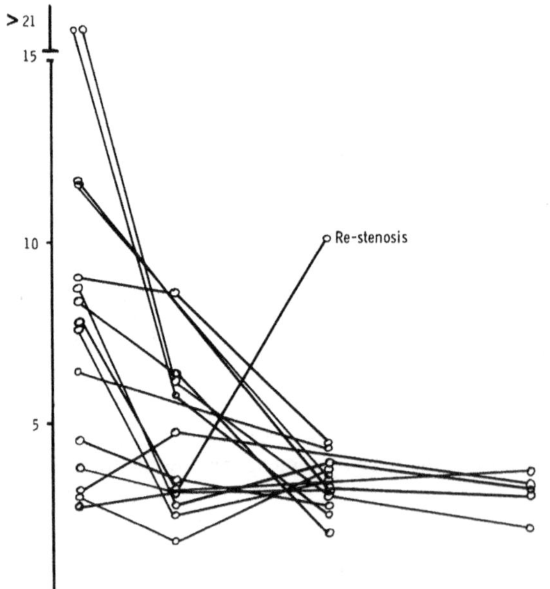

Fig. 8. Time to maximum in the radioisotope nephrogram. Shortening of the time after successful percutaneous transluminal renal angioplasty. $n = 13$ (15)

evident, therefore, that restenosis only occurred within the first 3 months. The incidence seems to have been higher among patients with fibromuscular disease.

The complication rate has been low up to now. Only one patient suffered an intimal lesion with temporary occlusion of the vessel; dilatation was nevertheless completed successfully. None of the patients had immediate thrombotic occlusion, since all were treated before, during, and after the procedure with 1.5 g aspirin per day.

There is no question about the fact that percutaneous transluminal angioplasty can be employed successfully in most renovascular hypertension patients [4, 7, 8, 10, 11–13]. Reoccurrence is rather frequent, but a second procedure can be carried out easily and with success.

Recanalization of a closed artery may be an important tool when the time interval between occlusion and reopening is short. The history of a 17-year-old girl who was completely anuric when she was referred to us is presented. She had undergone nephrectomy some years ago due to the presence of a small kidney on the left side, causing severe hypertension. Later on, a stenosis in the right renal artery was discovered. Three years later she developed hypertensive crisis, severe dyspnea, and fluid lung and gained 10 kg in weight. Dialysis was initiated and was continued for 3 weeks before she was transferred to our institution. As suspected, the right renal artery was occluded. A small branch to the upper pole of the kidney and collaterals to the main system were seen. A thrombus was recognized by the small contrast material depot within the artery.

A guide wire was gently pushed forward and a stronger one used to perforate the thrombus. Following this procedure a small channel in the renal artery was obtained. Then a 3.7-mm Grüntzig catheter was advanced without any problem and the artery was reopened by balloon inflations in successive segments. Contrast injection clearly showed displaced thrombus material in different locations in the artery. However, within minutes the intrinsic fibrinolytic elements in the blood acted to remove all the thrombus material. The vessel was widely opened to its full length. Despite an ischemic phase of nearly 3 weeks, urine production started immediately after the procedure and the serum creatinine dropped from 11 to 1.1 mg% within 10 days.

References

1. Bussmann W-D, Faßbinder W, Rummel D, Dowinsky S, Grützmacher P, Schöneberger A, Stark E, Kaltenbach M, Schoeppe W (1981) Transluminale Dilatation von Nierenarterienstenosen zur Behandlung der renovaskulären Hypertonie. Dtsch Med Wochenschr 106: 358
2. Bussmann W-D, Dowinsky S, Rummel D, Faßbinder W, Grützmacher P, Starke E, Kaltenbach M, Schoeppe W (1982) Percutaneous transluminal angioplasty in the treatment of renovascular hypertension. In: Kaltenbach M, Grüntzig A, Rentrop K, Bussmann W-D (eds) Coronary heart disease IV. Transluminal coronary angioplasty and intracoronary fibrinolysis.
3. Brecht HM (1978) Untersuchungen zur pathologischen Bedeutung des sympathischen Nervensystems, des Renin-Angiotensin-Aldosteron-Systems sowie der Na-Bilanz bei der essentiellen und renoparenchymatösen Hypertonie. Habilitationsschrift, Universität Frankfurt

4. Castaneda-Zunica WR, Formanek M, Tadavarthy M, et al. (1980) The mechanism of balloon angioplasty. Radiology 135: 565
5. Grüntzig A, Hopff H (1974) Perkutane Rekanalisation chronischer arterieller Verschlüsse mit einem neuen Dilatationskatheter. Modifikation der Dotter-Technik. Dtsch Med Wochenschr 99: 2502
6. Grüntzig A, Kuhlmann U, Vetter W, et al. (1978) Treatment of renovascular hypertension with percutaneous transluminal dilatation of a renal-artery stenosis. Lancet 1: 801
7. Hunt TC et al. (1974) Renal and renovascular hypertension: a reasoned approach to diagnosis and management. Arch Intern Med 133: 988
8. Katzen BT, Chang T, Lukowski GH, et al. (1979) Percutaneous transluminal angioplasty for treatment of renovascular hypertension. Radiology 131: 53
9. Kuhlmann U, Vetter W, Furrer T, et al. (1980) Renovascular hypertension. Treatment by percutaneous transluminal dilatation. Ann Intern Med 92: 1
10. Leu H, Grüntzig A (1978) Histopathologic aspects of transluminal recanalization. In: Zeitler E, Grüntzig A, Schoop W (eds) Percutaneous vascular recanalization. Springer, Berlin Heidelberg New York, pp 39
11. Motarjeme AJ, Keifer TW, Zuska AJ (1980) Percutaneous transluminal angioplasty and case selection. Radiology 135: 573
12. Schwarten DE, Yune HY, Klatte CE, et al. (1980) Clinical experience with percutaneous transluminal angioplasty (PTA) of stenotic renal arteries. Radiology 135: 601
13. Tegtmeyer CJ, Oyer R, Teates CD, et al. (1980) Percutaneous transluminal dilatation of the renal arteries. Radiology 135: 589

44. Renal Angioplasty in Hypertension: Technique, Radiological and Clinical Results, and Complications in 134 Dilatations

C. B. A. J. Puijlaert, G. G. Geyskes, J. H. J. Ruijs, H. P. J. Wüstefeld, and W. P. T. Mali

Method

In percutaneous transluminal renal angioplasty we use the following technique. On the contralateral side a 7-F pigtail catheter is introduced. The midstream is made. On the ipsilateral side a cobra is usually introduced, but sometimes a sidewinder. We try to pass the stenosis first with a J-wire with a very small J, then we try a J-wire with a withdrawn movable core, then a small pediatric J-guide-wire, which is changed for a bigger wire when the cobra has passed the stenosis. Finally, we try a straight wire with a flexible tip.

When the J-wire has passed the stenosis we anchor it in the peripheral renal vessels. A general midstream is made. The dilatation catheter is advanced through the stenosis. Contrast is injected through the dilatation catheter between catheter lumen and guide wire to make sure that the catheter is well placed. After the dilatation has been carried out the guide wire is left in place and the catheter is withdrawn. The midstream is made to check the results. When the result is not good enough the dilatation catheter can be advanced again or can be changed for a bigger one. Finally, the guide wire can be removed, a midstream can be made, and the final result can be assessed.

Complications

We will mention here only the complications that are really due to the dilatation technique and not the ones that come with every angiographic examination. Among our 134 cases there were two cholesterol embolizations: one of these was eventually fatal. There were two intraparenchymal contrast injections, probably without resulting damage. There were two intramural insertions of the coaxial renal balloon catheter, which destroyed the renal artery. Renal embolization was seen in six cases; three were probably permanent. In two cases perforation of the J-wire caused peripheral occlusion.

Results

The immediate technical results in 114 patients are given in Table 1. The clinical results in 80 patients after 6 months are given in Table 2. The criteria for

Percutaneous Transluminal Angioplasty
(ed. by C. T. Dotter, A. Grüntzig, W. Schoop, E. Zeitler)

Table 1. Renal artery dilatation in hypertension: immediate results and complications

Total dilations (in 114 patients)	134
Immediate good results	113
Good results after repeated dilatation	8
Direct technical failure	5
Insufficient dilatation	7
Entry impossible	3
Extravasations of parenchyma	2
Obstruction by spasm or thrombus of peripheral branch (3 permanent)	6

Table 2. Clinical results of renal artery dilatation in 80 patients (90 dilatations): follow-up > 6 months

Results		*n*	No change	Improved + cured
All patients		80	27	52 (64%)
Unilateral		59	19	39 (66%)
Bilateral	One side	7	2	5 (70%)
	Both sides	10	4	6 (60%)
Single kidney		2	0	2 (100%)
Segmental		3	2	1 (33%)
Fibromusculair		26	1	25 (95%)
Atheroma		52	25	26 (52%)

Table 3. Clinical results of renal artery dilatation in atheroma

	Patients (*n*)	BP unchanged	Improved + cured
Unilateral + bilateral	52	25 (48%)	26 (52%)
Age < 55	22	12 (54%)	10 (45%)
> 55	30	13 (43%)	16 (55%)
Serum creatinine			
< 120 μmol/l	23	11 (47%)	10 (53%)
> 120 μmol/l	29	13 (45%)	15 (50%)

BP, blood pressure

improved and cured are those of the Cooperative Study in the United States (Foster et al. 1975). In the group with atheromatous stenosis we examined the age and the serum creatinine level in order to identify subgroups that respond better to dilatation. These results are shown in Table 3.

References

1. Foster JH (1975) Renovascular occlusive disease. Results of operative treatment. JAMA 231:1043–1048

45. Percutaneous Transluminal Angioplasty of Renal Arteries – A Therapeutic Principle. Case Report of 128 Patients With Renovascular Hypertension

E. Löhr, H. C. Weichert, H. Hartjes, and A. Schrijvers

The nonoperative transluminal dilatation of renal arteries (percutaneous transluminal angioplasty, PTA) to correct arterial hypertension due to renal artery stenosis is a special form of interventional urologic radiology. Since this method was first described by Dotter and Judkins [4], multiple reports have been published by various investigators [1–3, 5, 8–11, 13–16]. Moreover, the first follow-up studies have been reported [15, 17]. The aim of PTA is twofold: to lower the arterial systemic pressure caused by stenosis of the renal arteries, and to save the affected kidney.

Materials and Methods

Arteriosclerosis is a more usual cause of renal hypertension than fibromuscular dysplasia. In 75% of our patients, renovascular hypertension was caused by arteriosclerosis. Before PTA was performed, renography, renal arteriography, and functional scintigraphic studies were carried out to detect any unilateral reduction of renal function and to exclude other forms of renovascular hypertension not based on renal artery stenosis [11]. Follow-up studies have been started, including isotope studies [5] and subtraction angiography.

Technique

Both the Grüntzig balloon catheter [6] and the coaxial catheter system [7, 8] were used. The choice of catheter system depended on the location and extent of the renovascular stenosis. Most arteriosclerotic lesions were at the orifice of the renal artery. Even with a 90% stenosis, dilatation with the balloon catheter was successful. In addition, the guided balloon technique was associated with a very small incidence of intimal laceration and rupture.

The main indications for the coaxial system is deduced by the extent of the proximal stenosis or by its peripheral location. During the first 2 years of our experience with the coaxial system in PTA of renal arteries, the material of the coaxial catheters was very stiff, so that the internal small balloon catheter could not be maneuvered very well. Since the development of new materials these problems no longer exist, however.

Percutaneous Transluminal Angioplasty
(ed. by C. T. Dotter, A. Grüntzig, W. Schoop, E. Zeitler)

Dilatation Technique and Intravasal Blood Pressure Measurements

In cases of renovascular stenosis due to arteriosclerosis, the dilatation of the vessel was performed at a pressure of 5 bar; in cases of fibrodysplasia the maximum pressure was reduced to 3–4 bar. This procedure should be repeated no more than three times, each cycle lasting no longer than 2 min. Small amounts of contrast medium injected into the artery after each dilatation make it possible to visualize the effect of dilatation and to observe complications such as intimal depots of contrast medium. Additional recording by video tape allows repeated inspection without further fluoroscopy.

Blood pressure curves were recorded continuously from the most peripheral point of the renal artery to the aorta. If the final pressure gradient across the stenosis did not exceed 5 mm Hg, the PTA was considered to have been optimal. If the pressure difference between the aorta and the renal artery was within the range of 25 mm Hg, it was regarded as successful.

Results

The results in 128 patients who had undergone PTA of the renal arteries are represented in Table 1. In 65 patients (50%) complete dilatation of the main renal artery or of segmental branches was achieved. The pressure difference was approximately 5 mm Hg. In 40 cases (31%) vascular dilatation could be considered to have been carried out successfully. In 23 cases our attempts failed or were not satifactory.

Table 1. Results of PTA in patients with renovascular hypertension

Results	No. of patients	%
Total PTAs attempted	128	100
PTAs successful	104	81
Optimal PTA[a]	65	50
PTA failed or not satisfactory	23	19

[a] Pressure difference between aorta and renal artery ca. 5 mm Hg

Table 2. Complications in patients with obliterations of the renal arteries treated by PTA

Complications	No. of patients	Surgery required
Subintimal dissection or hemorrhage	6	6
Rupture of the renal artery	2	2
Embolic obstruction of the main artery	1	1
Laceration of the brachial plexus	1	1
Anuria (transient)	2	–

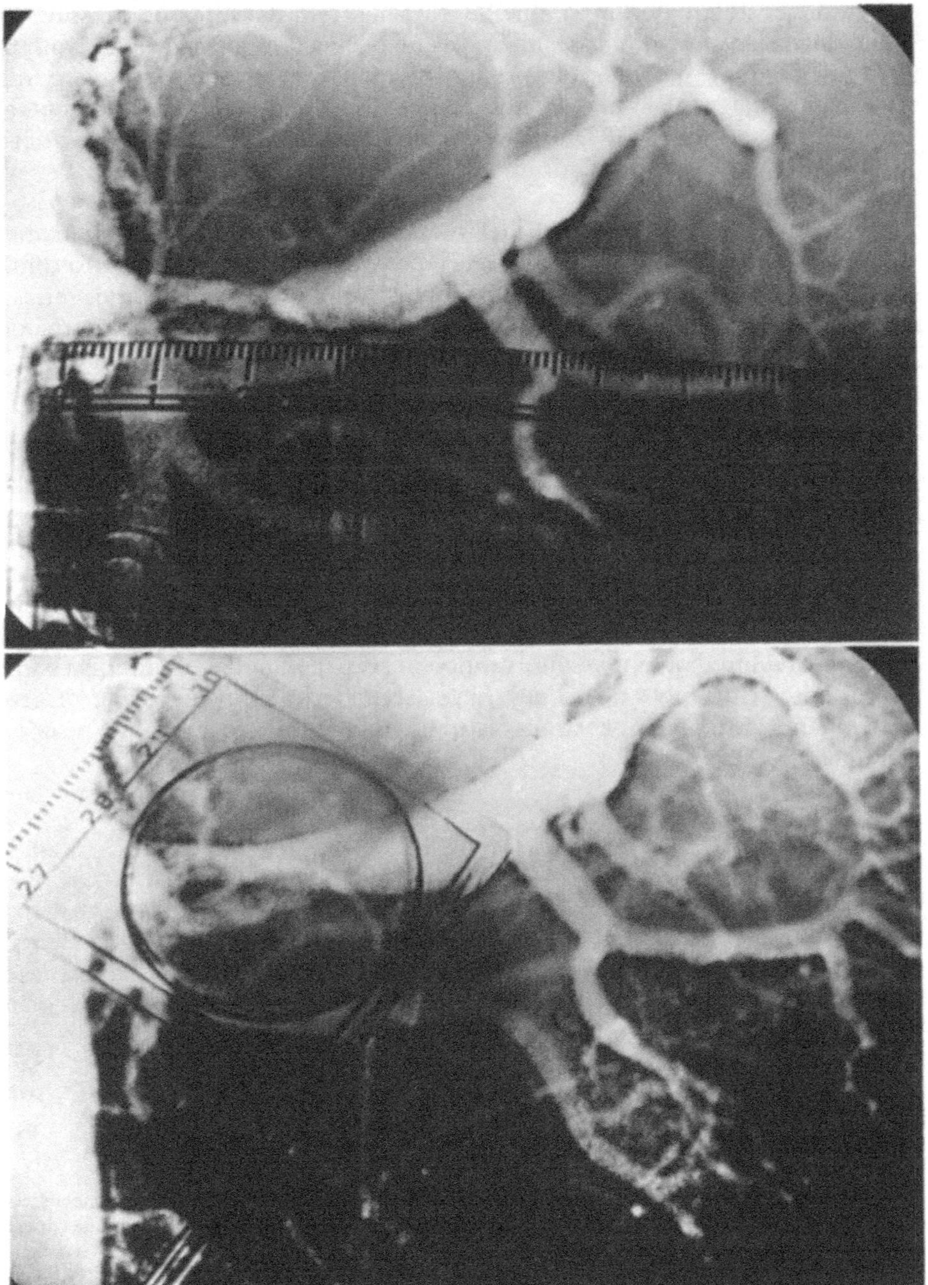

a

b

Fig. 1. Extended proximal arteriosclerotic stenosis of the main renal artery of a 56-year-old patient with a secondary solitary kidney. The balloon dilatation was entirely successful; the blood pressure reverted to normal values within 1 day. Visualization by electronically harmonized magnification

In the postdilatation phase the development of arterial blood pressure was quite different: in several cases the pressure declined to normal values with the first few hours, even when the primary systemic pressure had been very high over many years. In about 42% normal pressure could be retained without any antihypertensive drugs; 38% required reduced doses, and 38% still had arterial hypertension and required drugs in the same dosage as before PTA was attempted.

Recurrences were observed in three arteriosclerotic cases. In one patient supposed at first to be suffering a recurrence, an arteriosclerotic stenosis of the contralateral side developed within 8 months. A follow-up study of this series of patients undergoing PTA of renal arteries will collate detailed information concerning the relationship between blood pressure and kidney function.

Complications

The incidences of various complications are given in Table 2. Ruptures of the renal artery occurred in two cases, both in the early period. The kidneys (and the patients) were saved by immediate operation. In one case an arterial thrombosis developed. Laceration of the intima due to the stiff material of the first coaxial catheters required operative intervention in six patients. Patients at highest risk were those with only one kidney (most secondarily). In this group of seven patients no lasting complication occurred, though in two there was transient anuria (Fig. 1).

Conclusions

Percutaneous transluminal angioplasty of renal arteries must be acknowledged as a therapeutic means of curing hypertension due to fibrous dysplasia or arteriosclerosis. The further development of blood pressure is dependent on the caliber of the renal artery and the intrarenal vascular structures.

References

1. Bussmann WD, Fassbinder W, Rummel D, Dowinsky S, Grützmacher P, Schöneberger A, Stark E, Kaltenbach M, Schoeppe W (1981) Transluminale Dilatation von Nierenarterienstenosen zur Behandlung der renovaskulären Hypertonie. Dtsch Med Wochenschr 106: 358–363
2. Castañeda-Zuniga WR, Formanek A, Tadavarthy M, Vlodaver Z, Edwards JE, Zollikofer CH, Amplatz K (1981) The mechanism of balloon angioplasty. Radiology 135: 565–571
3. Colapinto RF (1980) Inadivertent percutaneous transluminal dilatation of renal artery with a four-year follow-up. Radiology 135: 605–606
4. Dotter CT, Judkins MP (1964) Transluminal treatment of arteriosclerotic obstruction. Description of a new technique and a preliminary report of its application. Circulation 30: 654–670

5. Funke-Völkers R, Strötges MW (1981) Veränderungen der Nierenfunktion nach Eingriffen an den Nierenarterien unter besonderer Berücksichtigung der Methode nach Dotter. Radiologe 21: 10–15
6. Grüntzig A, Hopf K (1974) Perkutane Rekanalisation chronischer arterieller Verschlüsse mit einem neuen Dilatationskatheter; Modifikation oder Dotter-Technik. Dtsch Med Wochenschr 99: 2502
7. Grüntzig A (1978) Percutaneous transluminal recanalization (PTR) with the double lumen catheter In: Zeitler E, Grüntzig A, Schoop W (eds) Percuaneous vascular recanalization. Springer, Berlin Heidelberg New York, pp 17–23
8. Grüntzig A, Kuhlmann U, Vetter W (1978) Treatment of renovascular hypertension with percutaneous transluminal dilatation of renal artery stenosis. Lancet 1: 801–802
9. Katzen BT, Chang J, Lukowsky GH, Abramson EG (1979) Percutaneous transluminal angiopasty for treatment of renovascular hypertension. Radiology 131: 53–58
10. Löhr E, Weichert HC, Kaul E, Eigler FW (1980) Nicht-Operative Gefäßdilation von Nierenarterien. Verh Dtsch Röntgen-Kongress Köln
11. Löhr E, Weichert HC, Funke-Völkers R, Strötges HW, Bildstein A (1982) Critical comments to PTA of renal arteries. Urol Radiol 4: 211–214
12. Löhr E, Langmack B (to be published) Zur Differenzierung der intrarenalen Gefäßstruktur bei Hypertonie-Patienten mittels des elektronischen Harmonisierungs- u. Vergrößerungsverfahrens. Radiologe
13. Lux E, Seybold D, Grosse-Vorholt R, Zeitler E, Gessler U (1980) Percutane transluminale Katheterdilatation von Nierenarterienstenosen bei Patienten mit renovaskulärer Hypertonie. Fortschr Med 98 (15): 563–566
14. Mathias K, Billmann P, Liebig R, Kröpelin T, Thierfelder K (1980) Behandlung der renovaskulären Hypertonie mit der Katheterdilatation. Radiologe 20: 494–499
15. Schwarten DE, Heun YY, Klatte CC, Grimm CE, Weinberger MH (1980) Clinical experience with percutaneous transluminal angioplasty (PTA) of stenotic arteries. Radiology 135: 601–604
16. Tegtmeier CJ, Dyer R, Teates C Ayers C, Carey RM, Wellons HA, Stanton LW (1980) Percutaneous dilatation of the renal arteries. Radiology 135: 589–599
17. Tegtmeier CJ, Teates CD, Crigler N, Gandee W, Ayers CR, Stoddard M, Wellons HA, Jr (1981) Percutaneous transluminal angioplasty in patients with renal artery stenosis: follow-up studies. Radiology 140 (2): 323–330
18. Zeitler E, Schoop W, Zahnow W (1971) The treatment of occlusive arterial disease by transluminal catheter angioplasty. Radiology 99: 19–26

46. Technique, Indications, Complications, and Results of Percutaneous Transluminal Renal Artery Dilatation

E.-I. Richter, E. Krönert, and E. Zeitler

Percutaneous transluminal renal artery dilatation (PTRD) was able to be seriously considered as a useful clinical method only after development of the coaxial and double-lumen balloon catheters by Grüntzig for coronary artery dilatation [9, 11, 12]. Not until a safe technique of passing a stenosis and dilating it with a balloon had been established one could speak of PTRD as an alternative to renal vascular surgery [3, 4, 9, 10, 15, 18, 22, 25, 27, 29, 30, 32, 33, 36, 41]. Between January 1978 and March 1982 we examined 70 patients (Table 1) with suspected renovascular hypertension with the objective of treating them by PTRD.

In two cases, angiography revealed renal artery occlusion which had developed from a renal artery stenosis in the interval between a previous angiogram and our repeat study. In contrast to other centers [23, 35], we did not treat totally occluded renal arteries. Seven patients had no pressure gradient between aorta and renal artery peripheral to the atheromatous wall deformation.

In a 21-year-old patient with fibromuscular renal artery stenosis who had previously undergone right nephrectomy, angiography demonstrated a high-grade renal artery stenosis on the left impossible to pass. He also had a fibromuscular stenosis in the superior mesenteric artery. This patient underwent vascular surgery.

Catheter passage failed in another four patients. A 70-year-old female with high-grade renal artery stenosis had an atrophic kidney. Two patients had aortic

Table 1. Patients considered as candidates for PTRD

No. of patients	M[a]	F[b]	Decision
70	45	25	
7	5	2	No PTRD because no pressure gradient
2	2		No PTRD because of renal artery occlusion
5	3	2	No PTRD because no passage through the stenosis (2 vascular surgery, 1 renal atrophy, 1 hypernephroma on contralateral side, 1 aortic aneurysm)
56 (91.8%)	35	21	PTRD

[a] Mean age 49.8 years (17–60); [b] mean age 34.5 (20–70)
In 61 out of 70 patients (91.8%) PTRD was indicated

Percutaneous Transluminal Angioplasty
(ed. by C. T. Dotter, A. Grüntzig, W. Schoop, E. Zeitler)

bifurcation grafts, and we used the transaxillary route in the same way as described by Tegtmeyer [38].

In the remaining 56 patients with a total of 68 renal artery stenoses (Table 2), it was possible to pass a catheter and perform balloon dilatation. Thus in our series dilatation was possible for 91.8% of the angiographically proven and hemodynamically significant stenoses and was possible in 63 out of stenoses (92.6%).

Fig. 1 shows that even dilatation on both renal arteries is possible. This 38-year-old man had high-grade left and right renal artery stenoses. The renin ratio was pathologically elevated, and blood pressure, in spite of antihypertensive medication, was about 190/120 mm Hg. The stenosis could be passed initially with the sidewinder 2 catheter. After three dilatations the poststenotic pressure on the left side was normal (Fig. 2). Thirty months after PTRD, this patient's blood pressure was able to be normalized by reduced antihypertensive medication. Only one patient required surgery for complications after renal dilatation. However, a second PTRD was necessary in 14 of our patients (26%): in 11 cases at the time of the first angiographic follow-up after 3 months; in 1 after 5 months; and in 2 cases, more than 1 year later.

Therefore, it follows that a control angiogram, if possible by means of digital subtraction angiography (DSA) [1, 5, 34], is indicated after 3 months and if hypertension persists or recurs. In cases of residual stenosis, recidivation of stenosis, or persistent hypertension, it is important to recheck the pressure gradient in the renal artery at the post-PTRD follow-up. The follow-up angiogram permits discovery of possible residual or recurrent stenoses [20, 24, 41] if the patient is not normotensive or continues to require antihypertensive drugs.

The primary success can be assessed angiographically and clinically in terms of decrease in the pressure gradient, improved perfusion on renal camera scintigraphy, and reduction in blood pressure. On average, the intraarterial systolic pressure gradient was reduced by PTRD primarily from 125 mm Hg to 28 mm Hg (Fig. 3).

Table 2. Location of stenoses and complications attending PTRD in 56 patients with 68 renal artery stenoses

Location		
Right	24	
Left	20	
Right and left	12	
Complications		4 (5.9%)
Perforation of a renal artery branch (CT control): no operation		2
Small intimal dissection: no operation		1
Thrombotic occlusion 4 days after PTRD (patient received no coumarin or ASS:		
successful vascular surgery		1 (1.5%)

CT, computer tomography; ASS, acetylsalicylic acid Percentages relate to no. of stenoses in group undergoing PTRD (68)

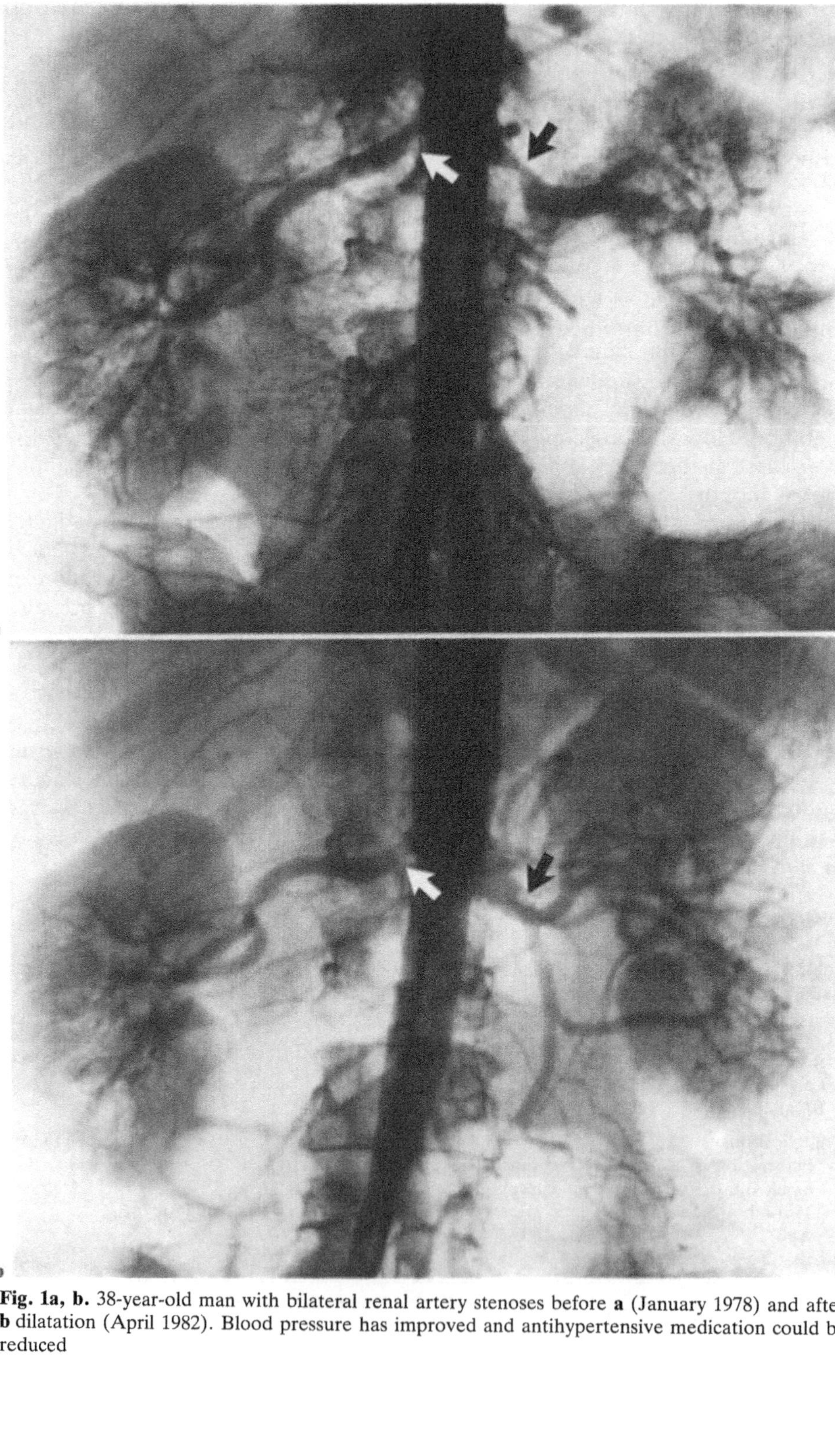

a

b

Fig. 1a, b. 38-year-old man with bilateral renal artery stenoses before **a** (January 1978) and after **b** dilatation (April 1982). Blood pressure has improved and antihypertensive medication could be reduced

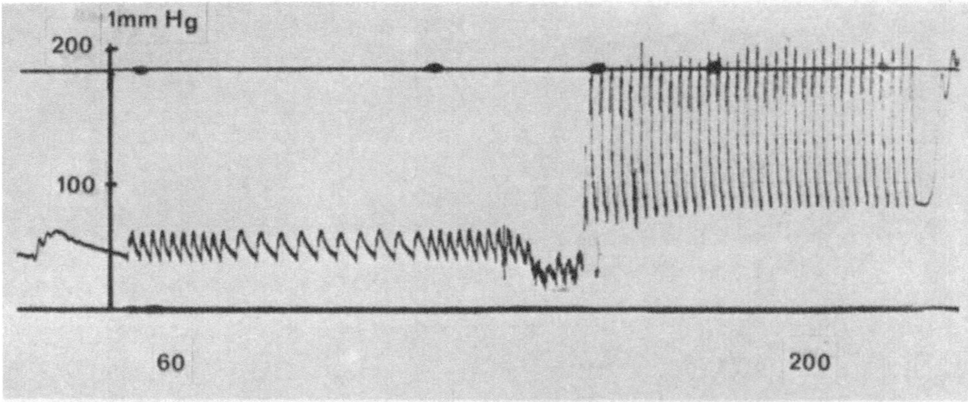

a

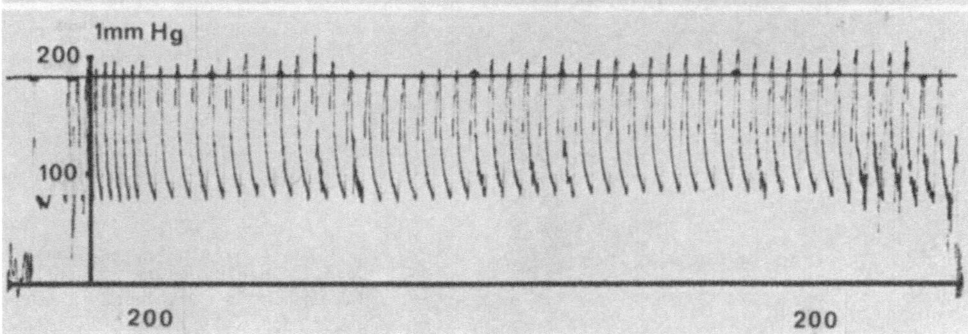

b

Fig. 2a, b. Intraarterial blood pressure control. **a** post- and prestenotic blood pressure before dilatation; **b** catheter withdrawal curve after dilatation without blood pressure gradient

In 41 patients renal function was evaluated by means of radionuclides before PTRD and repeatedly afterward [17]. In 17 cases regression of the initial rise was demonstrated (Fig. 4). In 18 further cases it had significantly decreased, and in 6 cases it remained unchanged after dilatation. Objective improvement of tubulosecretory function could be substantiated in only 65% of our patients.

The normalization of blood pressure and the reduced doses of antihypertensives required constitute the best and simplest measures of the efficacy of PTRD [2, 11, 15, 16, 19, 21, 22, 28, 30, 32, 33, 36, 37, 39, 41]. Differentiating between patients under 40 years and those over 45 (Table 3), we found that the pressure values always normalized in younger patients: drugs often were no longer necessary, and in the remaining cases the doses of the applied antihypertensives could be reduced. In 33% of the patients over 45, the blood pressure normalized without antihypertensives, and in another 33% drug therapy was still necessary. In the remaining third, however, the pressure values remained unchanged.

The first patient treated with the Grüntzig balloon catheter technique, in January 1978, was last seen at follow-up in March 1983. Initially, he had bilateral

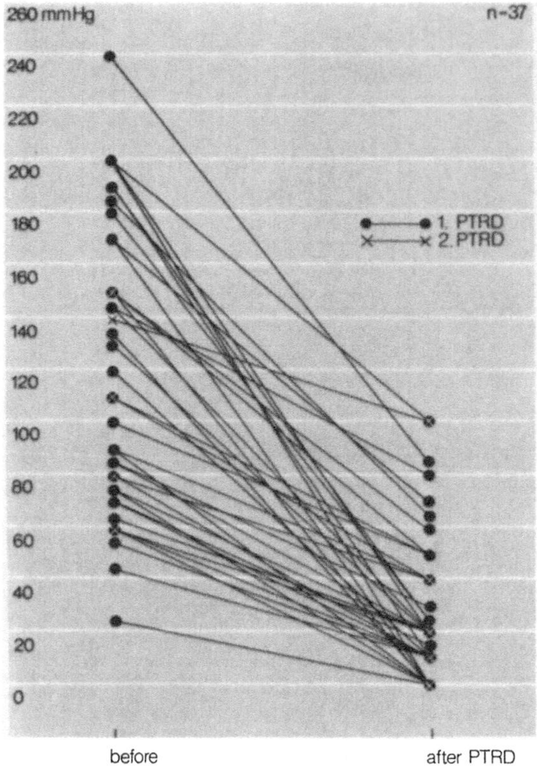

Fig. 3. Change in pressure gradient Δp after PTRD in 30 patients (37 stenoses). Mean value before PTRD, 125 mm Hg; mean value after, 28 mm Hg

Table 3. Change in blood pressure between PTRD and the last control (n = 30)

Under 40 years (n = 5)	41–45 years (n = 10)	over 45 years (n = 15)
4 normal blood pressure (80%) without drugs		5 normal blood pressure (33%) without drugs
1 normal blood pressure (20%) with drugs		5 normal blood pressure (33%) with drugs
5 normalized out of 5 (100%)	5 out of 10 with normalized blood pressure (50%)	5 unaffected hypertension (33%) in spite of drugs

Mean observation period: 12 months (2–39)

arteriosclerotic renal artery stenoses (Fig. 5). We dilated the left one in January 1978 and the right in March 1978. At that time we checked the pressure gradient on the left side. Now, 4 years later, the control angiogram shows normal renal arteries. The patient still needs antihypertensives, but at lower dosage. Instead of blood pressure values varying between 200/120 and 240/140 mm Hg, he now has values between 180/100 and 150/85 mm Hg.

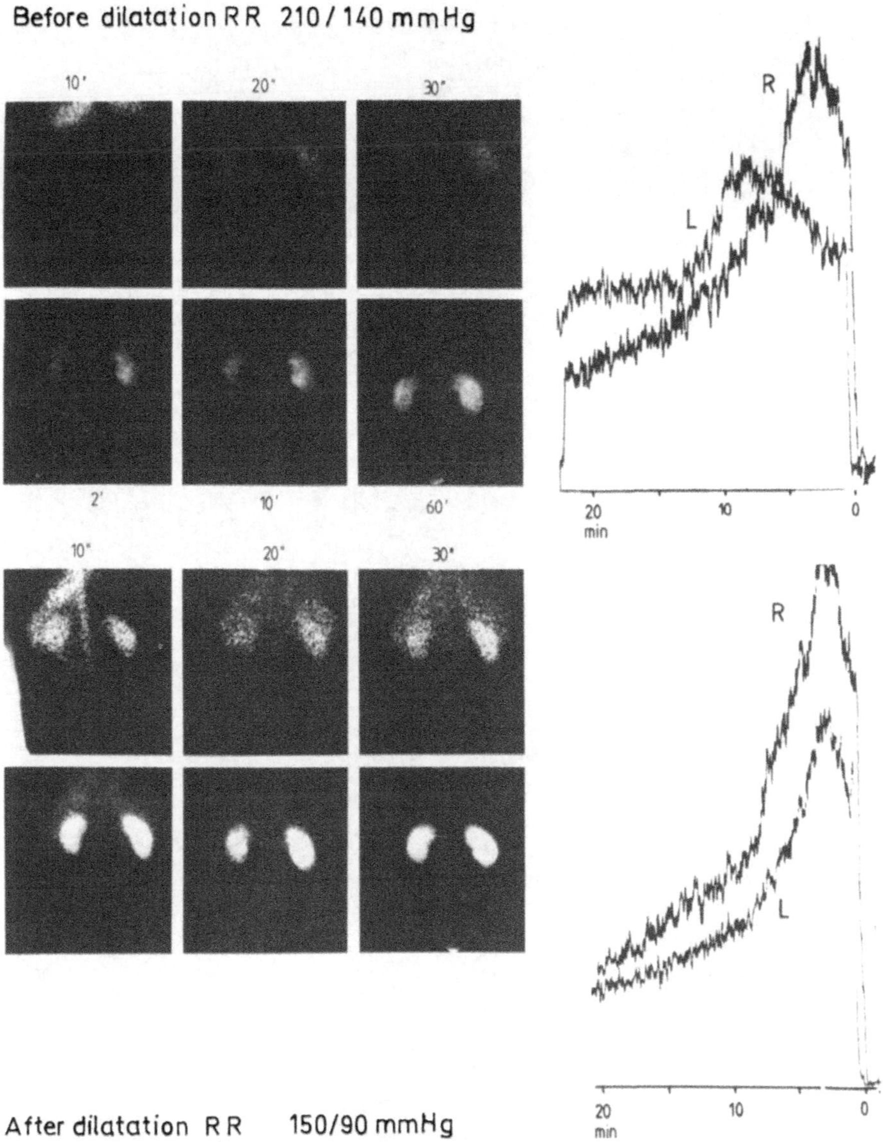

Fig. 4a, b. Sequence scintigram and isotope nephrogram. **a** before PTRD: amplitude difference as against the right side and also slight secretory disturbances; **b** control ING showing a normal course of the curve on both sides

Since the introduction of DSA [1, 5, 34] follow-up consists primarily of blood pressure measurement, monitoring of dosage and numbers of antihypertensives, and DSA performed after 3–6 months. If angiography shows residual stenoses or if hypertension has recurred, a second PTRD must be considered. If the renal artery diameter is not nearly normal and the patient remains hypertensive 3–6 months after repeated PTRD, surgical bypass technique must be considered for patients under 45 years.

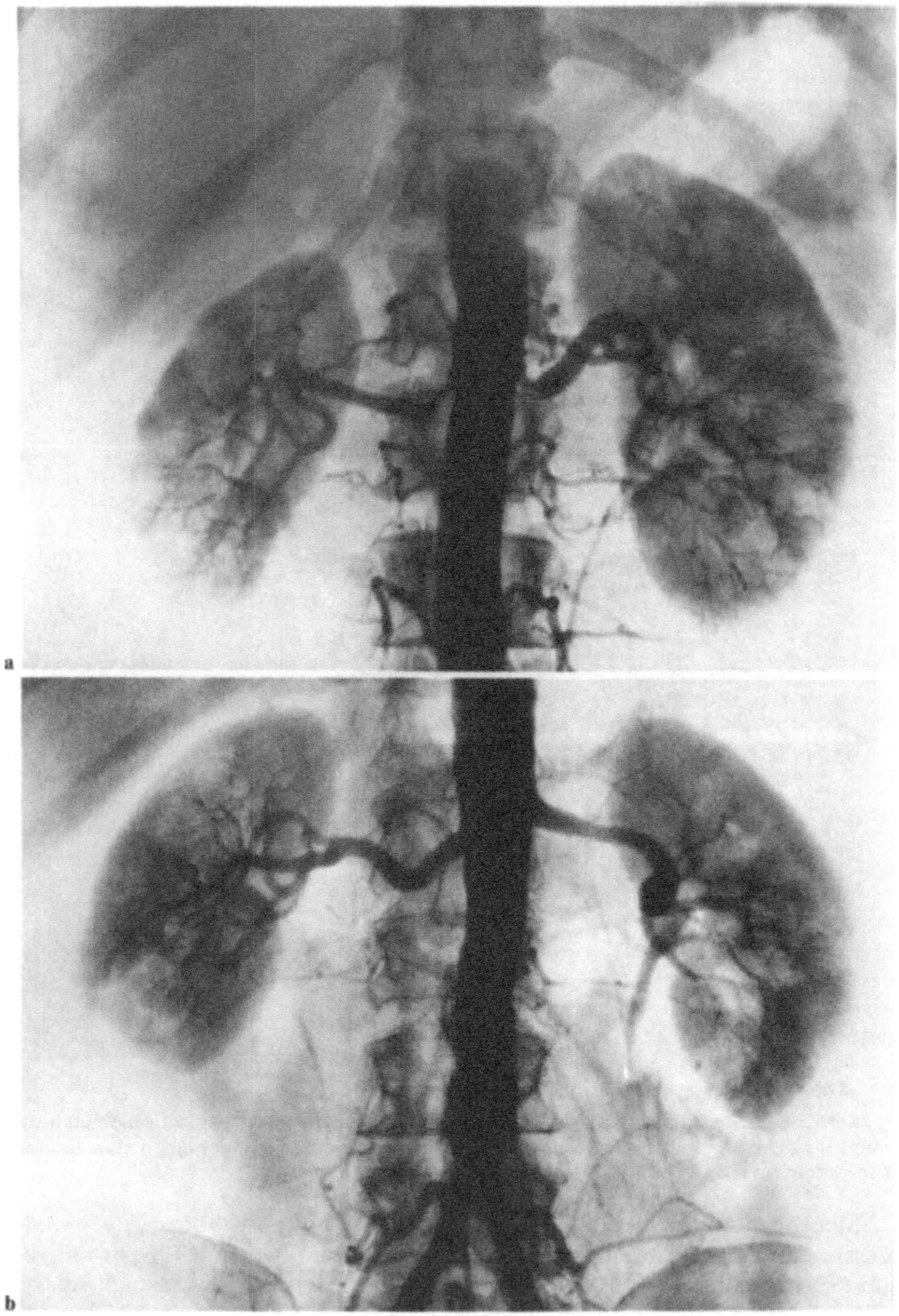

Fig. 5a, b. Bilateral arteriosclerotic renal artery stenoses in a 42-year-old man. **a** Before dilatation. **b** Four years after PTRD with Grüntzig balloon catheter; no stenoses provable. Blood pressure was normalized without antihypertensives

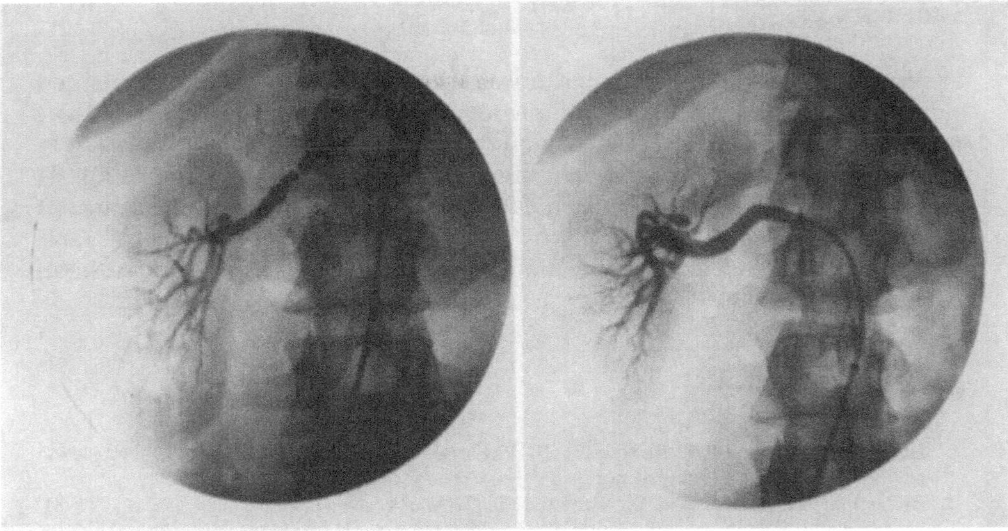
a b

Fig. 6a, b. Angiograms taken in a 36-year-old patient with fibromuscular dysplasia of the right renal artery, renovascular hypertension, and pathological right/left renin ratio. **a** before PTRD; **b** after dilatation (no stenosis)

The best results are obtained in patients under 40 years of age who suffer fibrous dysplasia [19, 20, 22, 24, 26, 28, 31, 32, 39]. Such patients were found in our series. As described above, one patient who had previously undergone right nephrectomy had fibromuscular stenoses of the left renal artery and the superior mesenteric artery which could not be passed at angioplasty. This patient was treated by means of a venous bypass graft. Another patient underwent successful dilatation but received neither aggregation inhibitors nor anticoagulants afterward. Thrombosis occurred at the site of the previous stenosis 4 days after the procedure, and a venous bypass was successfully performed. Both of these patients and the remaining cases of fibromuscular dysplasia undergoing dilatation became normotensive (Fig. 6).

A special problem is posed in the dilatation of renal artery stenoses in transplanted kidneys [3, 26]. Mathias and Sniderman [27, 36] were the first who reported such treatment. Stenoses of an aortorenal venous interposition can also be successfully dilated [14].

Among our patients were three cases of renal artery stenosis in a transplanted kidney. Dilatation was technically successful in two patients. In one of these the kidney was saved and the blood pressure better controlled by means of additional antihypertensive medication. The other patient experienced rejection independent of the arterial stenosis.

The findings to date allow us to state that results comparable to those of surgery are possible in patients with fibromuscular dysplasia who are under 45 years of age [6–8, 13, 40]. Future studies are necessary for definitive assessment of PTRD results with respect to success rate and complications.

Summary

The results of PTRD in 68 renal artery stenoses and stenoses of 3 transplanted kidneys, obtained during a mean follow-up of 15 months (range 1–51 months), show that PTRD is a very effective method. Without question, more and longer follow-up controls are necessary and should be compared to the good results of vascular surgery. So far, the 6-day death rate after PTRD is quite insignificant (below 1%). Complications which need vascular surgery are very rare. Nonetheless, close clinical observation for the first 2–3 days is required in all cases.

References

1. Buonocore E, Meaney TF, Borkowski GP, Pavlicek W, Gallagher J (1981) Digital substraction angiography of the abdominal aorta and renal arteries. Radiology 139: 281–286
2. Bussmann WD, Faßbinder W, Rummel D, Dowinsky S, Grützmacher P, et al. (1981) Transluminal Dilatation von Nierenarterienstenosen zur Behandlung der renovaskulären Hypertonie. Dtsch Med Wochenschr 106: 258–362
3. Casarella WJ (1979) Preliminary results with renal angioplasty. Combined meeting of the European College of Angiography and the American Society of Cardiovascular Radiology, Dublin, June 1979
4. Colapinto RF, Harries-Jones EP, Johnson KW (1980) Percutaneous transluminal dilatation and recanalization in the treatment of peripheral vascular disease. Radiology 135: 583–587
5. Crummy AB, Strother CM, Sacket JP, et al. (1980) Computerized fluoroscopy: digital substraction for intravenous angiocardiography and arteriography. AJR 1131–1140
6. Eigler FW, Jakubowski D, Schneiders H (1976) Early and late complications following surgical correction of renovascular hypertension. Contrib Nephrol 3: 104
7. Forster JH, Maxwell MH, Franklin SS, Bleifer KH, Trippel OH, Julian OC, Decamp PT, Varady PT (1975) Renovascular occlusive disease: results of operative management. JAMA 231: 1043–1048
8. Franklin SS, Young JD Jr, Maxwell MH, Forster JH, Palmer JM, Cerny J, Varady PD (1975) Operative morbidity and mortality in renovascular disease. JAMA 231: 1148
9. Grüntzig A (1976) Perkutane Dilatation von koronarstenoser Beschreibung eines neues Kathetersystems. Klin Wochenschr 54: 543
10. Grüntzig A, Kumpe DA (1979) Technique of percutaneous angioplasty with the Grüntzig balloon catheter. AJR 312: 547–552
11. Grüntzig A, Vetter W, Meier B, Kuhlmann U, Lütolf U, Siegenthaler W (1978) Treatment of renovascular hypertension with percutaneous transluminal dilatation of a renal artery stenosis. Lancet I: 801
12. Grüntzig A, Senning A, Siegenthaler W (1979) Nonoperative dilatation of coronary artery stenoses: percutaneous transluminal coronary angioplasty (PTCA). N Engl J Med 301: 61–68
13. Hunt JC, Strong CG (1973) Renovascular hypertension: mechanisms, natural history and management. Ann J Cardiol 32: 562–574
14. Ingrisch H, Härlin M (1980) Perkutane transluminale Angioplastik einer Stenose in einem aortorenalen Veneninterpositionstransplantat. ROEFO 133/5: 493–495
15. Ingrisch H, Holzgreve H, Middeke N, Frey KW (1980) Moderne röntgenologische Diagnostik und Therapie des Hochdruckes bei Nierenarterienstenosen. Klin Wochenschr 58: 1105–1115
16. Katzen BT, Chang J, Lukowsky G, Abramson E (1979) Percutaneous transluminal angioplasty for treatment of renovascular hypertension. Radiology 131: 53–58
17. Krönert E, Grosse-Vorholt R (1981) Nephrographie und Kamerasequence-Scintigraphie der Nieren zur Verlaufsbeobachtung und Therapiekontrolle von Kathetereingriffen an den

Nierenarterien. In: Schmidt HAE, Wolf F, Mahlstedt J (Hrsg.) Nuklearmedizin – Nuklearmedizin im interdisziplinären Bezug. Schattauer, Stuttgart, pp 508–511
18. Kuhlmann U, Grüntzig A, Vetter W, Furrer J, Lütolf U, Siegenthaler W (1978) Renovaskuläre Hypertonie: Therapie durch perkutane transluminale Dilatation von Nierenarterienstenosen. Schweiz Med Wochenschr 108/47: 1847–1859
19. Kuhlmann U, Vetter W, Furrer J, Lütolf U, Siegenthaler W, Grüntzig A (1980) Renovascular hypertension. Treatment by percutaneous transluminal dilatation. Ann Intern Med 92: 1
20. Kuhlmann U, Vetter W, Schneider E, Greminger P, Pouliadis G, Siegenthaler W (1982) Initial and long-term results after PTA in renal artery stenoses. VASA 11: 353–357
21. Lantz MT, Link DP, Lewis EL, Foerster JM, Lee G (1981) Renal artery blood flow assessed by video dilution technique before and after percutaneous transluminal angioplasty. Acta Radiol (Diagn) 22: 49–57
22. Lux E, Seybold D, Grosse-Vorholt R, Zeitler E, Gessler U (1980) Perkutane transluminale Katheterdilatation von Nierenarterienstnosen bei Patienten mit renovaskulärer Hypertonie. Fortschr Med 98/15: 563–658
23. Mahler F (1982) Transluminale Nierenarteriendilatation. Symposium, Lyon
24. Mahler F, Probst B (1982) Technique and complications of PTA in renal artery stenoses. VASA 11: 353–357
25. Mahler F, Krneta A, Haertel M (1979) Treatment of renovascular hypertension by transluminal renal artery dilatation. Ann Intern Med 90: 56–57
26. Martin EC, Diamond NG, Casarella WJ (1980) Percutaneous transluminal angioplasty in nonatherosclerotic disease. Radiology 135: 27–33
27. Mathias K, Rau W, Kauffmann G (1979) Katheterdilatation einer Arterienstenose nach Nierentransplantation. Dtsch Med Wochenschr 104: 437–438
28. Millan VG, Mast WE, Madias NE (1979) Nonsurgical treatment of severe hypertension due to renal-artery intimal fibroplasia by percutaneous transluminal angioplasty. N Engl J Med 300: 1371
29. Puijlaert C (1979) Preliminary report in dilatation of renal artery stenosis in hypertension with the aid of a balloon catheter. J Belge Radiol 62: 345–355
30. Richter E-I, Grüntzig A, Ingrisch H (1980) Percutaneous dilatation of renal artery stenoses. Ann Radiol (Paris) 23/4: 275–278
31. Saddekni S, Sniderman KW, Hilton S (1980) Percutaneous transluminal angioplasty of nonatherosclerotic lesions. AJR 135: 975–982
32. Schwarten DE (1980) Percutaneous transluminal angioplasty of renal artery. Cardiovasc Intervent Radiol 34: 197–206
33. Schwarten DE, Yune HY, Klatte EC, Grim CE, Weinberger MH (1980) Clinical experience with percutaneous transluminal angioplasty (PTA) of stenotic renal arteries. Radiology 135: 601–604
34. Seyferth W, Marhoff P, Zeitler E (1982) Transvenöse und arterielle digitale Video-Subtraktionsangiographie (DVSA). ROEFO 136: 3
35. Sniderman KW, Sos TA (1982) Percutaneous transluminal recanalization and dilatation of totally occluded renal arteries. Radiology 142: 607–610
36. Sniderman KW, Sos TA, Sprayregen S, et al. (1980) Percutaneous transluminal angioplasty in renal transplant arterial stenosis for relief of hypertension. Radiology 135: 23–26
37. Sörensen R, Grüntzig A, Apitzsch DE, Oelker W, Pellnitz W (1979) Transluminale Angioplastie von Nierenarterienstenosen zur Behandlung des renalen Hochdrucks. ROEFO 131: 575
38. Tegtmeyer CJ, Ayers CA, Wellons HA (1980) The axillary approach to percutaneous renal artery dilatation. Radiology 135: 775–776
39. Tegtmeyer CJ, Elson J, Glass TA, Ayers CR, Chevalier RL, Wellons HA, Studdard WE (1982) Percutaneous transluminal angioplasty: the treatment of choice for renovascular hypertension due to fibromuscular dysplasia. Radiology 143: 631–637
40. van Dongen RJAM (1971) Ergebnisse der Wiederherstellungschirurgie bei renovaskulärem Hochdruck. In: Denck H, Flora G, Hilbe G, Plza F (eds) Renovaskuläre Hypertonie. Wiener Med Akademie, Vienna, pp 223–229
41. Zeitler E, Grosse-Vorholt R, Lux E, Gessler U (1982) Percutaneous transluminal recanalization (angioplasty) in renal arteries (PTRDR). In: Kaltenbach S, et al. (eds) Transluminal coronary angioplasty and intracoronary thrombolysis. Springer, Berlin Heidelberg New York

XII. Indications for Percutaneous Transluminal Angioplasty

47. Special Indications for Angioplasty

F.-J. Roth and G. Cappius

Angioplasty has become an increasingly popular technique for treating stenoses and occlusions of the iliofemoral arteries [4, 18, 19, 23, 26–28], as well as the renal [7, 8, 11, 20, 22], the coronary [9], and the subclavian arteries [12–15].

Recent reports suggest a wide spectrum of applications for percutaneous transluminal angioplasty. Up to now stenoses of the visceral and the brachiocephalic arteries and of the abdominal aorta [17, 24, 29] have been described. Basically there are two less common applications of angioplasty: (a) nonatherosclerotic lesions and lesions following vascular surgery, and (b) atherosclerotic lesions with an unusual localization or an unusual radiographic appearance.

Nonatherosclerotic Lesions

Case Report

A 58-year-old woman suffered from severe claudication of both arms. She was no longer able to comb her hair. Arteriography revealed both brachial arteries (Fig. 1) to be duplicated, each with a significant stenosis in its proximal segment. Angioplasty was successfully attempted in both arms using the brachial approach (Fig. 1).

We also treated six brachial arteries in three other women with claudication of the arms due to an occlusion or a stenosis of the brachial arteries. In four cases we were successful and short-term follow-up (8–29 months) of two women demonstrated a good result. Both were asymptomatic, and the blood pressure and the oscillograms were normal.

Angioplasty of Venous Bypass Graft

If patients suffer from recurrent claudication following venous bypass graft, the arteriogram may reveal an occlusion of the graft, a stenosis of the graft, or occlusion of an artery proximal or distal to the bypass graft. In cases of long-standing occlusion of the graft angioplasty cannot usually be accomplished.

Percutaneous Transluminal Angioplasty
(ed. by C. T. Dotter, A. Grüntzig, W. Schoop, E. Zeitler)

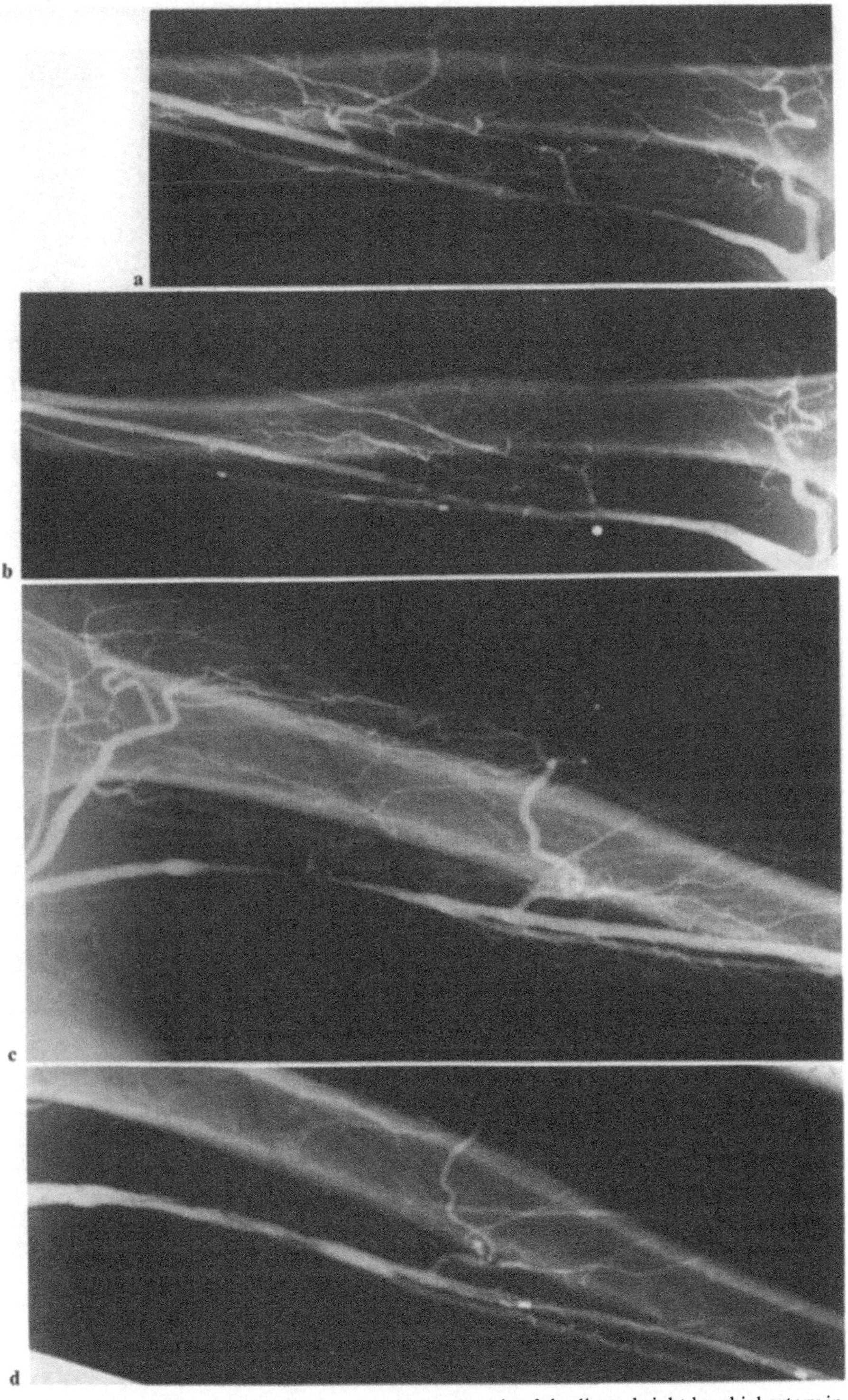

Fig. 1a–d. Arteriograms of brachial artery showing **a** stenosis of duplicated right brachial artery in the proximal segment, **b** patent right brachial artery after angioplasty, **c** stenosis of left duplicated brachial artery in the proximal segment, and **d** patent left brachial artery after angioplasty

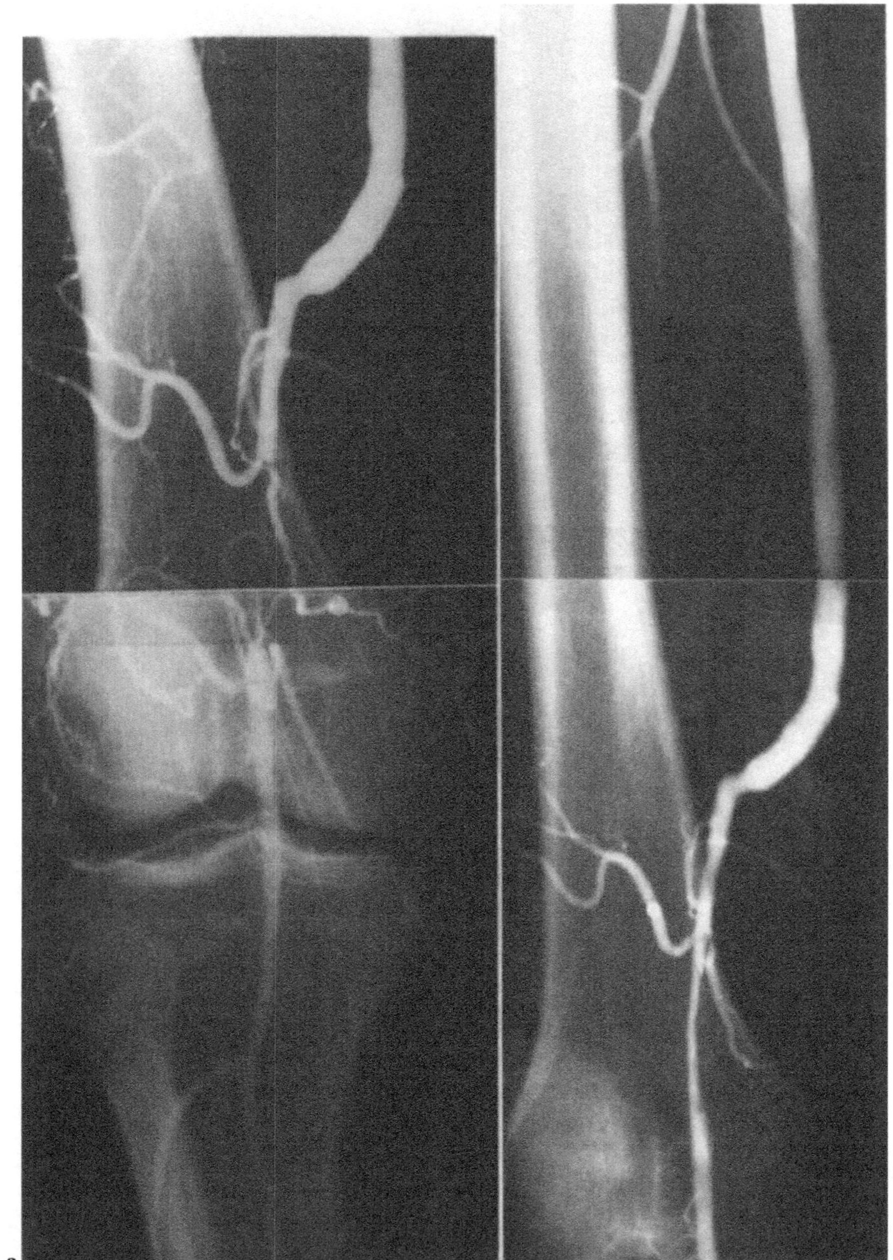

Fig. 2a, b. Arteriograms of the superficial femoral artery showing **a** patent femoropopliteal venous graft and occlusion of the popliteal artery distal to the venous graft, and **b** recanalized popliteal artery and venous graft still patent

If an artery proximal or distal to the bypass graft is occluded, routine angioplasty may be performed. In most of these instances the balloon catheter has to be advanced through the graft (Fig. 2). The stenosis of the venous bypass graft itself may be caused by an intimal thickening, fibrosis of the venous valve, fibrosis due to the surgical trauma, suture stenosis, or an atherosclerotic-like lesion [21].

No compressible core substance is found in stenoses of venous grafts except in the case of the atherosclerotic-like lesions. Therefore, the mechanism of angioplasty in venous grafts is believed to be localized overstretching of the graft by the maneuvring dilating catheter in most cases.

The technique used for angioplasty of venous grafts depends on the localization of the lesions. The venous graft should not be directly punctured as this may lead to further injury of the graft itself.

Case Reports

A 50-year-old man had a femoropopliteal venous graft because of severe claudication. When postoperative claudication occurred a year later, an arteriogram revealed two stenoses (Fig. 3a, b). The one in the proximal part of the graft was probably an atherosclerotic-like lesion and the one in the distal segment was thought to be a suture stenosis. Both were dilated by a balloon catheter using the common femoral approach (Fig. 3c, d).

A 44-year-old man had a femoropopliteal venous bypass graft because of an occlusion of the distal superficial femoral artery (Fig. 4a). The graft was accomplished by means of a duplicated saphenous vein. When postoperative claudication occurred 4 years later, both channels of the vein were found to be proximally stenotic. The two segments were satisfactorily dilated by means of a balloon catheter, using the crossover technique (Fig. 4b).

A 50-year-old man had a left nephrectomy and an aortorenal venous bypass graft on his right kidney because of a renal artery stenosis which caused renal hypertension. When recurrence occurred, a stenosis of the venous bypass graft was angiographically demonstrated (Fig. 5a, b). Angioplasty was successfully attempted and the patient became normotonic. One year later the patient suffered again from hypertension and an arteriogram (Fig. 5c, d) revealed a restenosis. Angioplasty of the aortorenal bypass graft was successfully repeated and the patient's blood pressure returned to normal again.

Atherosclerotic Lesions

Patients with atherosclerotic disease mostly suffer from claudication or gangrene of the lower and seldom of the upper extremities. Therefore, angioplasty of the upper extremity is not very often required. On the other hand, vascular surgery of the carotid artery or of the aorta gives good primary and long-term results. Nevertheless, angioplasty of the upper extremity or of the aorta sometimes has

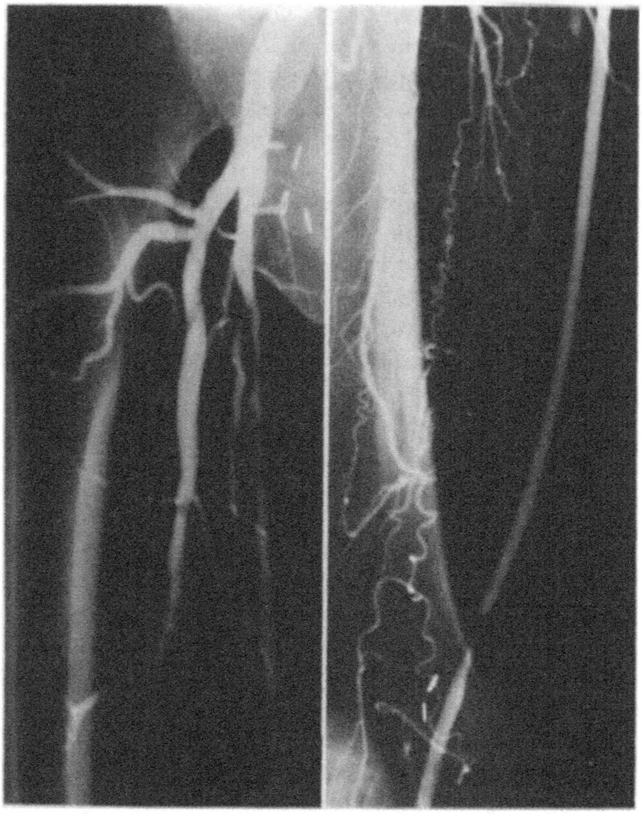

a b

Fig. 3a–d. Arteriograms of the superficial femoral artery showing **a, b** femoropopliteal venous bypass graft with a stenosis on its proximal and distal part, and **c, d** (after angioplasty) no stenosis in the proximal part but slight residual stenosis in the distal part of the venous graft. The patient was clinically improved after angioplasty

to be attempted because there are patients for whom surgery involves considerable riks. Angioplasty of the aorta is technically difficult. Some authors introduce two or even three balloon catheters at once in order to widen stenoses of this large vessel.

Case Reports

In a 72-year-old woman suffering from severe claudication of the left arm due to a stenosis of the axillary artery, angioplasty was carried out with a good primary result (Fig. 6a, b). The patient became free of symptoms and the blood pressure and oscillogram reverted to normal.

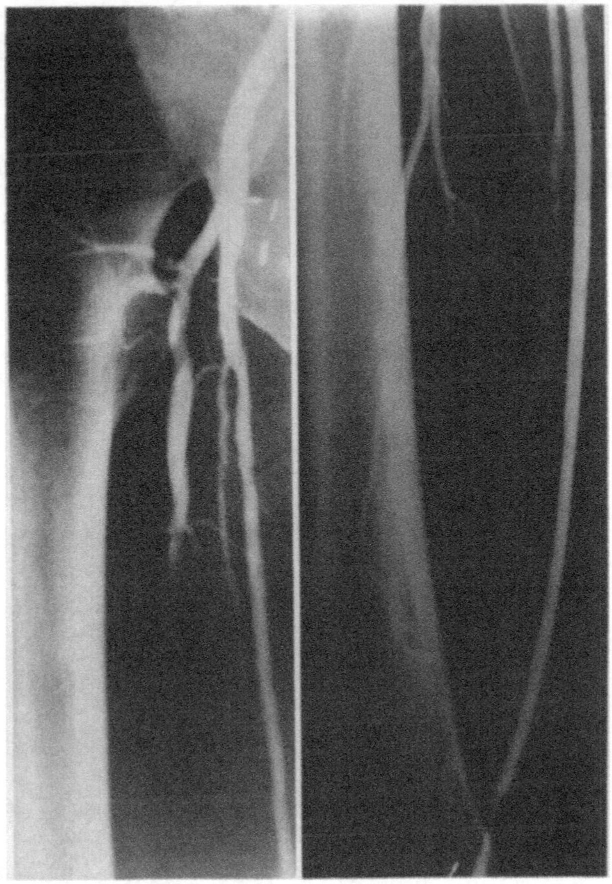

Fig. 3c, d

In a 58-year-old lady suffering from a defect of the mitral valve and severe claudication of both legs, an arteriogram revealed a significant atherosclerotic stenosis of the infrarenal aorta. A dissection of the aorta remaining from a former coronarography was well outlined (Fig. 7). The aortic stenosis was successfully widened by means of one 10-mm balloon catheter and using the common femoral approach. The patient improved clinically.

Discussion

Angioplasty is much more rarely applied for nonatherosclerotic lesions than for atherosclerotic ones [16, 17]. There are no reports of angioplasty for a

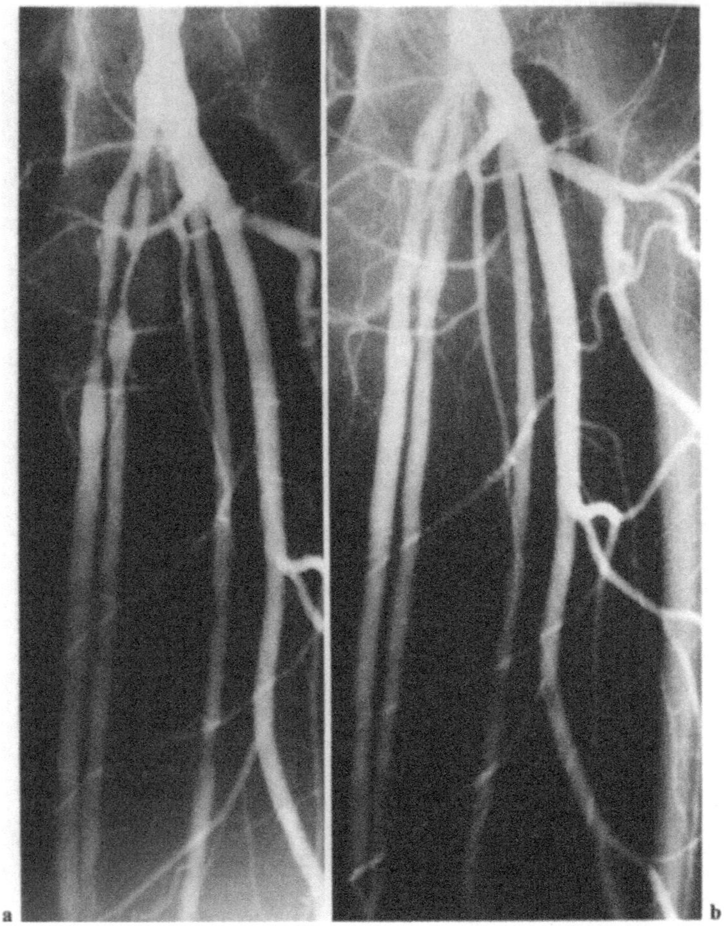

Fig. 4a, b. Arteriograms of the superficial femoral artery showing **a** femoropopliteal venous bypass graft performed by means of a duplicated saphenous vein, both channels stenotic at their proximal part, and **b** (after angioplasty) patent bypass graft with irregularities of the vessel wall in the area of the former stenoses

nonatherosclerotic lesion of the brachial artery to be found in the literature. We treated three patients bilaterally and succeeded completely in four arteries and partly in two. During short-term follow-up (8–29 months) of our four successfully treated arteries we found that all patients became free of symptoms, and the oscillogram as well as the blood pressure were normalized. Clinically, the women improved in both arms, even when angioplasty of the brachial artery had partly failed. In angioplasty of the brachial artery or of the aortic arch branches the brachial or axillary approach should be preferred in order to avoid neurological complications. We did not observe any severe complications in our patients. Because follow-up was short and the number of patients small, the question of the value of angioplasty in nonatherosclerotic lesions cannot yet be answered.

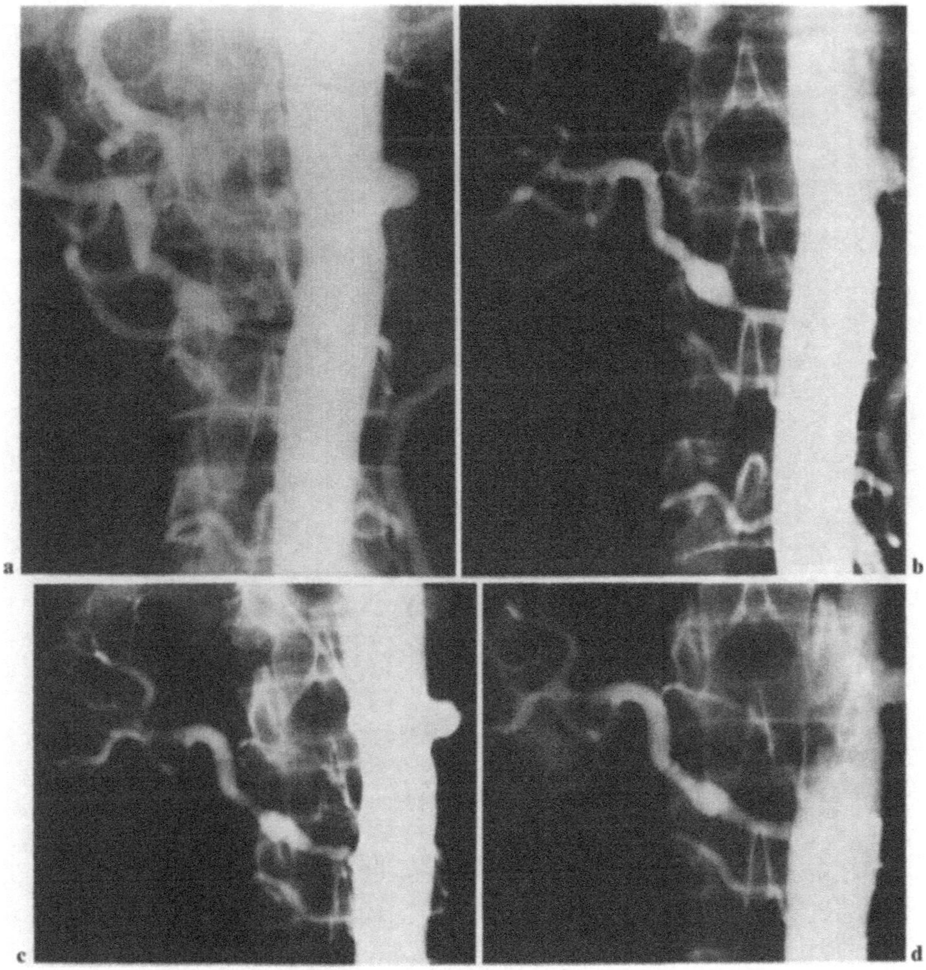

Fig. 5a–d. Aortograms showing **a** right kidney with significant stenosis of an aortorenal venous bypass graft and small vascular stump of the left renal artery following nephrectomy, **b** (after angioplasty) patent aortorenal bypass graft, **c** (at 1-year follow-up) restenosis of the aorotorenal venous bypass graft adjacent to the anastomosis, and **d** (after repeated angioplasty) patent venous graft

Angioplasty is useful in patients with recurrent disease after venous bypass graft surgery, and reoperation may be avoided [25]. Zajko and co-workers [25] have the most experience in this field. They gain good primary results by directly puncturing the venous graft, and have observed no severe complications. In our opinion the direct puncture of the venous graft should be aboided in order to prevent further damage to the graft itself. It is obvious that the mechanism of angioplasty of the venous graft is probably an overstretching of the graft wall, because the stenotic lesions are mostly caused by proliferation of the intima and media or by fibrosis as a result of instrumental damage or fibroplastic

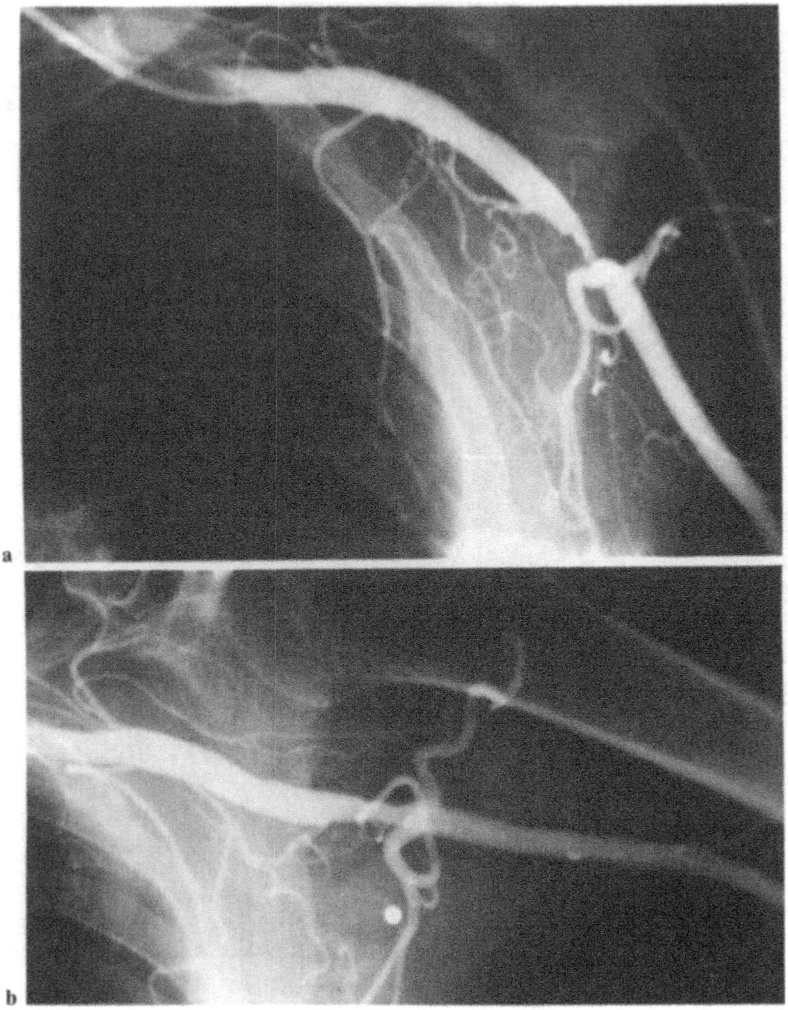

Fig. 6a, b. Arteriograms of the subclavian artery showing **a** stenosis of the axillary artery and **b** (after angioplasty) irregularities in the area of the former stenosis

organization of sequential mural thrombus. We performed angioplasty of five femoropopliteal and four aortorenal venal bypass grafts with good primary results. In all our cases recurrence occurred approximately 1 year after treatment. Possibly injury by the dilating balloon itself causes the restenosis. But our own experience of angioplasty of venous bypass grafts and that of other groups as reported in the literature is poor, and no long-term results are available. It is therefore not known whether patients with vein grafts will benefit from this therapeutic principle.

In the literature there are few case reports about angioplasty of stenosed abdominal aortas [6, 24, 29]. Velasquez et al. [24] and Zorn-Bopp et al. [29] use

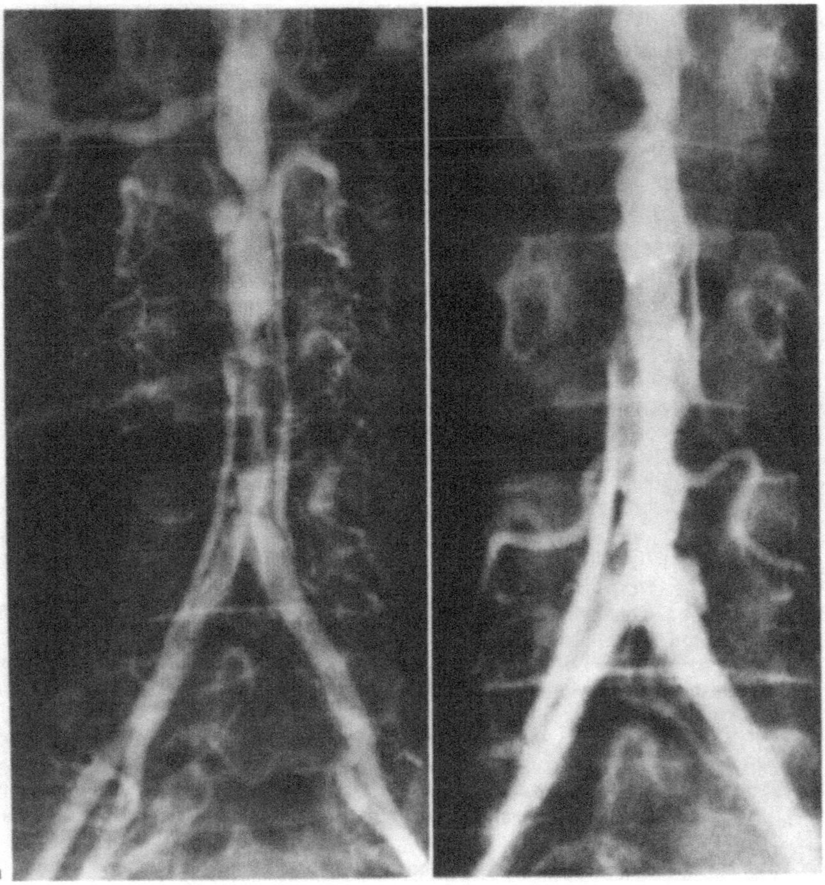

Fig. 7a, b. Aortograms showing **a** severe atherosclerotic stenosis of the infrarenal aorta and dissection of the aorta remaining from a former coronarography, and **b** (after angioplasty) patent aorta with irregularities of the vessel wall and slight residual stenosis

two balloon catheters in angioplasty of the aorta (kissing balloons). We used the single- and the two-balloon-catheter methods and feel that the single-catheter method should be preferred in order to avoid additional damage to the healthy arteries and reduce the risk of complications at the puncture site. We treated two patients using the single- and one patient using the two-balloon catheter method, each of them with good primary results.

Summary

To emphasize the potential application of transluminal angioplasty to the treatment of stenotic and occlusive lesions throughout the vascular system, some less common uses of the Dotter procedure are illustrated: nonatherosclerotic and unusual atherosclerotic lesions, and those following vascular surgery. The technique, the primary results, and the indications for angioplasty of the brachial artery, the aorta, and the venous bypass grafts are discussed. Long-term results are not yet available, either in the literature or as a result of our studies.

References

1. Bachmann DM, Kim RM (1980) Transluminal dilatation for subclavian steal syndrome. AJR 135: 995–996
2. Bollinger A (1979) Funktionelle Angiologie, Lehrbuch und Atlas. Thieme, Stuttgart, pp 88–136
3. Cope C (1980) Balloon dilatation of closed mesocaval shunt. AJR 135: 983–993
4. Dotter CT, Judkins MP (1964) Transluminal treatment of arteriosclerotic obstruction. Description of a new technic and a preliminary report of its application. Circulation 30: 654
5. Furrer J, Grüntzig A, Kugelmeier J, Goebel N (1979) Treatment of abdominal angina with percutaneous dilatation of an artery mesenterica superior stenosis. Cardiovasc Intervent 3: 61–68
6. Grollmann JH, Del Vicario M, Mittel AK (1980) Percutaneous transluminal abdominal aortic angioplasty. AJR 134: 1053–1054
7. Grüntzig A, Kuhlmann U, Vetter W (1978) Percutaneous transluminal dilatation of atherosclerotic renal artery stenosis. Circulation 213
8. Grüntzig A, Kuhlmann U, Vetter W, Lüthoff U, Meier B, Siegenthaler W (1978) Treatment of renovascular hypertension with percutaneous transluminal dilatation of a renal artery stenosis. Lancet 1: 801–802
9. Grüntzig A, Senning A, Siegenthaler WE (1979) Nonoperative dilatation of coronary artery stenosis. Percutaneous transluminal coronary angioplasty. N Engl J Med 303: 61–68
10. Hasso AN, Bird CR, Thompson JR, Hinshan DB (1980) Percutaneous angioplasty of the carotid artery. Presented at the annual meeting of the American Society of Neuroradiology, Los Angeles, March 1980
11. Katzer B, Chans J, Lukowsky G, Abramson EG (1979) Percutaneous transluminal angioplasty for treatment of renovascular hypertension. Radiology 131: 53
12. Mathias K (1981) Perkutane transluminale Katheterbehandlung supraaortaler Arterienobstruktionen. Angio 3: 47–50
13. Mathias K, Staiger J, Thron A, Spillner G, Heiss HW, Konrad-Graf S (1980) Perkutane Katheterangioplastik der Arteria subclavia. Dtsch Med Wochenschr 1: 16–18
14. Mathias K, Schlosser V, Reinke M (1980) Katheterrekanalisation eines Subklaviaverschlusses. ROEFO 132: 346–347
15. Mortarjeme A, Keifer JW, Zuska AJ (1982) Percutaneous transluminal angioplasty of the brachiocephalic arteries. AJR 138: 457–462
16. Novelline RA (1980) Percutaneous transluminal angioplasty: newer applications. AJR 135: 983–988
17. Saddekni S, Sniderman KW, Hilton S, Sos TA (1980) Percutaneous transluminal angioplasty of nonatherosclerotic lesions. AJR 135: 975–982
18. Schmidtke I, Zeitler E, Schoop W (1978) Spätergebnisse (5–8 Jahre) der perkutanen Katheterbehandlung (Dotter-Technik) bei femoropoplitealen Arterienverschlüssen im Stadium II. VASA 7/1: 4–15
19. Schoop W, Levy H, Cappius G, Mansjoer M, Zeitler E (1978) Early and late results of PTD in iliac stenosis. In: Zeitler E, Grüntzig A, Schoop W (eds) Percutaneous vascular recanalization. Springer, Berlin Heidelberg New York, pp 111–117
20. Schwarten DE (1980) Transluminal angioplasty of renal artery stenosis. AJR 135: 969–974
21. Szilagyi DE (1978) Atherogenesis in venous bypass grafts: In: Sawyer PN (ed) Vascular grafts. Appleton-Century-Crofts, New York, pp 243–260

22. Tegtmeyer CJ, Dyes R, Teates CD, Ayers CR, Carey RM, Wellons HA, Stanton LW (1980) Percutaneous transluminal dilatation of the renal arteries. Radiology 135: 589–599
23. van Andel GJ (1976) Percutaneous transluminal angioplasty. The Dotter procedure. Excerpta Medica, Amsterdam
24. Velasquez G, Castaneda-Zuniga W, Formanek A, Zollikofer C, Barreto A, Nicoloff D, Amplatz K, Sullivan A, (1980) Nonsurgical aortoplasty in Leriche syndrome. Radiology 134: 359–360
25. Zajko AB, McLean GK, Freiman DB, Oleaga JA, Ring EJ (1981) Percutaneous puncture of venous bypass grafts for transluminal angioplasty. AJR 137: 799–802
26. Zeitler E (1974) Leistungsfähigkeit der perkutanen Beseitigung arterieller Obliterationen mit der Dotter-Technik. In: Ehringer H (ed) Fortschritte der konservativen Therapie der peripheren arteriellen Verschlußkrankheit. Aktuelle Probleme in der Angiologie, vol 24. Huber, Bern, pp 70
27. Zeitler E, Schmidtke I, Schoop W, Giessler R, Dembski J, Mansjoer H (1976) Ergebnisse nach perkutaner transluminaler Angioplastik bei über 700 Behandlungen. Röntgenpraxis 29: 78
28. Zeitler E, Grüntzig A, Schoop W (eds) (1978) Percutaneous vascular recanalization. Technique, application, clinical results. Springer, Berlin Heidelberg New York
29. Zorn-Bopp E, Ingrisch H, Mietaschk A, Frey KW (1981) Transluminale Gefäßdilatation der distalen Bauchaorta, der Arteria iliaca communis und externa. ROEFO 134/5: 471–475

48. Results of Percutaneous Transluminal Angioplasty of the Deep Femoral Artery – a Preliminary Study

H. Rieger*, F.-J. Roth, and W. Schoop

There have been only sporadic reports of successful treatment of stenoses of the deep femoral artery by the Dotter procedure [1, 2]. These few cases, however, indicate that in high-risk situations this method can be helpful. Between the beginning of 1979 and December 1980 we attempted dilatation of the deep femoral artery in 29 patients with high-grade stenoses (1977, $n = 5$; 1978, $n = 6$; 1979, $n = 6$; 1980, $n = 12$). The average age was 63.5 years (45–81). These patients were of a quite different type from those described in our report on iliac stenoses. Most of them were high-risk patients. More than 80% were suffering from advanced stages of peripheral occlusive disease (Table 1), 41% showed strong signs of coronary heart disease, and nearly 30% also had reduced flow in the cerebral vessels. In all cases there was complete occlusion of the superficial femoral artery, often combined with popliteal occlusion (41% of the patients) and with further occlusions of two or three lower leg arteries (69% of the patients).

In 22 patients (76%) the procedure was successful from the radiological point of view. Three treatments failed to improve the clinical picture. Somewhat impressive was the observation that a good many of the patients immediately showed a clinical improvement, often leading to a change in clinical stage (see Table 2): in 86.1% of the successful dilatations a better clinical stage was attained. Of the successfully treated patients one had moved away, three could not be located, two had undergone surgery, nine had died, and seven were

Table 1. Distribution of clinical stage, risk factors, and types of disease or obstruction in 29 patients who underwent treatment of the deep femoral artery by the Dotter procedure. CHD, coronary heart disease; COD, cerebral occlusive disease; FO, femoral occlusion; PO, popliteal occlusion; LLAO, lower leg arterial occlusion

	Stages				Risk factors				Disease/obstruction				
	IIa	IIb	III	IV	nic	hyp	diab	lip	CHD	COD	FO	PO	LLAO
%	14	27	21	38	58	55	52	21	41	28	100	41	69
		(IIb–IV) 86%											

* Supported by grants of the Verein zur Bekämpfung von Gefäßkrankheiten e.V., D-5250 Engelskirchen

Percutaneous Transluminal Angioplasty
(ed. by C. T. Dotter, A. Grüntzig, W. Schoop, E. Zeitler)

Table 2. Changes in clinical stage in 22 patients in whom the Dotter procedure was successful from the technical point of view

II → I	: $n =$ 0 (0%)	
IIa → IIa	: $n =$ 4 (18.1%)	86% (IIa → IIa to IV → II)
IIb → IIa	: $n =$ 7 (31.8%)	
III → II	: $n =$ 4 (18.1%)	
IV → II	: $n =$ 4 (18.1%)	
Technical + clinical Ø	: $n =$ 3 (13.9%)	
Total	: $n =$ 22 (100%)	

Table 3. Angiographically controlled stenoses of the deep femoral artery before, immediately after, and 1–2 years after dilatation by the Dotter procedure. The percentage of reduction in cross section was approximately calculated according to the formula $\frac{A - B}{A} \cdot 100$ (A = diameter of the normal vessel, B = diameter of the stenotic segment)

Pat. no.	Before PTD	After PTD	Late result
1145/80	63%	50%	0%
2308/79	57%	20%	30%
2659/80	56%	23%	28%
168/80	65%	28%	0%
2562/79	72%	28%	27%
2621/80	65%	29%	29%
1284/77	68%	34%	Occluded

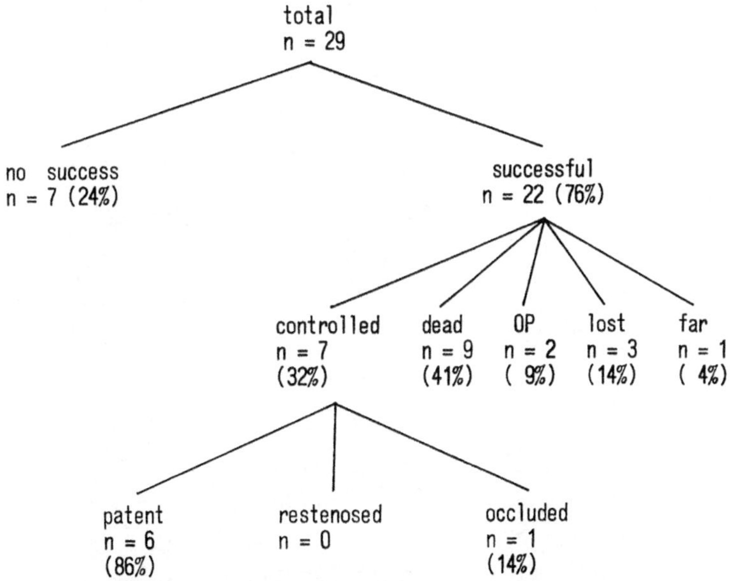

Fig. 1. Synopsis of technical successes and failures ($n = 22$) of the Dotter technique. *Far*, patient had moved; *lost*, could not be located; *OP*, undergone surgery

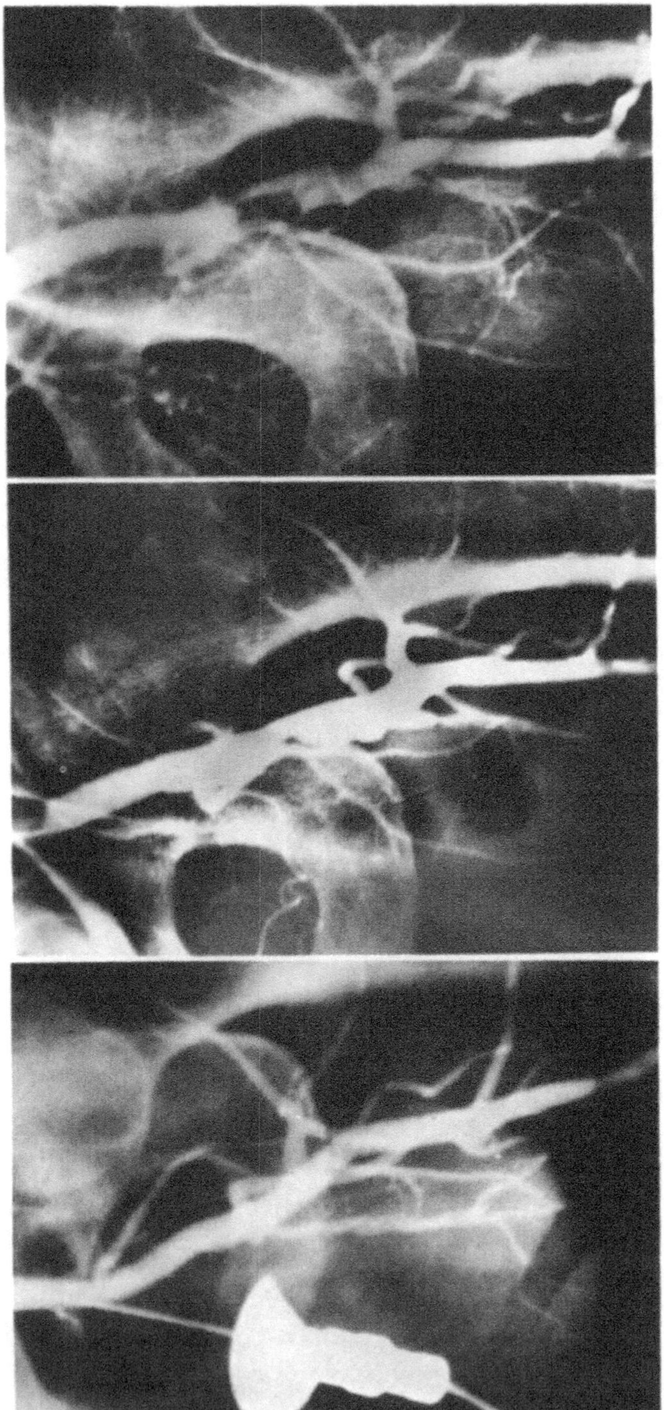

a

b

c

Fig. 2a–c. Deep femoral artery, **a** before dilatation, **b** immediately after catheter dilatation, showing a residual stenosis of ca. 50%, and **c** 2 years later, showing that the stenosis had spontaneously disappeared reexamined (Fig. 1). In the light of the fact that the deep femoral artery does not easily allow direct clinical assessment, and because of the frequency of long occlusions, including lower leg and popliteal arteries, neither the Doppler ultrasound technique nor oscillography were reliable diagnostic means. We therefore relied on monitoring of symptoms and the performance of angiographic controls. The results are given in Table 3. It is noteworthy that in two cases (1145/80 and 168/80), stenoses of 50% and 30% remained after the Dotter procedure but had spontaneously and completely disappeared by 2 years later (see Fig. 1).

We can thus conclude that the dilatation of a high-grade stenosis of the deep femoral artery (reduction in cross section of more than 60%) by the Dotter technique can represent a viable alternative to surgery.

References

1. Mahler F, Grüntzig A, Schlumpf M (1978) Transluminal dilatation of a stenosis in the deep femoral artery. In: Zeitler E, Grüntzig A, Schoop W (eds) Percutaneous vascular recanalization. Springer, Berlin Heidelberg New York
2. Schoop W (1978) Indications for PTR from the angiologic point of view. In: Zeitler E, Grüntzig A, Schoop W (eds) Percutaneous vascular recanalization. Springer, Berlin Heidelberg New York

49. Percutaneous Transluminal Angioplasty as a Complement to Surgery

A. Motarjeme, J. W. Keifer, A. J. Zuska, and P. Nabavi

Introduction

Transluminal angioplasty, a nonsurgical technique described by Dotter and Judkins in 1964 [1], is now widely used as a substitute for reconstructive vascular surgery in the management of atherosclerotic occlusive disease. A double-lumen catheter designed by Grüntzig and Hopff 1974 [2] is now frequently used in dilatation of many arteries and even in the abdominal aorta [3–14]. Successful dilatation of arterial occlusions may alleviate the need for lengthy and costly reconstructive vascular surgery, but this is not applicable in every case and surgery is still the primary treatment in the majority of patients. The patency of an arterial bypass is directly related to adequate inflow and proportionate outflow. Any hemodynamically significant occlusive lesion, proximal or distal to an arterial bypass, endangers the patency of the graft; if not relieved it will eventually lead to graft thrombosis. Arterial dilatation can easily be used in both pre- and postsurgical stages to treat these lesions, thus preventing graft occlusion.

The major reconstructive vascular surgeries, such as aortic bifurcation grafts, are not tolerated well by many elderly patients with poor general health. In some instances this major transabdominal surgery can be modified to a simpler procedure, such as a femorofemoral graft, with the aid of transluminal angioplasty. We have used arterial dilatation in conjunction with surgery, as a pre- and postsurgical technique as well as intraoperatively, with a high rate of success.

Materials and Methods

Seventy-two arteries were treated in 59 patients. Fifteen patients were treated prior to surgery, 15 patients were treated postsurgically, and 29 patients were treated intraoperatively. Arteries dilated included 36 iliac, 2 common femoral, 18 superficial femoral, 6 deep femoral, 7 popliteal, and 2 common carotid, and there was 1 venous graft. There were 34 men and 25 women, ranging in age from 46 to 86. Stenotic lesions of the iliac arteries with significant gradient were dilated prior to a femoropopliteal graft, six totally occluded superficial femoral arteries were recanalized, and five severely stenotic arteries were dilated intraoperatively during an aortic bifurcation femoral graft (Fig. 1).

Percutaneous Transluminal Angioplasty
(ed. by C. T. Dotter, A. Grüntzig, W. Schoop, E. Zeitler)

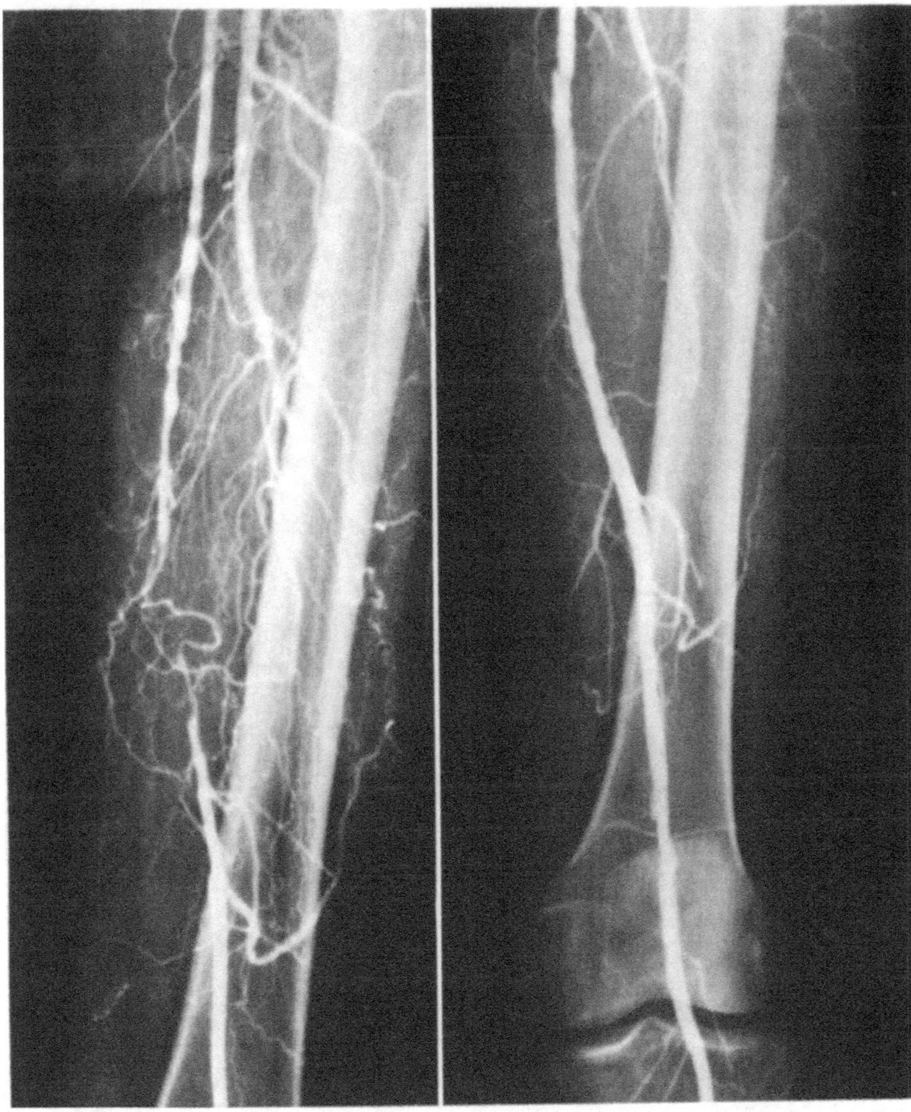

a b

Fig. 1a, b. A 66-year-old woman with severe claudication of both legs and weak femoral pulse bilaterally. There were no palpable or pedal pulses on either side. **a** In addition to severe stenotic lesions of both iliac arteries (not shown), a left femoral arteriogram showed a 9-cm total occlusion of the superficial femoral artery. **b** Recanalization of the superficial femoral artery during aortic bifurcation graft

In the postsurgical group there were three patients with arterial stenosis or total occlusion proximal to the graft and one with stenosis of the aorta proximal to an aortoiliac graft. Eight patients had stenosis distal to the graft, three had stenosis at anastomosis of the aortoiliac graft (Fig. 2), and three had stenosis of the popliteal artery distal to the femoropopliteal graft (fig. 3). Two patients with

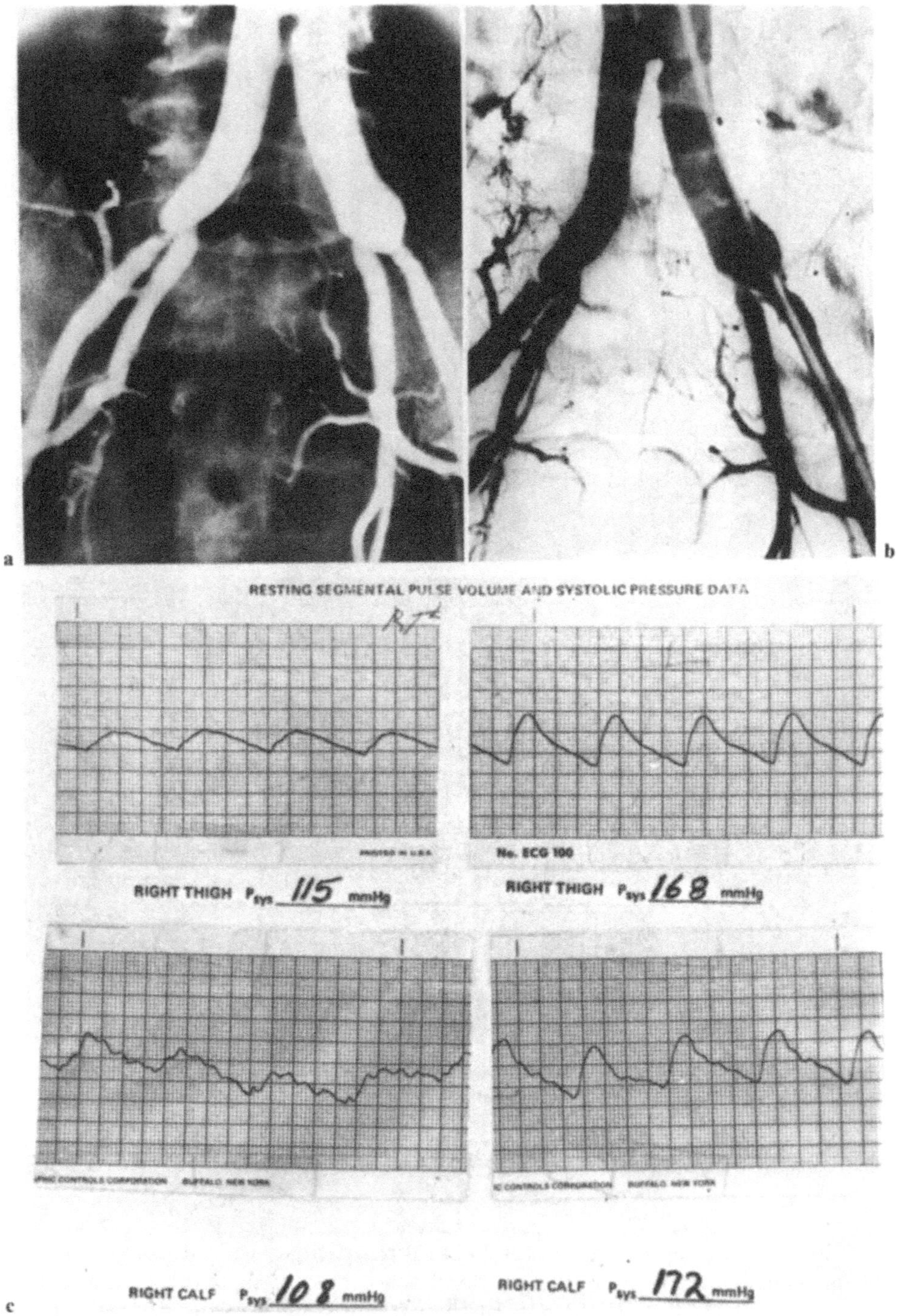

Fig. 2a–c. A 48-year-old man complaining of severe claudication of the right leg for the past few months. Aortic bifurcation graft had been performed 2 years earlier. **a** abdominal aortogram showing an 80% stenosis of the right iliac artery, just distal to anastomosis; **b** abdominal aortogram after angioplasty showing satisfactory dilatation of the right iliac artery; **c** pulse volume recording before and after angioplasty

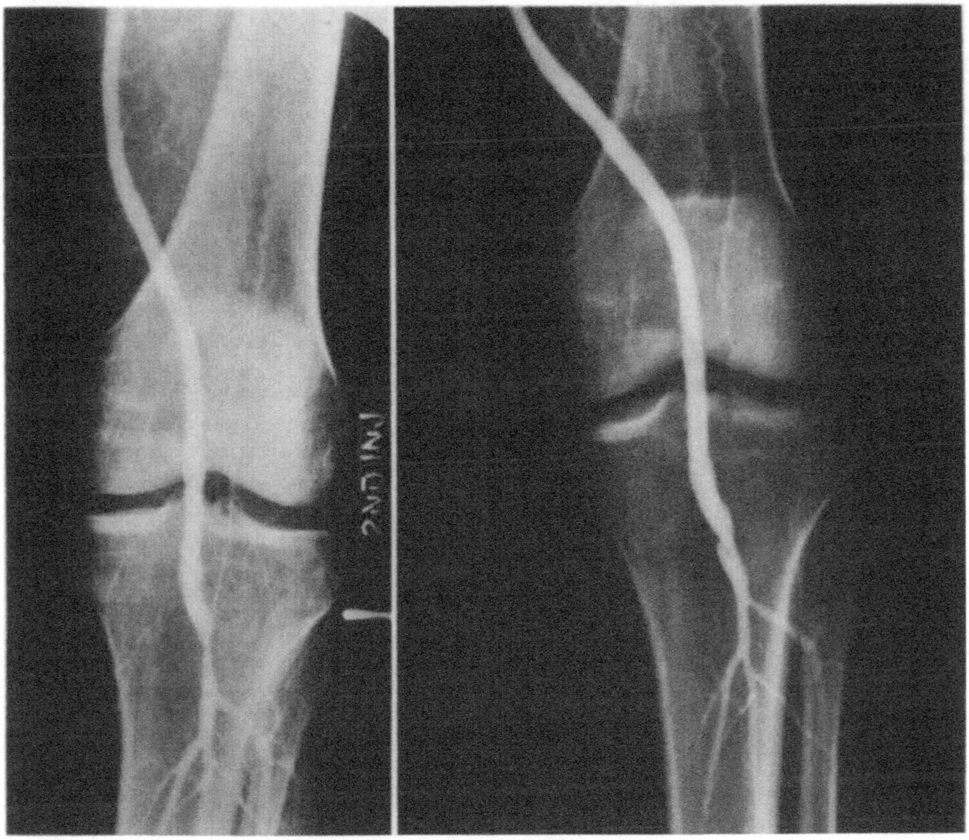

a b

Fig. 3a, b. A 40-year-old man complaining of severe claudication of the left mid-calf. A femoropopliteal graft below the knee had been performed 6 months earlier. **a** femoral arteriogram showing severe stenosis of the popliteal artery, just distal to the anastomosis; **b** left femoral arteriogram 6 months after angioplasty, showing patency of the popliteal artery

aortofemoral graft had stenosis of the deep femoral artery just distal to the graft (Fig. 4). Six patients in need of aortic bifurcation femoral graft had total occlusion of one iliac artery and severe stenosis of the other. These patients were not able to tolerate this major transabdominal surgery due to old age and/or poor general health. Dilatation of one of the ilicac arteries made it possible to treat them with femorofemoral grafts, three under local anesthesia. One patient whose right leg had been amputated had multiple stenoses of both iliac arteries in addition to total occlusion of the left common femoral artery. This patient underwent an endarterectomy of the femoral artery and intraoperative dilatation of the iliac arteries.

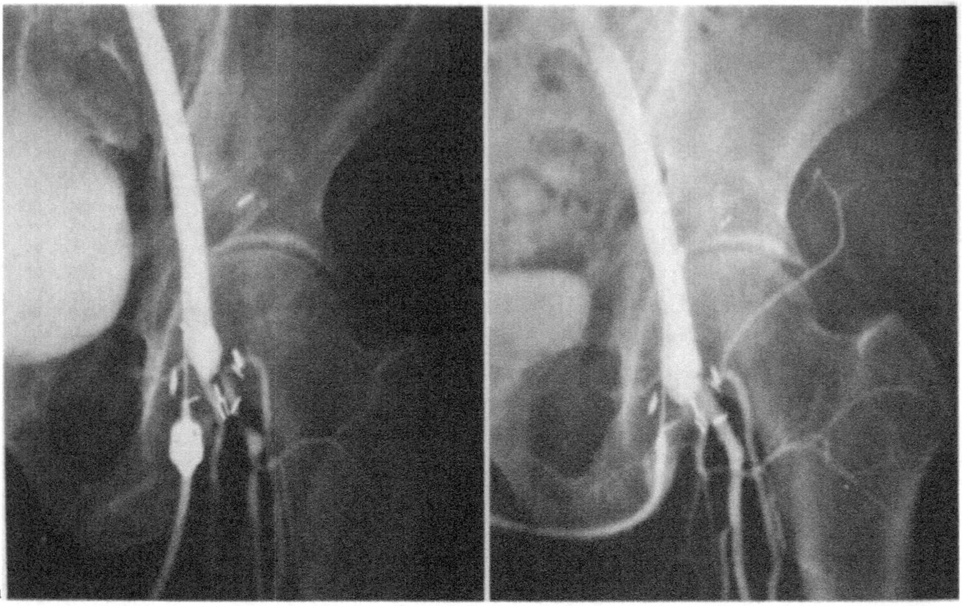

a b

Fig. 4a, b. A 64-year-old nondiabetic man had severe claudication of the left leg. He had had a previous aortic bifurcation and femoral graft, but refused further vascular surgery. **a** Patent aortofemoral graft, total occlusion of the left superficial femoral and severe stenosis of the deep femoral arteries. **b** Six-week follow-up arteriogram, showing a dilated deep femoral artery. There was a significant decrease in claudication

Technique

The Seldinger technique was used to obtain abdominal aortograms and bilateral femoral arteriograms via the femoral artery on the asymptomatic or less symptomatic side; this was done in one procedure by means of a contralateral approach. Furthermore, the common femoral artery of the symptomatic side was preserved for recanalization of the occluded superficial femoral or popliteal arteries using the antegrade approach.

A pigtail catheter was used for angiographic examination and the symptomatic iliac artery was catheterized using the same catheter as described by Bachmann et al. [15]. After injection of 5,000 units heparin through the catheter, the stenotic lesion was traversed by the guide wire, and while the wire was kept in place, the angiographic catheter was exchanged for a balloon catheter of the proper size. The balloon was located within the stenosis and inflated by hand, using a 6-ml syringe and a 50% dilution of the contrast material.

After deflation and removal of the balloon from the dilated segment, a postangioplasty arteriogram was obtained. Pulse volume recordings were made using a plethysmography machine, both on the day of angioplasty and the day after. Patients were treated with vasodilators, such as Persantine (dipyridamole,

50–75 mg three times daily), and if a totally occluded artery was successfully recanalized, the patient was treated with heparin and then Coumadin (wafarin sodium) for a period of not less than 6 months. Patients were examined in the Angioplasty Clinic for follow-up every 3 months.

Operative transluminal angioplasty is performed by a vascular radiologist with the vascular surgeon's assistance. An intraoperative angioplasty requires a radiolucent operating table (usually glass) and a portable C-arm fluoroscopy unit. Most of the glass tables available are wider than the standard operating table and not comfortable for vascular surgeons. Upon our request, one of the manufacturers (A.D.C. Medical) has designed a table to our specifications [20 in (50.8 cm) wide and capable of being elevated or lowered].

The intraoperative iliac artery dilatation is performed via the ipsilateral femoral artery. A J-guide-wire is first inserted through the arteriotomy incision and (under fluoroscopic control) the stenosis is traversed. The insertion of the balloon catheter and dilatation is performed according to the usual method. Dilatation and recanalization of the femoral and popliteal arteries is performed in the same manner but using the antegrade approach. Intraoperative arteriography can be performed after completion of the angioplasty, but fluorsocopic observation is adequate in most instances.

Results

Fifty-nine patients underwent percutaneous transluminal angioplasty (PTA) in addition to surgery. Potential occlusion of the graft was avoided in 13 patients by dilatation of the stenotic arteries proximal and distal to the graft, and in one patient by dilatation of the venous femoropopliteal graft. In one patient a superficial femoral artery totally occluded proximal to the femoropopliteal graft was recanalized (Fig. 5).

The chances of success of bypass surgery were improved in 28 patients by increasing the inflow or outflow prior to bypass surgery. The need for transabdominal surgical procedures was avoided in seven elderly, high-risk patients. Six of these patients underwent femorofemoral bypass after dilatation of the iliac artery, three of them under local anesthesia. In the seventh, femoral endarterectomy and intraoperative dilatation of the iliac arteries were performed. In one patient, the femoropopliteal graft below the knee was modified to a graft above the knee, which has a more favorable prognosis. The outcome of the aortic bifurcation graft was conserably improved by recanalization or dilatation of the femoral arteries in 11 patients. The rate of success in this carefully selected group is higher than in our previously reported cases [16]. There were only 2 failures out of 72 attempts; both were intraoperative. One of these occurred in recanalization of a long-segment occlusion of the superficial femoral artery and the other in dilatation of a hard stenosis of the left common iliac artery. The duration of follow-up ranges from 5 to 40 months. Five patients were lost to follow-up. A 78-year-old man who underwent dilatation of the left iliac artery and femorofemoral graft had thrombosis of the graft after 1 year. He

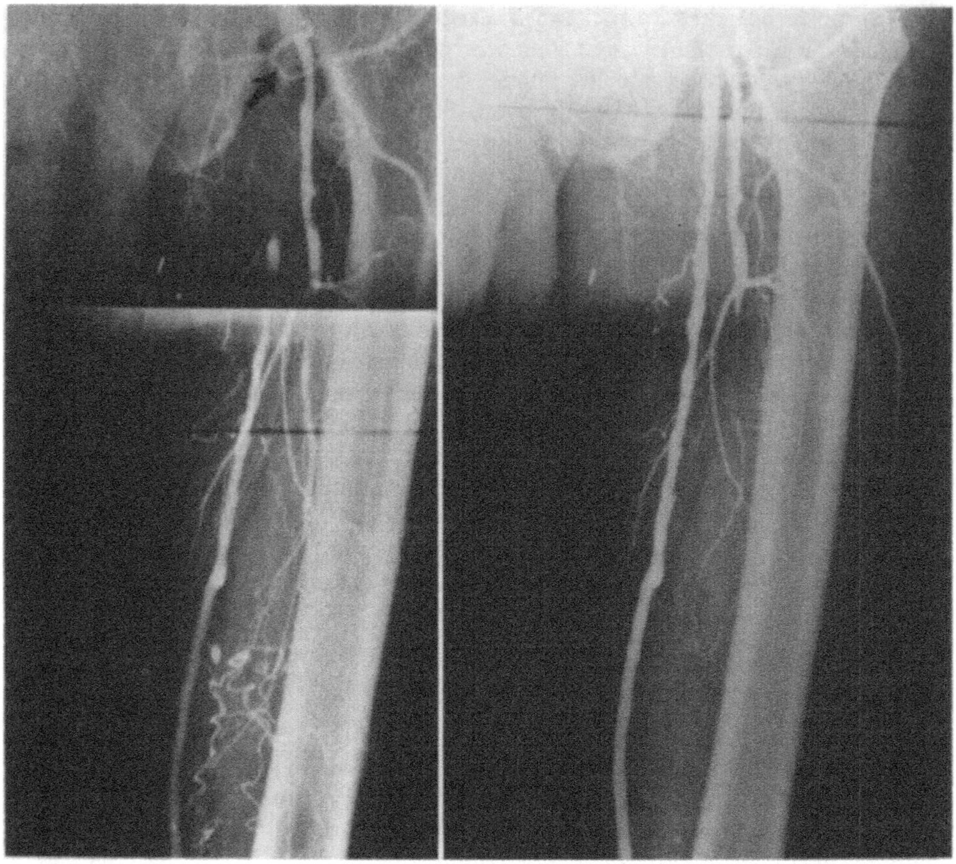

a b

Fig. 5a, b. A 62-year-old man complaining of claudication of the left calf. Femoropopliteal graft had been performed years earlier. **a** Patent femoropopliteal graft but total occlusion of the superficial femoral artery proximal to the graft *(arrows);* **b** postangioplasty arteriogram showing patent superficial femoral artery proximal to the graft

died shortly after amputation of the right leg. There was one reocclusion of a superficial femoral artery 5 months after recanalization. The remainder of the arteries remain patent to date.

Complications

There were two large local hematomas at the puncture site that did not require surgical treatment. There was, however, one intraabdominal hematoma due to bleeding from a high puncture site in the common femoral artery; this required an emergency laparotomy and suturing of the bleeding point.

Discussion

Percutaneous transluminal angioplasty has been proved to be an effective nonsurgical treatment of atherosclerotic disease. Long-term follow-up studies, in carefully selected cases, have shown a patency rate comparable with that following surgery [17]. The application of PTA has a wide spectrum of indications, ranging from reconstruction of a totally occluded artery to a means of palliation. PTA is not meant to replace surgery in every instance, but should be recognized as an alternative to surgery in selected cases. Application of PTA does not preclude subsequent surgery, should the PTA be unsuccessful. We have shown that a nondesirable surgical procedure can be modified to a more favorable procedure by the use of PTA, and PTA can easily be performed along with surgery to improve the outcome. In the hands of a skilled and experienced angiographer, PTA is a safe procedure with few complications. The treatment is fairly painless, hospitalization and recuperation are short, and there is no need for general anesthesia. Intraoperative arterial dilatation does not burden the patient with additional physical and psychological discomfort. Vascular surgeons not familiar with this technique are often reluctant to accept its validity, but there is now enough evidence to prove its effectiveness as an aid to surgery in the treatment of arterial occlusive disease in particular cases. It can even be effective in some cases where surgery has already failed. Case selection is the key to success, as it is with surgery.

Summary

Transluminal angioplasty, a nonsurgical treatment of atherosclerotic acclusive disease, was performed on 72 arteries in 59 patients inconjunction with reconstructive vascular surgery. Fifteen patients were treated prior to and 15 patients after surgery, and 29 patients were treated intraoperatively. Some arteries were dilated to increase arterial inflow to the graft or to improve the distal runoff. In other cases, a major reconstructive surgical procedure was modified to a less traumatic or more favorable one. The long-term patency rate is still under investigation. The rate of success was 95%.

References

1. Dotter CT, Judkins MP (1964) Transluminal treatment of arteriosclerotic obstruction. Circulation 30: 654–670
2. Gruentzig A, Hopff H (1974) Perkutane Rekanalisation chronischer arterieller Verschlüsse mit einem neuen Dilatationskatheter. Modifikation der Dotter-Technik. Dtsch Med Wochenschr 99: 2502–2510
3. Gruentzig A, Myler R, Stertzer S, et al. (1978) Coronary percutaneous transluminal angioplasty: preliminary report. Circulation 57: 211
4. Gruentzig A, Kuhlmann U, Vetter W, Lutlof U, Meier B, Siegenthaler W (1978) Treatment of renovascular hypertension with percutaneous transluminal dilatation of renal-artery stenosis. Lancet 1: 801–802

5. Tegtmeyer CJ, Dyer R, Teates CR, et al. (1980) Percutaneous transluminal dilatation of the renal arteries. Radiology 135: 589–599
6. Schwarten DE, Yune HY, Klatte EC, Grim CE, Weinberger MH (1980) Clinical experience with percutaneous transluminal angioplasty (PTA) of stenotic renal arteries. Radiology 135: 601–604
7. Motarjeme A, Keifer J, Zuska AJ (1980) Percutaneous transluminal angioplasty of the deep femoral artery. Radiology 135: 613–617
8. Motarjeme A, Keifer JW, Zuska AJ (1981) Percutaneous transluminal angioplasty of the vertebral arteries. Radiology 139: 715–717
9. Block PC (1980) Percutaneous transluminal angioplasty. AJR 135: 955–959
10. Motarjeme A, Keifer JW, Zuska AJ (1980) Percutaneous transluminal angioplasty of the iliac arteries: 66 experiences. AJR 135: 937–944
11. Schwarten DE (1980) Transluminal angioplasty of renal artery stenosis: 70 experiences. AJR 135: 937–944
12. Motarjeme A, Keifer JW, Zuska AJ (1981) Percutaneous transluminal angioplasty of the brachiocephalic arteries. Presented at 1981 American Roentgen Ray Society Meeting, San Francisco
13. Waltman AC (1980) Percutaneous transluminal angioplasty: iliac and deep femoral arteries. AJR 135: 921–925
14. Sniderman KW, Sos TA, Sprayregen S, et al. (1980) Percutaneous transluminal angioplasty in renal transplant arterial stenosis for relief of hypertension. Radiology 135: 23–6
15. Bachmann DM, Casarella WJ, Sos TA (1979) Percutaneous iliofemoral angioplasty via the contralateral femoral artery. Radiology 130: 617–621
16. Motarjeme A, Keifer JW, Zuska AJ (1980) Percutaneous transluminal angioplasty and case selection. Radiology 135: 573–581
17. Van Andel GJ (1980) Transluminal iliac angioplasty: long-term results. Radiology 135: 607–611

50. The Place of Percutaneous Transluminal Angioplasty in the Therapy of a Clinic for Vascular Diseases

M. Köhler, C. Demmer, and F.-J. Roth

Percutaneous transluminal angioplasty (PTA) is rapidly becoming an accepted mode of therapy for stenotic and occlusive arterial disease. Recently, many symposia have dealt with the problems and successes of angioplasty. But how valuable is this method in the field of angiology? And how often is PTA indicated? In order to answer these questions we have analyzed data on 1609 consecutive patients with peripheral arterial disease hospitalized in 1981 in our clinic for vascular diseases. The present chapter reports the first findings of this extensive study, which was undertaken with a view to establishing the theapeutic possibilities.

Results

In 1981, 2,737 patients with vascular diseases were admitted to our clinic, 1,609 of them suffering from disorders of the arteries. Angioplasty was carried out in 335 patients (20.8%); 157 (9.8%) underwent surgery; and 492 (30.6%) were treated by blood-vessel-opening procedures. This reveals that in approximately one-third of the patients with vascular diseases invasive methods were used to improve circulation, the remaining 69.4% receiving conservative treatment.

It was predominantly patients with femoral occlusions (34.3%) who were treated by means of PTA. However, a high percentage (24.4%) of patients with iliac stenoses were also able to be treated by this method. Furthermore, femoral stenoses (14.0%) and disturbances of circulation in the popliteotibial area (9.9%) were significantly represented. Table 1 presents more detailed data on localization.

The severity of the vascular disease varied and was accordingly graded on a scale from 1 to 4. The majority (80.3%) of patients for whom angioplasty was

Table 1. Case material (patients admitted during 1981)

Patient group	No.	
Total	2737	
Arterial disease	1609	(100%)
PTA	335	(20.8%)
Vascular surgery	157	(9.8%)
Conservative treatment	1117	(69.4%)

Percutaneous Transluminal Angioplasty
(ed. by C. T. Dotter, A. Grüntzig, W. Schoop, E. Zeitler)

Table 2. Localizations of PTA ($n = 335$)

Localization	No.	%
Iliac		
Occlusion	6	1.8
Stenosis		
Unilateral	85	25.4
Bilateral	13	3.9
Common femoral	15	4.5
Deep femoral	3	0.9
Femoral		
Occlusion		
Unilateral	115	34.3
Bilateral	0	0
Stenosis		
Unilateral	47	14.0
Bilateral	1	0.3
Popliteal/tibial	33	9.9
Other arteries	17	5.1
Total	335	100

Table 3. Degree of severity

	No.	%
Stage II (int. claud.)	269	80.3
Stage III (rest pain)	22	6.6
Stage IV (ulcer. lesion)	44	13.1
Total	335	100

necessary suffered from interittent claudication, so their ability to walk was not insignificantly hampered. A total of 66 out of the 335 patients (19.7%) in a late stage (rest pain or ulcer) required angioplasty. Table 2 shows the numbers of patients in the varying stages of disease.

Discussion

From the clinical-angiological point of view it is important to know how often treatment by menas of angioplasty is possible for patients with peripheral arterial occlusion or stenosis. We know of no published studies providing an answer to this question. We have therefore processed the date on patients treated at our clinic during 1981 and have been able to establish a first analysis. This investigation shows that out of 1,609 patients suffering from vascular diseases,

20.8% of all cases were required to undergo PTA. Our figures shows that conservative treatment indeed remains the basic therapy. Further work on our data will give an indication of how often treatment by angioplasty was necessary for the individual.

Summary

Our results point out the important role of angioplasty in treatment of stenotic and occlusive arterial disease today. Although conservative treatment remains the basic therapeutic method in patients suffering from arterial diseases, our experiences have shown that in 20% angioplasty is indicated.

51. Indications for Percutaneous Transluminal Angioplasty from the Surgeon's Point of View

H. Denck

As early as 1976 and 1977 I had the opportunity of reporting on the surgeon's point of view regarding percutaneous transluminal angioplasty (PTA). At that time PTA was already regarded as an alternative to surgery in certain circumstances, recognition being given to the concept as well as the results. However, at that time we were able to report only on a few patients, and these had been under observation for a comparatively short time. In the meantime our experience in terms of number of patients and follow-up period has increased, and we may summarize our present "surgical" point of view as follows:

Every patient technically suited for PTA who suffers from disease of stages II–IV presents primarily an indication for PTA, and that to the same extent as an indication for surgical intervention. Consequently, we have had a rapid increase in the percentage of PTA candidates among our primarily surgical patients (Fig. 1). The percentage (1.4%) of PTA candidates among our patients in 1976 had risen to 18% by May 1982. These figures are sufficient to reflect our experiences with and our opinion of PTA.

From the total of 461 of Olbert's PTA patients, we have selected the patients treated in 1981, for these best reflect the distribution of lesions suitable for treatment by this method. Table 1 shows that the main indication for PTA was still the short femoropopliteal occlusion, which we treated during late stage II as well as during stage III and stage IV (Table 2). Four times distal occlusions were

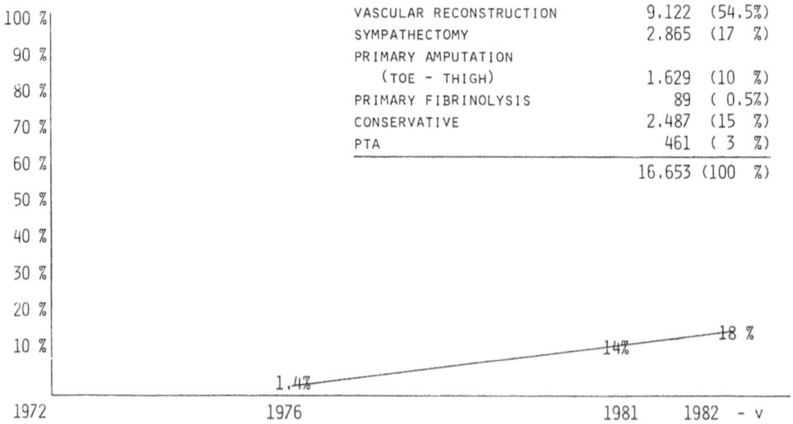

Fig. 1. Increase in the number of PTAs performed in our department between 1972 and 1982

Percutaneous Transluminal Angioplasty
(ed. by C. T. Dotter, A. Grüntzig, W. Schoop, E. Zeitler)

Table 1. Patients selected for PTA in 1981: distribution of obliterations

Artery	Total no. of cases	No. of PTAs	No. of failures
Popliteal	17	1 (5.8%)	
Femoropopliteal	222	53 (23%)	3
Aortoiliac	1	1 (4× Streptokinase)	1
Aortoiliofemoral	201	9 (4.4%)	
Renal	9	3 (33.3%)	
Subclavian	13	3 (23%)	

Table 2. Indications for PTA and stages of disease: 1981 patients ($n = 69$)

	n	II	III	IV
Popliteal artery	1		1	
Femoropopliteal	53		17 (32%)	36 (68%)
Aortoiliac	9	4	5	

Table 3. Reoperations after PTA

Femoropopliteal ($n = 53$)	Acute	2 (3.7%)	9.3%
	Later	3 (5.6%)	
Aortoiliac ($n = 9$)	Acute	0	
	Later	1 (11%)	

treated with simultaneous administration of streptokinase; two of these cases were treated successfully and the extremities were saved.

Altogether we had to repeat the procedure six times after PTA; in the femoropopliteal region an acute reintervention was necessary in two cases and three patients underwent reoperation within the first half year; in the aortoiliac region a reoperation was necessary in one case within the first half year (Table 3).

It is true that long-term results after PTA are not always as good as those after surgical intervention, but they are not significantly worse, and we should like to stress again our opinion that PTA should be performed when it is technically feasible and when it promises success. Special indications, such as stenoses of the subclavian artery or of the renal arteries, brought 100% good results in our patients, so that a valuable area of indication has been opened up here during recent years (Fig. 2).

Of particular interest is the combination of reconstructive vascular surgery with transluminal dilatation in cases of multiple occlusions. My collaborator Hagmüller has compiled 18 such cases: in 5 a reconstruction of the iliac artery was combined with PTA of the femoral artery; in 7 a PTA of the ipsi- or contralateral iliac artery was combined with reconstruction of the ipsi- or

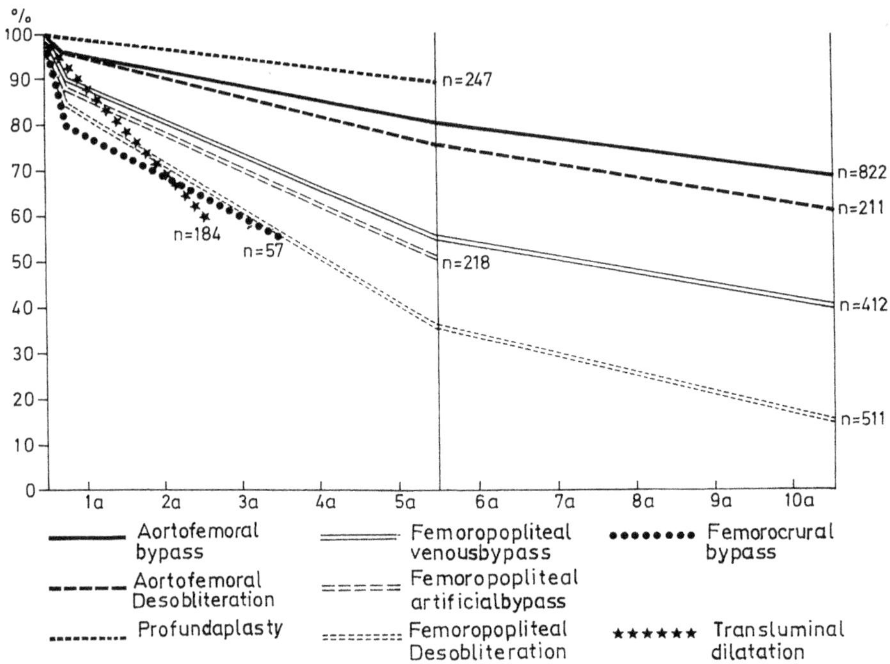

Fig. 2. Long term results of vascular reconstructions and PTA

contralateral femoropopliteal artery; in 6 cases combinations distally from the inguinal ligament with profunda patch plasty and PTA of the femoropopliteal artery were performed; and in 1 case a PTA of the central subclavian artery was combined with surgery of the brachial artery. The hemodynamic result were – as Hagmüller has shown – completely equal to those achieved by multiple surgical reconstruction; the same ist rue of long-term results.

Our experiences and results thus make it clear that PTA represents a true alternative to surgical reconstruction. For patients of advanced age and those in poor general condition, PTA has the advantage of causing less stress, especially in cases of multiple surgery (combination with small surgical interventions). From the economic point of view, it must be borne in mind that PTA involves much lower costs because of the markedly reduced hospitalization period.

52. Indications for Percutaneous Transluminal Angioplasty: The Nephrologist's View

E. Lux and D. Seybold

There are two reasons for treating renovascular hypertension: first, to normalize blood pressure; and secondly, to prevent or improve renal failure due to renal artery stenosis, especially in patients with a solitary kidney, bilateral renal artery stenoses, or damaged contralateral kidney. There is no established way of distinguishing patients with progressive from those with stable disease.

Suitable Candidates for Percutaneous Transluminal Angioplasty in Renal Artery Stenosis

1. Patients in whom operative revascularization is indicated, provided that the chances of successful treatment are not harmed by unsuccessful percutaneous transluminal angioplasty (PTA). Controlled studies have yet to demonstrate whether the long-term results with respect to blood pressure normalization and recurrence are comparable to those of surgical treatment.
2. Patients representing a high operative risk whose blood pressure cannot be controlled by drug therapy alone. As certain complications may require immediate surgical intervention, there should not be any absolute contraindications to operation.
3. Patients representing a high operative risk: PTA may be employed as an alternative to drug treatment. This also has to be investigated in controlled studies.
4. Patients with transplant renal artery stenosis and hypertension.
5. Patients with renal insufficiency: PTA may be performed not only to cure hypertension but also to improve renal function. Because the kidney behind the stenosis is protected against high blood pressure, recovery of renal function is possible with improvement of total renal function. Even after total occlusion of the renal artery over a period of 38 days successful revascularization has been reported [18].

One could speculate that if PTA were useful in the very early phase of disease, the screening program for renovascular disease would certainly have to be altered.

Up to now it has been generally accepted that patients under the age of 40 with fibromuscular dysplasia and elevated blood pressure should be operated on because of low operative mortality (2.4%) and good long-term results regarding

Percutaneous Transluminal Angioplasty
(ed. by C. T. Dotter, A. Grüntzig, W. Schoop, E. Zeitler)

blood pressure normalization [3]. Unfortunately, there exists no test to predict the effect of surgery in every patient with renovascular hypertension. Factors which influence blood pressure response to surgical treatment are the age of the patient, duration of hypertension, bilateral renal artery stenoses, extrarenal arterial lesions, and preoperative systolic blood pressure [17].

The following facts contribute to a high mortality among patients undergoing surgical treatment: coronary heart disease, previous myocardial infarction, cerebrovascular insufficiency, advanced age, renal insufficiency, bilateral stenoses, and solitary kidney. The prognosis for patients with uncontrolled hypertension is poor, so operative intervention has seemed to be justified. However, the mortality among such patients is high, the short- and long-term results with regard to blood pressure reduction are moderate, and the late survival rates are not essentially better than for those patients receiving drug therapy. In patients with coronary heart disease or impaired renal function, Franklin et al. found a mortality of 22%, versus 5% in patients without these complications [7]. Recent studies, however, report somewhat better results: 77 patients between 50 and 65 years old showed a mortality of 1%–2%, with benefit from operation (cured or improved) in 80%–87% [2]. Laroche reports on a group of 12 patients with no mortality; all high-risk patients showed improvement of hypertension and/or renal function [12].

Recently, antihypertensive drugs have been developed which block the renin-angiotensin system (RAS), which is thought to be involved in the pathogenesis of renovascular hypertension. The question therefore arises: Can captopril (an orally acting converting enzyme inhibitor) compete with PTA in the treatment of renovascular hypertension, especially in high-risk patients? A large number of studies have demonstrated the efficacy of captopril in moderate and severe hypertension due to renal artery stenosis. Nonetheless, there are case reports regarding patients with renal artery stenoses treated with captopril, usually in combination with diuretics, in whom reversible acute renal failure occurred [1, 6, 20]. A possible explanation might be that the fall in systemic blood pressure reduces perfusion behind the stenosis and, since captopril blocks the intrarenal effect of angiotensin II, it might prevent its constrictory effect on the vas afferens [10]. Therefore, the treatment with captopril of patients with significant stenoses (bilateral stenoses or solitary kidney) without removal of the stenosis bears the risk of acute renal failure and seems not to be an appropriate alternative to PTA in every case.

Case Report

A 50-year-old patient with bilateral renal artery stenoses and high blood pressure was treated with captopril in combination with other antihypertensive drugs. Immediately on starting the treatment with captopril serum creatinine rose to 6 mg%. After PTA and withdrawal of captopril, blood pressure fell and renal function improved. After normalization of serum creatinine, captopril was given again and no impairment of renal function was observed (Fig. 1).

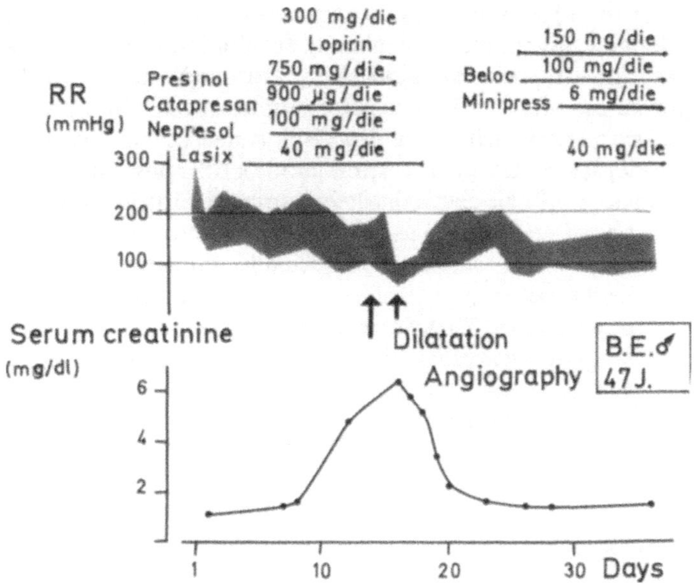

Fig. 1. Reversible acute renal failure in a 50-year-old patient with bilateral renal artery stenoses during treatment with captopril before and after PTA

The Role of PTA in the Treatment of Transplant Renal Artery Stenosis

Despite intensive medication blood pressure sometimes can not be controlled, and deterioration of renal function occurs. The frequency of hypertension in renal transplant patients is about 60% in adults, and it is estimated that in 1%–12% of these patients renal artery stenosis is the cause of elevated blood pressure [5, 8, 11, 13, 14]. Surgical repair of arterial stenosis bears the risk of graft loss. As shown in the study by Whiteside, three of eight patients operated on for renal artery stenosis lost their graft [19]. Where PTA is technically possible, short-term results are therefore encouraging, and it may prove to be the initial treatment of choice in such patients [9, 15, 16].

Management of Patients Before and Shortly After PTA

In animal studies blood pressure falls rapidly after reversal of renal artery stenosis. If plasma renin activity (PRA) was elevated, it returns to normal. Sodium and fluid excretion increases, but not in all cases, so that factors other than the RAS and sodium balance seem to play a role in the fall of blood pressure [4]. In most studies antihypertensive medication was discontinued at least 12 h prior to PTA.

If blood pressure rose, short-acting antihypertensive agents like nitroprusside were given, but hydralazine or clonidine could be used alternatively. As some investigators have observed a dramatic fall of blood pressure within the first hours after PTA, a careful monitoring of the patient with frequent blood pressure checks within the first 24 h is necessary. Patients who are volume- and salt-depleted and have a stimulated RAS consequent to prior treatment with diuretics might be particularly endangered. Intravenous replacement of salt and water or, if necessary, vasoconstricting agents can prevent a further fall in blood pressure, which might be especially dangerous for patients with general arteriosclerosis.

In conclusion, PTA seems to be as effective and safe a method as medication and surgical treatment, thus offering a new therapeutic option for selected patients in whom it is necessary to improve renovascular hypertension and preserve renal function.

References

1. Collste P, Haglund K, Lundgren G, Magnusson G, Östman J (1979) Reversible renal failure during treatment with captopril. Br Med J 2: 612
2. Dean RH, Foster JH (1977) Surgical management of renovasulcar hypertension in older patients. Med Clin North Am 61: 643
3. Denecke H (1980) Renovaskulärer Hochdruck – Spätprognose nach Operation. Urban and Schwarzenberg, Munich
4. Dietz R, Mast GJ, Schömig A, Lüth JB, Rascher W (1978) Reversal of renal hypertension: effects on renin, salt and water balance. Klin Wochenschr [Suppl I] 56: 23
5. Doyle TJ, McGregor WR, Fox PS, Maddison FE, Rodgers RE, Kauffman HM (1975) Homotransplant renal artery stenosis. Surgery 77: 53
6. Farrow PR, Wilkinson R (1979) Reversible renal failure during treatment with captopril. Br Med J 1: 1680
7. Franklin SS, Young JD, Maxwell MH, Foster JH, Palmer JM, Cerny J, Varady D (1975) Operative morbidity and mortality in renovascular disease. JAMA 231: 1148
8. Goldman MH, Tilney NL, Vineyard GC, Laks H, Kahan MG, Wilson RE (1975) A twenty-year survey of arterial complications of renal transplantation. Surg Gynecol Obstet 141: 758
9. Harries-Jones EP, Wilson DR, Colapinto RF, Fenton SSA (1980) Percutaneous transluminal angioplasty in a renal transplant recipient for stenosis of the grafted renal artery. Can Med Assoc J 123: 761
10. Kirchertz EJ, Scheler F (1982) Captopril bei Nierenateriensteno sen und Niereninsuffizienz. Internist (Berlin) 23: 237
11. Ladefoged J, Nerstrøm B (1978) Significance of renin determinations in selecting transplanted patients for bilateral nephrectomy in treatment of hypertension. Dial Transplant 7: 737
12. Laroche GP, Lachance JG, Lebel M (1980) Renal revascularisation as treatment for malignant hypertension. Can J Surg 23: 329
13. Lindsey ES, Garbus SB, Golladay ES, McDonald JD (1975) Hypertension due to renal artery stenosis in transplanted kidneys. Ann Surg 181: 604
14. Margules RM, Belzer FO, Kountz SL (1973) Surgical correction of renovascular hypertension following renal allotransplantation. Arch Surg 106: 13
15. Mathias K, Rau W, Kauffmann G (1979) Katheterdilatation einer Arterienstenose nach Nierentransplantation. Dtsch Med Wochenschr 104: 437
16. Sniderman KW, Sos TA, Sprayregen S, Saddekni S, Cheigh JS, Tapia L, Tellis V, Vieth FJ (1980) Percutaneous transluminal angioplasty in renal transplant arterial stenosis for relief of hypertension. Radiology 135: 23

17. Vetter W, Vetter H, Tenschert W, Kuhlmann U, Stucher H, Glänzer K, Pouliadis G (1979) Renovaskuläre Hypertonie. Klin Wochenschr 57: 863
18. Wasser WG, Krakoff LR, Haimov M, Glabman S, Mitty HA (1981) Restoration of renal function after bilateral renal artery occlusion. Arch Intern Med 141: 1547
19. Whiteside CI, Cardella CJ, Yeung H, de Veber GA, Cook GT (1982) The role of percutaneous transluminal dilatation in the treatment of transplant renal artery stenosis. Clin Nephrol 17: 55
20. Woodhouse K, Farrow PR, Wilkinson R (1979) Reversible renal failure during treatment with captopril. Br Med J 2: 1146

53. Indications for Percutaneous Transluminal Angioplasty: The Angiologist's Point of View

W. Schoop

Angiologically, there are only two different standpoints that come into consideration as far as the indication for percutaneous transluminal angioplasty (PTA) is concerned, this depending on whether the angiologist operates himself or lets someone else carry out the treatment. In the following chapter, I am going to take the internist's point of view. He is the one who evaluates the patient's case, who treats him using conservative clinical procedures, and who refers him for invasive therapy if he considers it necessary; this of course after consulting the surgeon in the case of surgery, or the radiologist in the case of PTA.

Although PTA may be indicated, the following factors must be considered before it is selected.

1. The results to be expected in terms of:
   a) Early results
   b) Complications
   c) Late results
2. The extent of the expected improvement in blood flow, and therefore in general condition

The more promising the situation appears to be, the quicker one will decide on a PTA. Most stenoses and recent short occlusions of not more than 5 cm in length in the femoropopliteal region are very promising vascular lesions. The chances of success are smaller but good for somewhat longer occlusions in the femoral region (up to 10 cm). Less promising, but not hopeless, are the longer occlusions of the femoral artery, as well as those of the iliac artery, common femoral artery, deep femoral artery, and the lower leg arteries. Since the planned PTA often fails for different reasons, even in cases which appear to be most promising, PTA must be considered an initial therapeutic trial. One almost always has the possibility of a reconstructive operation after treatment failure.

Complications are generally unavoidable. Their occurrence and severity depend on the physician's experience and skill, as well as on his readiness to take a risk. With a conservative attitude, which is advisable in most cases, serious complications seldom occur as a direct result of the procedure. The angiologist referring the patient must know that peripheral emboli often result from fresh thromboses. The average number and severity of the complications are far below those after reconstructive arterial surgery, even in higher-risk patients, such as those of clinical stages III–IV.

It is important to consider the clinical situation, especially when trying to avoid complications during PTA. The radiologist should not only have specific

Percutaneous Transluminal Angioplasty
(ed. by C. T. Dotter, A. Grüntzig, W. Schoop, E. Zeitler)

clinical radiological knowledge but should also keep in touch with the clinical angiologist during the procedure. In questionable situations, the clinicians will probably decide to minimize risk rather than to attempt treatment unlikely to be successful.

The evaluation of a recanalization very much depends on how long it is going to last. As after operative reconstruction, the late results are markedly better after PTA in the iliac region than after PTA in the femoropopliteal region. With regard to the patency rate after surgery and after PTA, the late results seem to be about the same in patients with iliac stenoses and those with short femoropopliteal occlusions. This assumes, of course, similar postoperative or postprocedural treatment and follow-up. But the evaluation of the late results should not be limited to the patency rate! The fate of those stricken with a reobliteration raises the questions: What does the recurrence mean? Does the same state occur as before treatment? Is it better or worse than before?

The femoropopliteal region is of primary interest, since it is the one which most often obliterates, is recanalized, and reobliterates. It is understandable that an acute occlusion or bypass of a reopened artery will put the leg in danger, since now there is usually no efficient collateral circulation present.

Our own studies showed that even slow reobliteration after surgical reconstruction of the femoral artery creates a bad situation due to the distal lengthening of the occlusion with deficient collateral vessels. Similar studies involving 38 patients showed the following results after 45 occlusions were opened successfully. In 50% of the cases, the reocclusion corresponded with the condition before PTA; fewer than 25% of the reobliterations showed a distal lengthening and, therefore, a worsening of the hemodynamic situation.

One must bear in mind that even reobliteration after PTA can cause a worsening of the circulation in comparison to the condition before treatment, although this happens less often than after reconstructive surgery of the artery. In connection with this, I would like to remark that besides the actual postoperative complications, other discomforts – usually cicatricial – can occur, which may cause deterioration in the condition of some patients despite successful treatment. The following special indications are conclusions drawn from the previously stated facts and considerations.

Stage I

If there are no subjective symptoms, it does not seem wise to open an arterial occlusion, but the dilatation of a severe stenosis could be of prophylactic value. The tendency for spontaneous occlusion is greater in the femoropopliteal region and in the large pelvic arteries than it is after PTA. But we still do not have the results of any comparative tests including antiaggregational prophylaxis capable of slowing down or even preventing the tendency toward occlusion in the femoropopliteal regions.

Until now, conclusive arguments for a preventive dilatation of arterial stenoses have been lacking, but the whole matter may be judged differently when those patients unable to tolerate antiaggregational medication are taken into consideration. Occasionally, it may be wise to widen by catheter a narrow area which has been obstructed, in order to avoid an acute thrombosis.

Stage II

The main aim in stage II disease is to increase the restricted load capacity. If the patient has not previously felt restricted, essentially little can be gained by a successful PTA. In these cases we see no indication for a PTA, even if objective findings lead one to believe that a severe hemodynamic disorder is present. On the other hand, we think it is justifiable to try a PTA in all patients where an improvement is probable, and where complications or worsening of the condition due to treatment are not to be expected.

We believe that an expected reocclusion in 20%–30% of the cases during the following 2–3 years is no longer an unequivocal contraindication, since this only occasionally worsens the previous condition. In cases of reobliteration, we consider the ameliorated condition between the time of PTA and reobliteration as a temporary success of treatment, this being the goal sought by an internist as far as many illnesses are concerned. Since we believe that the occurrence of postoperative early and late complications is higher, we are of the opinion that there is an indication for PTA but seldom one for surgery in stage II patients – especially those with occlusions in the femoropopliteal region.

When fresh occlusions compensated by rest are involved, catheter lysis is a possibility. It is better to wait 3 months before doing a PTA because the occlusive material will then have time to get harder, thus diminishing the chances of embolic complications. Very often, the compensation improves the condition to such an extent that treatment is no longer necessary.

Stages III–IV

In cases of rest pain or tropic lesions, a successful recanalization is of high value, even if it is incomplete and temporary. When both the PTA and reconstructive surgery appear to be promising, we always try the PTA first without taking any higher risk. We pursue an aggressive approach if the loss of the extremity can be avoided by PTA. The use of catheter lysis and PTA makes it possible to treat acute thrombosis successfully without undertaking a high risk.

Aortic Arch Branches

Recent observations have been encouraging but not satisfactory enough to justify PTA in these cases. More evidence is needed that the risk is acceptably low.

XIII. Percutaneous Transluminal Angioplasty Today and in the Future

54. Percutaneous Transluminal Angioplasty: State of the Art and Future Perspectives

A. Bollinger, E. Schneider, U. Kuhlmann, G. Pouliadis, and U. Brunner

The data included in this volume and the articles published recently in the literature leave no doubt that the question should no longer be whether percutaneous transluminal angioplasty (PTA) is established, but where it is established.

Renal Artery Stenoses

The aim of renal artery dilatation is lowering or normalization of increased blood pressure and, especially in bilateral disease, improvement of impaired renal function. The first goal is reached in a high percentage of patients with fibromuscular dysplasia. About 80%–90% of cases respond favorably to PTA. In this type of lesion renal PTA is actually the first choice of treatment.

In arteriosclerotic renal artery stenoses, however, the primary and long-term results are less favorable. A good blood pressure response is obtained in only 60%–70% of patients. In this group the complication rate is higher and recurrence of stenosis or occlusion relatively common. Therefore, the value of PTA in atherosclerotic renal artery stenoses remains uncertain. Efforts should be made to define patients with optimal response. It seems that older patients with a long duration of hypertension are poor candidates and that younger patients with recent onset of hypertension and lateralization of renin levels in the renal veins are most likely to show a favorable response.

In several cases, renal function has been improved by PTA. However, the value of this therapy in patients with renal insufficiency remains to be established. Astonishing results in single patients encourage further research. The same holds true for PTA of stenosed arteries of a transplanted kidney.

Peripheral Arterial Occlusive Disease

From a clinical point of view the indications may be classified according to the stages of Fontaine. In stage I, occlusive disease without subjective symptoms, no active treatment is necessary. In early stage II, intermittent claudication and a restricted walking distance of more than 200 m, PTA should be performed when all the following criteria are fulfilled:

Percutaneous Transluminal Angioplasty
(ed. by C. T. Dotter, A. Grüntzig, W. Schoop, E. Zeitler)

1. The patient should be seriously limited in his activities (profession requiring physical work, important hobbies).
2. The arterial lesion should be optimal for PTA (short stenoses of the femoral or iliac arteries, short occlusions of the distal femoral artery).
3. The patient has to accept vigorous treatment of his individual risk factors.

Late stage II (walking distance of 200 m and less) is the field of generally accepted rules: stenosed iliac and femoropopliteal arteries should be dilated and femoral arteries with occlusions up to 10 cm in length recanalized. Surgery is preferred in iliac artery occlusions and long femoropopliteal occlusions.

In stages III and IV (rest pain and gangrene) the extremity is threatened. Before amputations are performed, the possibilities of PTA and reconstructive arterial surgery should be considered in every patient. The morphological pattern of the disease (shown by arteriography) facilitates the decision as to what procedure should be tried first. The rules outlined for stage II are no longer valid. PTA may succeed even in long occlusions or in the proximal calf region. A conference should be held to discuss treatment options and should include an experienced vascular surgeon. Combined procedures may be used in special cases.

Cerebrovascular Disease

Attempts have been made to treat proximal stenoses of the subclavian artery with or without subclavian steal, proximal stenoses of the vertebral artery, and stenoses at the carotid bifurcation. PTA for cerebrovascular disease is still experimental. Caution is especially advised in internal carotid artery stenoses, where small emboli may provoke strokes.

Future Developments

What direction will future research take? Four developments seem important and necessary:

1. More physicans should be trained to perform PTA. In many centers this therapy is not yet available. Close cooperation between internist, radiologist, and surgeon is necessary.
2. Results in patient subgroups should be studied to gain information on the outcome of PTA where the indication is not established. Examples are renal artery stenoses due to different forms of atherosclerosis, the combination of PTA with local fibrinolysis, and the controversy as to whether PTA (cross over technique) or surgery should be preferred for the treatment of stenoses in the femoral bifurcation.
3. Studies should be designed to improve the long-term patency rates after successful PTA. Secondary prophylaxis of reocclusion has been achieved mainly by use of anticoagulants. The value of different antiplatelet drugs is far from being established. It will probably be possible to increase long-term patency in the femoropopliteal segment by 10%–15%.
4. Better balloon catheters should be developed. Less compliant balloons are needed to allow the higher dilatation pressures helpful in treating calcified stenoses.

55. Transluminal Angioplasty: Results and Future Outlook

C. T. Dotter

Results

At a symposium in Nuremberg, Germany on 15 May 1982, a number of workers from North America and Europe who have had extensive experience with transluminal angioplasty provided the collective results shown in Table 1.

These demonstrate that, where it is feasible, transluminal angioplasty is a useful and often superior alternative to traditional vascular surgery. It is not irresponsible, but conservative, to argue that it often warrants a primary therapeutic role. The sale of perhaps 100,000 dilating catheters in the United States in 1981 shows the extent of interest it has earned. If only a tenth of those catheters were used as successful alternatives to iliac surgery, about 500 lives and $100 Million in health care costs were saved. Abrams' recent, as yet unpublished, painstaking statistical study bears out this rough estimate. The enthusiasm for transluminal angioplasty on the part of patients and those who indirectly pay is understandable; the expressed disapproval of some vascular surgeons has been disappointing.

Future Prospects

Selective clot lysis is finally gaining acceptance as a valuable adjunct to catheter angioplasty. It appears likely that percutaneous, image-guided techniques for

Table 1. Transluminal angioplasty – collective summary of results

	Treated	Immediate success	Long-term success	Complications needing op.	Deaths within 7 days
Femoro-popliteal	2337	87%	69% (5y)	2.0%	3
Iliac	1725	93%	84% (3y)	1.2%	1
Renal	792	FMD:[a] 95%	78% (2–4y)	2.1%	0
Total		AS:[b] 91%	57%		

[a] Fibromuscular disease
[b] Arteriosclerosis

Percutaneous Transluminal Angioplasty
(ed. by C. T. Dotter, A. Grüntzig, W. Schoop, E. Zeitler)

embolectomy, photovaporization of atheromatous occlusions, and transluminal sleeve graft placement will play important roles in the future management of vascular disease. It has already been shown that percutaneous catheter obliteration of variceal bleeding in portal hypertension can be of real, if limited, clinical value. It has an inherent weakness since hemorrhage is controlled at the cost of further obstruction to portal flow, increased portal pressure, and consequent recurrent bleeding. To make matters worse, the combination of sluggish portal flow and the trauma of portal catheterization pose a significant risk of complicating portal vein thrombosis. Pioneer experimental work by Rösch and recently published clinical trials indicate the likelihood that variceal obliteration will in the near future be combined with a potentiated endoprotheses by the simultaneous percutaneous creation of a fistula between intrahepatic portal and hepatic veins. A safer and more easily achieved alternative to traditional high-mortality portosystemic surgical shunting should allow more patients to live longer. We are presently exploring in pigs the use of a specially designed laser catheter for this purpose.

The combined attention of angiographers and cardiovascular surgeons in this and other sophisticated, relatively noninvasive means for treating deep-seated lesions will surely lead to progress in yet unthought of applications.

Appendix

56. Transluminal Angioplasty: A Comprehensive, Chronological Bibliography 1964–1982

C. T. Dotter and E. J. Ruble

This is, the authors believe, a comprehensive, chronologically ordered bibliography on the subject of transluminal angioplasty. A few publications may have been overlooked, either inadvertently or because their nature was not apparent to us during our search of the literature. In assembling this material, a weekly computer word and author citation search of current literature was used. Abstracts and editorials were generally not included unless considered to be of historical importance.

References

Dotter CT, Judkins MP (1964) Transluminal treatment of arteriosclerotic obstruction: Description of a new technique and a preliminary report of its application. Circulation 30: 654–670 (November)

Dotter CT, Judkins MP (1965) Percutaneous transluminal treatment of arteriosclerotic obstruction. Radiology 84: 631–643 (April)

Dotter CT, Krippaehne WW, Judkins MP (1965) Transluminal recanalization and dilatation in atherosclerotic obstruction of the femoral popliteal system. Am Surg 31: 453–459 (July)

Dotter CT, Judkins MP, Frische LH, Hutchins T (1965) Transluminal recanalization, In: XIth International congress of radiology, Rome, September 1965. International congress series, no 89. Excerpta Medica, Amsterdam, p 71

Dow J, Hardwick C (1966) Transluminal arterial recanalization. Lancet: 73–74 (January 8)

Dotter CT, Judkins MP, Frische LH, Mueller R (1966) The "non-surgical" treatment of ilio-femoral arteriosclerotic obstruction. Radiology 86: 871–875 (May)

Dotter CT, Judkins MP, Frische LH (1967) Transluminal catheter treatment of arteriosclerotic observation (Abstr). Proceedings of VIII congress of international CV society, Vienna, Sept 1967. J Cardiovasc Surg, 224–225

Dotter CT, Judkins MP, Frische LH, Rösch J (1967) Nonoperative treatment of arterial occlusive disease: A radiologically facilitated technique. Radiol Clin North Am 5: 531–542 (December)

Andresen I, Gjemdal T (1967) Transluminal Behandling av arteriosclerosis obliterans. Tidsskr Nor Laegeforen 87: 1057–1060

Porstmann W, Wierny L (1967) Intravasale Rekanalisation inoperabler arterieller Obliterationen. Zentralbl Chir 92 (26): 1586–1591

Dotter CT, Judkins MP, Frische LH, Rösch J (1968) Tratamiento Transluminal de La Obstruccion Arteriosclerotica. Rev Argent Angiol II: 27–36 (March)

Dotter CT (1968) Therapeutic catheter systems. Proceedings of the Fifth annual rocky mountain bioengineering symposium. Reprinted from: IEE conference record. Fifth annual rocky mountain bioengineering symposion, May 6–7, 1968. IEEE Trans Biomed Eng 102–104 (May)

Dotter CT, Judkins MP, Rösch J (1968) Nichtoperative, transluminale Behandlung der arteriosklerotischen Verschlußaffektionen. ROEFO 109: 125–133 (August)

Percutaneous Transluminal Angioplasty
(ed. by C. T. Dotter, A. Grüntzig, W. Schoop, E. Zeitler)

Dotter CT, Rösch J, Judkins MP (1968) Transluminal dilatation of atherosclerotic stenosis. Surg Gynecol Obstet 127: 794–804 (October)

Staple TW (1968) Modified catheter for percutaneous transluminal treatment of arteriosclerotic obstructions. Radiology 91: 1041–1043 (November)

Dotter CT, Judkins MP (1969) Transluminal dilatation for atherosclerotic ischemia of the lower extremity. Geriatrics 24: 108–111 (February)

Dotter CT, Rösch J, Judkins MP (1969) Transluminální Dilatace (Transluminal dilatation). Cesk Radiol 23: 15–19 (February)

Dotter CT, Judkins MP, Rösch J (1969) Transluminal angioplasty in arteriosclerotic obstruction of the lower extremities. Med Times 97 (7): 95–108 (July)

Zeitler E, Muller R (1969) Erste Ergebnisse mit der Katheter-Rekanalisation nach Dotter bei arterieller Verschlußkrankheit. ROEFO 111 (3): 345–352 (September)

Palayew MJ, Sedlezky I, Sigman HH, Sheiner NM (1969) Occlusive peripheral arteriosclerosis: Treatment by percutaneous transluminal recanalization – "The Dotter procedure". Can Med Assoc J 101: 672–672 (November)

Berglund G, Bodvall B, Eldh J, Yden S (1969) Nytt behandlingsalternative vid artiell insufficiens i benen. Lakartidningen 66: 129–138

Brahme F, Swedenborg J, Tibel B (1969) Evaluation of transluminal recanalisation of the femoral artery. Acta Chir Scand 135: 679–684

Dotter CT (1970) Arteriosclerosis. Semin Roentgenol 5: 228–244 (July)

Zeitler E, Maresta A (1970) Ricanalizzazione Transluminale Percutanea delle Occlusioni e delle Stenosi Arteriose nella Arteriopatia Aterosclerotica Obliterativa. G Clin Med 51: 381

Freeney P (1971) Transluminal angioplasty. Bull Mason Clin 31 (1): 9–15 (Spring)

Zeitler E, Schoop W, Zahnow W (1971) The treatment of occlusive arterial disease by transluminal catheter angioplasty. Radiology 99 (1): 19–26 (April)

Zeitler E (1971) Angiographische Probleme zur Diagnostik und Therapie der renovaskulären Hypertonie. In: Denck H, Flora G, Hilbe G, Piza F (eds) Renovasculäre Hypertonie. Wiener Medizinische Akademie, Vienna, pp 113–117

Zeitler E (1971) Perkutane transluminale Verschlußrekanalisation und Stenosedilatation bei Angiopathia obliterans. Aktuel Chir 6: 143–154

Zeitler E, Hüring HG, Schoop W, Schmidtke I (1971) Mechanische Behandlung von Beckenarterienstenosen mit der Perkutanen Kathetertechnik. Verh Dtsch Ges Herz Kreislaufforsch 37: 402–407

Dotter CT (1971) Clinical indications for transluminal dilatation in the management of atheromatous leg ischema. Cardiovasc Clin 3 (1): 104–111

Dotter CT, Rösch J (1971) Transluminal angioplasty: The catheter treatment of peripheral arterial obstruction. In: Dale WA (ed) Management of arterial occlusive disease, Chapt 15. Yearbook Publishing Company, Chicago, pp 257–267

Catalano D (1972) L'angioplastica transluminale alla Dotter. Reparto radiologico ospedale San Gennaro. Dal Palasciano 1 (1): 3–11

Degni M, Deucher GP, Marques M de B (1972) Apresentaçâo de Nova Tecnica de Dilataçâo Arterial Para Tratamento das Estenoses Arteriais de Origem Ateroesclerótica. Rev Bras Cardiovasc 8 (4): 355–374

Kohler M (1972) Konservative Behandlungsmöglichkeiten bei arteriellen Durchblutungsstörungen. Herz/Kreislaufforsch 4 (4): 127–133 (April)

Zeitler E (1972) Transluminale Verschlußrekanalisation mit Angiographiekatheter. Herz/Kreislaufforsch 4 (4): 138–143 (April)

Eie H, Ro J, Amundsen E, Osvik K (1972) Combined thrombolytic and Dotter treatment in arterial occlusive disease. J Oslo City Hosp 22: 141–148 (September)

Peeters FLM (1972) Een niet operatieve methode voor de behandeling van claudicatieklachten, de zogenammde catheter augioplastiek. Med Tijdschr Geneeskd 116: 1977

Zeitler E, Schoop W, Schmidtke I, Hennings D, Rotter A (1972) Ergebnisse der Katheterbehandlung (Dotter-Technik) arterieller Obliterationen an den unteren Extremitäten. Verh Dtsch Ges Inn Med 78: 631

Zeitler E (1972) Die perkutane Rekanalisation arterieller Obliterationen mit Katheter nach Dotter (Dotter-Technik). Dtsch Med Wochenschr 97: 1392–1394

Wierny L, Plass R, Porstmann W (1973) Langzeitbeobachtungen nach transluminaler Katheterrekanalisation arterieller Obliterationen nach Dotter und Judkins. Zentralbl Chir 98 (50): 1761–1772

Bean WJ, Smith SL, Corcoran JR (1973) Transluminal popliteal artery dilatation. J La State Med Soc 125 (3): 91–92 (March)

Zeitler E, Schmidtke J, Schoop W (1973) Die perkutane Behandlung von arteriellen Durchblutungsstörungen der Extremitäten mit Katheter. VASA 2 (4): 401–408

Sobbe A, Martin M, Trubestein G (1973) Besondere Aspekte der transluminalen Katheterrekanalisation und ihrer Rezidivbehandlung. ROEFO 118: 682–690 (June)

Zeitler E (1973) Die perkutane Behandlung von arteriellen Durchblutungsstörungen der Extremitäten mit Katheter. Radiologe 13 (8): 319–324

Porter JM, Eidemiller LR, Dotter CT, Rösch J, Vetto M (1973) Combined arterial dilatation and femorofemoral bypass for limb salvage. Surg Gynecol Obstet 137: 409–412 (September)

Dotter CT, Rösch J, Bilbao MK (1973) Transluminal angioplasty. In: Abstracts, XIIIth international congress of radiology, Madrid, October 1973. International congress series, no 301. Excerpta Medica, Amsterdam, p 145

Kikkis D, Zeitler E (1973) Durchblutungsmessung vor und nach Katheterrekanalisation mit der Xe-133-Clearancemethode. In: Zeitler E (ed) Aktuelle Probleme in der Angiologie: 19, Diagnostik mit Isotopen bei arteriellen und venösen Durchblutungsstörungen der Extremitäten. Huber, Bern, pp 79–82

Porstmann W (1973) Ein neuer Korsett-Ballonkatheter zur transluminalen Rekanalisation nach Dotter unter besonderer Berücksichtigung von Obliterationen an den Beckenarterien. Radiol Diagn (Berl) 2: 239–244

Sobbe A, Martin M, Zeitler E (1973) Besondere Aspekte der transluminalen Katheterrekanalisation nach Dotter. ROEFO Beiheft: 252

Wierny L, Plass R, Porstmann W (1973) Langzeitbeobachtungen nach transluminaler Katheterrekanalisation arterieller Obliterationen nach Dotter und Judkins. Zentralbl Chir 98 (50): 1761–1772

Zeitler E, Reichold J, Schoop W, Loew D (1973) Einfluß von Acetylsalicylsäure auf das Frühergebnis nach perkutaner Rekanalisation arterieller Obliterationen nach Dotter. Dtsch Med Wochenschr 98: 1285–1288

Dotter CT (1974) Catheter technics in diagnosing and treating femoral artery atherosclerosis. Geriatrics 29: 93–102 (March)

Dotter CT, Rösch J, Seaman AJ (1974) Selective clot lysis with low-dose streptokinase. Radiology 111: 31–37 (April)

Stanley JC, Fry WJ, Seeger JF, Hoffman GL, Gabrielsen TO (1974) Extracranial internal carotid and vertebral artery fibrodysplasia. Arch Surg 109: 215–221 (August)

Eidemiller ER, Porter JM, Rösch J, Dotter CT, Krippaehne WW (1974) Surgical treatment of bilateral iliac artery occlusive disease in high-risk patients. Am Surg 40: 511–517 (September)

Grüntzig A, Schlumpf M, Wellauer J, Bollinger A (1974) Results of transluminal vascular canalization after Dotter surveillance using Doppler ultrasonic pressure measurement (Abstract). ASCA 249–251 (September)

Wierny LR, Plass R, Porstmann W (1974) Long-term results in 100 consecutive patients treated by transluminal angioplasty. Radiology 112 (3): 543–548 (September)

Dotter CT, Rösch J, Anderson JM, Antonovic R, Robinson M (1974) Transluminal iliac artery dilatation – nonsurgical catheter treatment of atheromatous narrowing. JAMA 230: 117–124 (October)

Grüntzig A, Hopff H (1974) Perkutane Rekanalisation chronischer arterieller Verschlüsse mit einem neuen Dilatationskatheter. Dtsch Med Wochenschr 99: 2502

Grüntzig A, Wellauer J, Bollinger A (1974) Rekanalisation arterieller Verschlüsse nach Dotter. Erste Erfahrungen. In: Ehringer H (ed) Fortschritte der konservativen Therapie der peripheren arteriellen Verschlußkrankheit. Aktuelle Probleme in der Angiologie, vol 24. Huber, Bonn, p 87

Zeitler E (1974) Die perkutane Behandlung arterieller Obliterationen mit Kathetern. In: Heberer G, Rau G, Schoop W (eds) Angiologie. Grundlagen, Klinik & Praxis, 2nd edn. Thieme, Stuttgart, pp 298

Zeitler E (1974) Leistungsfähigkeit der perkutanen Beseitigung arterieller Obliterationen mit der Dotter-Technik. In: Ehringer H (ed) Fortschritte der konservativen Therapie der peripheren arteriellen Verschlußkrankheit. Aktuelle Probleme in der Angiologie, vol 24. Huber, Bern, pp 70

Hohn P, Wagner R, Zeitler E (1975) Histologische Befunde nach der Katheterbehandlung arterieller Obliterationen nach Dotter und ihre Bedeutung. Herz/Kreislaufforsch 7 (1): 13–23

Schmidtke I, Zeitler E, Schoop W (1975) Langzeitergebnisse der perkutanen Katheterbehandlung (Dotter-Technik) bei femoro-poplitealen Arterienverschlüssen im Stadium II. VASA 4 (3): 210–226

Brunner U, Gruntzig A (1975) Das Dilatationsverfahren nach Dotter in gefäßchirurgischer Sicht. VASA 4 (4): 334–337

Zeitler E (1975) Behandlung mit Kathetern bei peripheren arteriellen Durchblutungsstörungen. Med Welt 26: 1863–1869 (October 10)

Olbert F, Kumpan W, Ogris E, Denck H, Weidinger P, Hugeneck J, Jonas M, Russe O (1975) Die percutane, transluminale Dilatation nach Dotter – eine radiologische Methode zur Wiederherstellung der arteriellen Strombahn. Ost Ärzteztg 30 (19): 1226

Giessler R, Zeitler E (1975) Gefäßschäden bei transkutaner Katheterdilatation nach Dotter. 6. Jahrestagung Österr Ges Gefäßchirurgie (Iatrogene Gefäßschäden), Klagenfurt 1973. Karger, Basel, pp 95–97

Horvath L, Illes I (1975) A combveroer-elzarodas kezelese kateteres modszerrel: transluminalis angioplastica es kozverlen erdmenyei. Magy Radiol 27: 203–211

Van Andel GJ (1975) Transluminale angioplastiek volgens Dotter. Ned Tijdschr Geneeskd 119: 343–344

Van Andel GJ (1975) Transluminal angioplasty according to Dotter-Judkins. Radiol Clin 44: 228

Zeitler E (1975) Die „Dotter-Technik" – ein klinisches Modell zur Prüfung antithrombotischer Substanzen. Ther Ber Bayer 47: 23

Wallace S (1976) Interventional Radiology. Cancer 37 (1): 517–531 (January)

Grüntzig A (1976) Die perkutane Rekanalisation chronischer arterieller Verschlüsse mit einem neuen doppellumigen Dilatationskatheter. ROEFO 124: 80 (February)

Zeitler E (1976) Wirkung verschiedener Medikamente zur Verhütung des Reverschlusses nach Katheter-Desobliteration nach Dotter. Med Welt 27 (28): 1377–1380 (July)

Grüntzig A (1976) Perkutane Dilatation von Koronarstenosen. Beschreibung eines neuen Kathetersystem. Klin Wochenschr 54: 543–545

Grüntzig A, Turina MI, Schnieder JA (1976) Experimental percutaneous dilatation of coronary artery stenosis. Circulation 54 (4): 81–85 (October)

Grüntzig A, Reidhammer HH, Turina M, Rutishauser W (1976) Eine neue Methode zur perkutanen Dilatation von Koronarsternosen – tierexperimentelle Prüfung. Verh Dtsch Ges Kreislaufforsch 42: 282–285

Chudacek Z (1976) Our first experiences with the intraluminal recanalization (Abstr). In: Proceedings of IV congress of Czechozlovakian and international radiologists. Bratislave, 1976

Hopfner R, Wagner V (1976) Intraoperativ angewandte transluminale Katheter-Rekanalisation nach der Dotter-Technik. Fortschr Med 94: 624

Zeitler E, Schmidtke I, Schoop W, Giessler R, Dembski J, Mansjoer H (1976) Ergebnisse nach perkutaner transluminaler Angioplastik bei über 700 Behandlungen. Röntgenpraxis 29: 78–81

Van Andel GJ (1976) Percutaneous transluminal angioplasty. The Dotter procedure: a manual for the radiologist. Excerpta Medica, Amsterdam, pp 179

Zeitler E (1976) Transluminale Katheterrekanalisation und Fibrinolyse. In: Lohmann FW (ed) Chronische arterielle Durchblutungsstörungen der Extremitäten. Witzstrock, Baden-Baden, pp 78–94

Eguchi S, Takeuchi T, Ohtani SI (1977) Transvenous instrumental dilatation for obstruction of the hepatic portion of the inferior vena cava. J Cardiovasc Surg 18 (5): 493–499 (September–October)

Grüntzig A, Schneider HJ (1977) Die perkutane Dilatation chronischer Koronarstenosen – Experiment und Morphologie. Schweiz Med Wochenschr 107: 1588 (October)

Mathias K, Rau WS, Rohrbach R, Neff U (1977) Percutaneous transluminal angioplasty of carotid artery stenosis: experimental studies and possible application in patients. XIV Congress of radiologie, Rio de Janeiro, 23–29 Oct 1977. Excerpta Medica, Amsterdam, pp 45

Lawson JD, Boerth R, Foster JH, Dean RH (1977) Diagnosis and management of renovascular hypertension in children. Arch Surg 112: 1307–1316 (November)

Horvath L (1977) Az alsovegtag-arteriak rontgenvizsgalata es a katheteres (Dotter-fele) angioplastica. Radiologiai Közlemenyek Különlenyomet

Porter JM, Eidemiller LA, Hood RW, Wesche EH, Dotter CT, Rösch J (1977) Transluminal angioplasty and distal arterial bypass. Am Surg 43: 695–701

Grüntzig A (1977) Die perkutane transluminale Rekanalisation chronischer Arterienverschlüsse mit einer neuen Dilatationstechnik. Witzstrock, Baden-Baden

Grüntzig A (1977) Die perkutane transluminale Rekanalisation, ein Vergleich der Dotter- und Dilatationstechnik. In: Alexander K, Cachovan M (eds) Diabetische Angiopathren. Witzstrock, Baden-Baden

Marshall M, Hess H (1978) New findings concerning pathogenesis and nonsurgical treatment of peripheral arterial diseases. VASA 7: 49–53 (January)

Mathias K (1977) Ein neuartiges Kathetersystem zur perkutanen transluminalen Angioplastie von Karotisstenosen. Fortschr Med 95 (15): 1007–1011

Preter B, Grüntzig A, Greminge P (1978) (GE) Percutaneous transluminal recanalization after trauma. RÖFO 129 (6): 787–789 (January)

Schmidtke L, Zeitler E, Schoop W (1978) Spätergebnisse (5–8 Jahre) der perkutanen Katheterbehandlung (Dotter-Technik) bei femoro-poplitealen Arterienverschlüssen im Stadium II. VASA 7 (1): 4–15

Daskalakis MK (1978) Fibromuscular hyperplasia of external iliac arteries. West J Med 128 (4): 345–346 (April)

Dotter CT, Rösch J, Robinson M (1978) Fluroroscopically aided femoral artery puncture: technical note. Radiology 127: 266–267 (April)

Grüntzig A, Kuhlmann U, Vetter W, Lütolf U, Meier B, Siegenthaler W (1978) Treatment of renovascular hypertension with percutaneous transluminal dilatation of a renal artery stenosis. Lancet 1: 801–802 (April 15)

Walter JF, Bookstein JJ, Kramer RA, Cannon WB, Trollope MD, Jamplis RW (1978) Therapeutic angiography. Arch Surg 113: 432–439 (April)

Annexton M (1978) Burrowing through blocked arteries with a balloon 'relocates' plaques. JAMA 240: 1117–1119 (September)

Grüntzig A, Hirzel H, Goebel N, Gattiker R, Turina M, Myler R, Stertzer S, Kaltenbach M (1978) Die perkutane transluminale Dilatation chronischer Koronarstenosen. Schweiz Med Wochenschr 108: 1721–1723 (November)

Hess H, Muller-Fassbender H, Ingrisch H, Mietaschk A (1978) Verhütung von Wiederverschlüssen nach Rekanalisation obliterierter Arterien mit der Kathetermethode. Dtsch Med Wochenschr 103 (50): 1994–1997 (December)

Jester HG, Mellmann J (1978) Langzeitergebnisse nach transluminaler Rekanalisation arterieller Obliterationen. Med Klin 73 (40): 1389–1391

Kuhlmann U, Grüntzig A, Vetter W, Siegenthaler W (1978) Renovaskuläre Hypertonie: Therapie durch perkutane transluminale Dilatation von Nierenarterienstnosen. Schweiz Med Wochenschr 108: 1847–1850 (December)

Denck H, Hold M, Russe O, Kobinia G (1978) Indikationen zur transluminalen Arteriendilatation (Dotter) aus chrirugischer Sicht. VASA 7: 16–21

Grüntzig A (1978) Nonoperative dilatation of coronary artery stenosis: Percutaneous transluminal angioplasty (PTA). In: Kaltenbach et al. (eds) Coronary heart disease. Stuttgart, pp 325–343

Kuhlmann U, Grüntzig A, Vetter W, Lütolf U, Meier B, Siegenthaler W (1978) Percutaneous transluminal dilatation: A new treatment of renovascular hypertension? Klin Wochenschr 56: 703–707

Leu HJ (1978) Im Labyrinth von Minos – in angiologischer Sicht. VASA 7: 3

Rentrop P, DeVivie ER, Karsch KR, Kreuzer H (1978) Acute coronary occlusion with impending infarction as an angiographic complication relieved by a guide-wire recanalization. Clin Cardiol 1: 101–106
Zeitler E, Martin M (1978) Dotter-technique and subsequent SK-treatment. In: Zeitler E (ed) Aktuelle Probleme in der Angiologie: 37 new concepts in streptokinase dosimetry. Huber, Bern, pp 70–74
Zeitler E, Grüntzig A, Schoop W (eds) (1978) Percutaneous vascular recanalization. Springer, Berlin Heidelberg New York
Bollinger A (1978) Appraisal of the therapy. In: Zeitler E et al. (eds) Percutaneous vascular recanalization. Springer, Berlin Heidelberg New York, chapt 32, pp 194–195
Bollinger A, Grüntzig A, Schlumpf M, Casty M (1978) Ultrasound techniques for followup of hemodynamic changes after transluminal dilatation or recanalization. In: Zeitler E et al. (eds) Percutaneous vascular recanalization. Springer, Berlin Heidelberg New York, chapt 12, pp 78–85
Brunner U, Grüntzig A (1978) Vascular surgery and transluminal dilatation/recanalization: Complementary procedures for the reconstruction of peripheral occlusive diseases. In: Zeitler E et al. (eds) Percutaneous vascular recanalization. Springer, Berlin Heidelberg New York, chapt 26, pp 160–166
Dembski JC, Zeitler E (1978) Selective arterial clot lysis with angiography catheter. In: Zeitler E et al. (eds) Percutaneous vascular recanalization. Springer, Berlin Heidelberg New York, chapt 25, pp 157–159
Denck H, Hold M, Russe O, Kobinia G (1978) Indications for PTR from the surgical point of view. In: Zeitler E et al. (eds) Percutaneous vascular recanalization. Springer, Berlin Heidelberg New York, chapt 30, pp 183–188
Dotter CT, Grüntzig A, Schoop W, Zeitler E (1978) Introduction. In: Zeitler E et al. (eds) Percutaneous vascular recanalization. Springer, Berlin Heidelberg New York, chapt 1, pp 1–2
Dotter CT (1978) Transluminal angioplasty – pathologic basis. In: Zeitler E et al. (eds) Percutaneous vascular recanalization. Springer, Berlin Heidelberg New York, chapt 2, pp 3–12
Giessler R (1978) Surgical aspects of vascular reconstruction after PTR. In: Zeitler E et al. (eds) Percutaneous vascular recanalization. Springer, Berlin Heidelberg New York, chapt 27, pp 160–171
Grüntzig A (1978) Percutaneous transluminal recanalization (PTR) with the double-lumen dilatation catheter. In: Zeitler E et al. (eds) Percutaneous vascular recanalization. Springer, Berlin Heidelberg New York, chapt 4, pp 17–23
Grüntzig A (1978) Transluminal dilatation of coronary artery stenosis – experimental report. In: Zeitler E et al. (eds) Percutaneous vascular recanalization. Springer, Berlin Heidelberg New York, chapt 9, pp 57–65
Grüntzig A, Zeitler E (1978) Cooperative study of results of PTR in twelve different clinics. In: Zeitler E et al. (eds) Percutaneous vascular recanalization. Springer, Berlin Heidelberg New York, chapt 17, pp 118–119
Heidler R, Zeitler E, Gessler U (1978) Percutaneous transluminal dilatation of stenosis behind AV-fistulas in hemodialysis patients. In: Zeitler E et al. (eds) Percutaneous vascular recanalization. Springer, Berlin Heidelberg New York, chapt 21, pp 142–144
Hopfner R, Wagner V (1978) Intraoperative transluminal angioplasty by Dotter's method. In: Zeitler E et al. (eds) Percutaneous vascular recanalization. Springer, Berlin Heidelberg New York, chapt 28, pp 172–174
Horváth L, Illés I, Varró J (12978) Complications of the transluminal angioplasty excluding the puncture site complications. In: Zeitler E et al. (eds) Percutaneous vascular recanalization. Springer, Berlin Heidelberg New York, chapt 19, pp 126–139
Jester HG, Sinapius D (1978) Morphologic alterations after percutaneous transluminal recanalization of chronic femoral atherosclerosis. In: Zeitler E et al. (eds) Percutaneous vascular recanalization. Springer, Berlin Heidelberg New York, chapt 8, pp 51–56
Kramann B, Christen N, Feuerbach S, Wagner V (1978) Transvenous xeroarteriography, an appropriate method for angiographic follow-up after PTR. In: Zeitler E et al. (eds) Percutaneous vascular recanalization. Springer, Berlin Heidelberg New York, chapt 13, pp 86–90
Leu HJ, Grüntzig A (1978) Histopathologic aspects of transluminal recanalization. In: Zeitler E et al. (eds) Percutaneous vascular recanalization. Springer, Berlin Heidelberg New York, chapt 7, pp 39

Mahler F, Grüntzig A, Schlumpf M (1978) Transluminal dilatation of a stenosis in the deep femoral artery. In: Zeitler E et al. (eds) Percutaneous vascular recanalization. Springer, Berlin Heidelberg New York, chapt 20, pp 141

Martin M, Zeitler E (1978) Percutaneous transluminal recanalization (PTR) and fibrinolysis: Fibrinolytic treatment of femoral reocclusions subsequent to PTR procedures. In: Zeitler E et al. (eds) Percutaneous vascular recanalization. Springer, Berlin Heidelberg New York, chapt 24, pp 152–156

Mathias K, Rohrbach R, Neff W, Ensinger H (1978) Percutaneous transluminal dilatation (PTD) of carotid artery stenosis. In: Zeitler E et al. (eds) Percutaneous vascular recanalization. Springer, Berlin Heidelberg New York chapt 10, pp 66–72

Müller-Fassbender H, Hess H (1978) Percutaneous transluminal recanalization combined with fibrinolysis. In: Zeitler E et al. (eds) Percutaneous vascular recanalization. Springer, Berlin Heidelberg New York, chapt 23, pp 148–151

Olbert F, Hanecka L (1978) Transluminal vascular dilatation with a modified dilatation catheter. In: Zeitler E et al. (eds) Percutaneous vascular recanalization. Springer, Berlin Heidelberg New York, chapt 6, pp 32–38

Schmidtke L, Zeitler E, Schoop W (1978) Late results of percutaneous catheter treatment (Dotter's technique) in occlusion of the femoropopliteal arteries, Stage II. In: Zeitler E et al. (eds) Percutaneous vascular recanalization. Springer, Berlin Heidelberg New York, chapt 15, pp 96–110

Schoop W, Levy H, Cappius G, Mansjoer H, Zeitler E (1978) Early and late results of PTD in iliaca stenosis. In: Zeitler E et al. (eds) Percutaneous vascular recanalization. Springer, Berlin Heidelberg New York, chapt 16, pp 111–117

Schoop W (1978) Indications for PTR from the angiologic point of view. In: Zeitler E et al. (eds) Percutaneous vascular recanalization. Springer, Berlin Heidelberg New York, chapt 29, pp 175–182

Zeitler E (1978) Appraisal of the techniques. In: Zeitler E et al. (eds) Percutaneous vascular recanalizaton. Springer, Berlin Heidelberg New York, chapt 31, pp 189–193

Van Andel GJ (1978) Transluminal dilatation with separate teflon catheters. In: Zeitler E et al. (eds) Percutaneous vascular recanalization. Springer, Berlin Heidelberg New York, chapt 3, pp 13–16

Van Andel GJ (1978) Review of the results of the Dotter procedure. In: Zeitler E et al. (eds) Percutaneous vascular recanalization. Springer, Berlin Heidelberg New York, chapt 14, pp 91–95

Zeitler E (1978) Dilatation technique of iliac artery stenoses with balloon catheters. In: Zeitler E et al. (eds) Percutaneous vascular recanalization. Springer, Berlin Heidelberg New York, chapt 5, pp 24–32

Zeitler E (1978) Drug treatment before and after PTR. In: Zeitler E et al. (eds) Percutaneous vascular recanalization. Springer, Berlin Heidelberg New York, chapt 11, pp 73–77

Zeitler E (1978) Complications in and after PTR. In: Zeitler E et al. (eds) Percutaneous vascular recanalizaton. Springer, Berlin Heidelberg New York, chapt 18, pp 120–125

Zeitler E (1978) PTR in iliac vein thrombosis. In: Zeitler E et al. (eds) Percutaneous vascular recanalization. Springer, Berlin Heidelberg New York, chapt 22, pp 145–147

Peeters FLM (1979) A non-surgical method for the treatment of intermittent claudication: so-called catheter angioplasty. Radiol Clin 41 : 350–359

Mahler F, Krneta A, Haertel M (1979) Treatment of renovascular hypertension by transluminal renal artery dilatation. Ann Intern Med 90 (1) : 56–57 (January)

Mathias K, Nöldge G, Knorad-Graf S, Kiefer S (1979) Perkutane transluminale Katheterrekanalisation eines posttraumatischen Popliteaverschlusses. Dtsch Med Wochenschr 104 (2) : 60–61 (January 12)

Engel TR, Meister SG (1979) Coronary percutaneous transluminal angioplasty. Ann Intern Med 90 (2) : 268–269 (February)

Grüntzig A, Myler R, Stertzer S, Kaltenbach M, Bentivoglio LG (1979) Percutaneous transluminal coronary angioplasty – a cooperative Study (abstr). Am J Cardiol 43 (2) : 384 (February)

Bachman DM, Casarella WJ, Sos TA (1979) Percutaneous iliofemoral angioplasty via the contralateral femoral artery. Radiology 130 : 617–621 (March)

Geyskes GG, Puylaert CBAT, Oei HY, Boomsma JHB (1979) Intraluminal dilatation of renal artery stenosis. Clin Sci 57: 441–443 (March)

Katzen BT, Chang J (1979) Percutaneous transluminal angioplasty with the Grüntzig balloon catheter. Radiology 130 (3): 623–626 (March)

Mathias K, Rau W, Kauffmann G (1979) Katheterdilatation einer Arterienstenose nach Nierentransplantation. Dtsch Med Wochenschr 104 (12): 437–438 (March)

Grüntzig A, Kumpe DA (1979) Technique of percutaneous transluminal angioplasty with the Grüntzig balloon catheter. AJR 132: 547–552 (April)

Katzen BT, Chang J, Lukowsky GH, Abramson EG (1979) Percutaneous transluminal angioplasty for treatment of renovascular hypertension. Radiology 131 (1): 53–58 (April)

Mathias K, Spillner G, Staiger J, Ahmadi A, Werner JP (1979) Percutane transluminale Revaskularisation von Unterschenkelarterien. Chirurg 50: 158–163 (April)

Millan VG, Madias NE (1979) Percutaneous transluminal angioplasty for severe renovascular hypertension due to renal artery medial fibroplasia. Lancet I: 993–995 (May)

Richter EI, Grüntzig A, Ingrisch H, Mahler F, Mathias K, Roth FJ, Sörensen A, Zeitler E (1979) Percutaneous dilatation of renal artery stenoses. Ann Radiol 23: 275–278 (May)

Temkin LP (1979) Percutaneous transluminal coronary angiography – Can cardiac catheterization be therapeutic? Ariz Med 36: 353–355 (May)

Millan VG, Mast WE, Madias NE (1979) Nonsurgical treatment of severe hypertension due to renal artery intimal fibroplasia by percutaneous transluminal angioplasty. N Engl J Med 300 (24): 1371–1373 (June)

Puijlaert GBAJ (1980) Historical introduction. In: Veiga-Pires JA, da Silva H, Oliva L (eds) Intervention Radiology. Proceedings of 1st international symposium on interventional radiology. Algarve, Portugal, May 29–June 2, 1979. Excerpta Medica, Amsterdam, pp 25–28

Rentrop XP, Blanke H, Karsch KR, Kreuzer H (1979) Initial experience with transluminal recanalization of the recently occluded infarct-related coronary artery in acute myocardial infarction – Comparison with conventionally treated patients. Clin Cardiol 2: 92–105 (June)

Sörensen VR, Gruntzig A, Apitzsch DE, Oelkers W, Pellnit W (1979) Transluminal Angioplastie von Nierenarterienstenosen zur Behandlung des renalen Hochdrucks. ROEFO 131 (6): 575–580

Katzen BT, Chang J (1979) Percutaneous transluminal angioplasty (PTA) with the Grüntzig balloon catheter: Technical problems encountered in the first forty patients. Cardiovasc Intervent Radiol 2: 3–7 (July)

Black TJ (1979) Percutaneous transluminal angioplasty, a nonoperative treatment of occlusive vascular disease. J Maine Med Assoc 70 (8): 318–332 (August)

Freiman DB, Ring EJ, Oleaga JA, Berkowitz H, Roberts B (1979) Transluminal angioplasty of the iliac, femoral, and popliteal arteries. Radiology 132 (2): 285–288 (August)

Glenn JF, Williams KR (1979) Percutaneous transluminal angioplasty. Bryn Mawr Hosp Bull 1 (1): 26–31 (Autumn)

Turina M, Grüntzig A, Krayenbühl C, Senning A (1979) The role of the surgeon in percutaneous transluminal dilation of coronary stenosis. Ann Thorac Surg 28: 103–112 (August)

Udoff EJ, Barth KL, Harrington DP, Kaufman SL, White RI (1979) Hemodynamic significance of iliac artery stenosis: Pressure measurements during angiography. Radiology 132: 289–293 (August)

Van Andel GJ, Krepel VM (1979) De behandeling van stenosen in de arteriae iliacae met dilatatiecatheters (Dotter-Methode). Ned Tijdschr Geneeskd 123: 873–878 (August)

Houck WS (1979) Renovascular hypertension secondary to arterial fibrodysplasia: treatment by dilation using a Fogarty balloon. JAMA 242 (13): 1396–1397 (September)

Tegtmeyer CJ, Moore TS, Chandler JG, Wellons HA, Rudolf LE (1979) Percutaneous transluminal dilatation of a complete block in the right iliac artery. AJR 133: 532–535 (September)

Rentrop P, Blanke H, Wiegand V, Karsch KR (1979) Wiedereröffnung verschlossener Kranzgefäße im akuten Infarkt mit Hilfe von Kathetern. Dtsch Med Wochenschr 104 (40): 1401–1405 (October)

Weinberger MH, Yune HY, Grim CE, Luft FC, Klatte C, Donohue JP (1979) Percutaneous transluminal angioplasty for renal artery stenosis in a solitary functining kidney; an alternative to surgery in the high-risk patient. Ann Intern Med 91: 684–688 (November)

Alpert JR, Ring EJ, Berkowitz HD, Freiman DB, Oleaga JA, Gordon R, Roberts B (1979) Treatment of vein graft stenosis by balloon catheter dilation. JAMA 242 (25): 2769–2771 (December 21)

Diamond NG, Casarella WJ, Hardy MA, Appel GB (1979) Dilatation of critical transplant renal artery stenosis by percutaneous transluminal angioplasty. AJR 133: 1167–1169 (December)

Katzen BT, Chang J, Knox WG (1979) Percutaneous transluminal angioplasty with the Grüntzig balloon catheter – a review of 70 cases. Arch Surg 114: 1389–1399 (December)

Schlosser V, Spillner G, Mathias K (1979) Komplikationen nach perkutaner transluminaler Gefäßrekanalisation (PTR) und ihre chirurgische Behandlung. VASA 8: 324–328 (December)

Thomson KR, Goldin AR (1979) Angiographic techniques in interventional radiology. Radiol Clin North Am 17: 375–391 (December)

Katzen BT, Chang J (1979) Percutaneous transluminal angioplasty with the Grüntzig balloon catheter. Radiology 130: 623–626

Porstmann VW, Parsi RA, Romaniuk P, Pech HJ (1979) Die perkutane transluminale Koronar-Angioplastik – ein Katheterverfahren zur Behandlung singularer Koronararterienstenosen. Dtsch Gesundheitswes 34 (26): 1224–1229

Rentrop P, Blanke H, Karsch KR et al. (1979) Wiederöffnung des Infarktgefäßes durch transluminale Rekanalisation und intrakoronäre Streptokinase-Applikation. Dtsch Med Wochenschr 104: 1438

Schmidtke I, Roth FJ, Schoop W, Cappius G (1980) Perkutane transluminale Katheterbehandlung bei Kranken mit arteriellen Durchblutungsstörungen im Stadium II und IV. In: Müller-Wiefel H, Barras JP, Ehringer H, Krüger M (eds) Mikrozirkulation und Blutrheologie. Therapie der peripheren arteriellen Verschlußkrankheit. Witzstrock, Baden-Baden, pp 411–420 (September)

Puijlaert CBAJ (1979) Transluminale percutane catheter desobstructie van arteriosclerotische arterien: de Dotter-procedure. Bohn, Scheltema and Holkema, Utrecht, pp 407–419

Horvath L, Illes I (1979) The use of Grüntzig balloon catheter in obstructive arterial disease. Intervention radiology. Proceedings of the first international symposium on intervention radiology, Algarve, Portugal

Turina M, Grüntzig A, Krayenbuhl C, Senning A (1979) Percutaneous transluminal dilatation of coronary artery stenosis. Thorac Cardiovasc Surg 27: 199–201

Stertzer SH, Myler RK, Bruno MS, et al. (1979) Transluminal coronary artery dilatation. Pract Cardiol 5: 25–32

Rentrop KP, Blanke H, Karsch KR, Wiengand V, Kostering H, Oster H, Leitz K (1979) Acute myocardial infarction: intracoronary application of nitroglycerine and streptokinase. Clin Cardiol 2: 354–363

Ford W, Wholey MH, Zikria EA, Miller WH, Samadani SR, Koimattur AG, Sullivan ME (1980) Percutaneous transluminal angioplasty in the management of occlusive disease involving the coronary arteries and saphenous vein bypass grafts. Preliminary results. J Thorac Cardiovasc Surg 79: 1–11 (January)

Hartzler GO, Smith HC, Vlietstra RE, Oberle DA, Strelow DA (1980) Coronary bloodflow responses during successful percutaneous transluminal coronary angioplasty. May Clin Proc 55: 45–49 (January)

Kuhlmann U, Vetter W, Furrer J, Lütolf U, Siegenthaler W, Grüntzig A (1980) Renovascular hypertension: treatment by percutaneous transluminal dilattation. Ann Intern Med 92 (1): 1–6 (January)

Lee G, Ikeda RM, Joye JA, Bogren H, DeMaria AN, Mason DT (1980) Evaluation of transluminal angioplasty of chronic coronary artery stenosis: value and limitations assessed in fresh human cadaver hearts. Circulation 61 (1): 77–83 (January)

Mathias K, Staiger J, Thron A, Spillner G, Heiss HW, Konrad-Graf S (1980) Perkutane Katheterangioplastik der Arteria Subclavia. Dtsch Med Wochenschr 105 (1): 16–18 (January)

Podlas H, Snychess FD (1980) Successful transluminal recanalization in legs. S Afr Med J 57 (1): 15–17 (January)

Kaltenbach M, Kober G, Schere D (1980) Mechanische Dilatation von Koronararterienstenosen (Transluminale Angioplastie) Z Kardiol 69: 1–10 (February)

Kaufman SL (1980) Femoral puncture using Doppler ultrasound guidance: Aid to transluminal angioplasty and other applications. AJR 134: 402 (February)

Morettin LB, Schreiber MH (1980) Interventional radiology: An alternative to surgery. Tex Med 76 (2): 4344 (February)

Sinnott RC, Rich NM, Collins GJ, Clagett GP, Collins JT (1980) Percutaneous transluminal angioplasty: Report of the first two cases at Walter Reed army medical center. Milit Med 145 (2): 91–92 (February)

Velasquez G, Castaneda-Zuniga W, Formanek A, Zollikofer C, Barreto A, Nicoloff D, Amplatz K, Sullivan A (1980) Nonsurgical aortoplasty in Leriche syndrome. Radiology 134 (3): 359–360 (February)

Wallsh E, Franzone AJ, Clauss RH, Bruno MS, Steichen F, Stertzer SH (1980) Transluminal coronary angioplasty during saphenous coronary bypass surgery. A preliminary report. Ann Surg 191: 234–237 (February)

Alderman EL (1980) PTCA: Clinical studies. In: Proceedings of the workshop on percutaneous coronary angioplasty, Bethesda, June 1979. NIH Publ 80-2030, pp 179–180

Bentivoglio LG (1980) Clinical Experience: Philadelphia. In: Proceedings of the workshop on percutaneous coronary angioplasty, Bethesda, June 1979. NIH Publ 80-2030, pp 49–52

Block PC (1980) Histological and ultrastructural studies in animals. In: Proceedings of the workshop on percutaneous coronary angioplasty, Bethesda, June 1979. NIH Publ 80-2030, pp 155–156

Dotter CT (1980) Transluminal angioplasty: Background and rationale. In: Proceedings of the workshop on percutaneous coronary angioplasty, Bethesda, June 1979. NIH Publ 80-2030, pp 5–6

Grüntzig A (1980) Clinical experience: Zurich, Switzerland. In: Proceedings of the workshop on percutaneous coronary angioplasty, Bethesda, June 1979. NIH Publ 80-2030, pp 9–13

Grüntzig AR (1980) PTCA technique with a double-lumen dilatation catheter. In: Proceedings of the workshop on percutaneous coronary angioplasty, Bethesda, June 1979. NIH Publ 80-2030, pp 123–126

Kaltenbach M, Kober G, Schere D (1980) Clinical experience: Frankfurt, West Germany. In: Proceedings of the workshop on percutaneous coronary angioplasty, Bethesda, June 1979. NIH Publ 80-2030, pp 53–62

Kent KM, Bonow RO, Rosing DR, Lipson LC, Bacharach SL, Green VM, Epstein SE (1980) Improved myocardial perfusion and function following percutaneous transluminal coronary angioplasty. In: Proceedings of the workshop on percutaneous coronary angioplasty, Bethesda, June 1979. NIH Publ 80-2030, pp 39–40

Krayenbuehl HP (1980) Patient selection and complications. In: Proceedings of the workshop on percutaneous coronary angioplasty, Bethesda, June 1979. NIH Publ 80-2030, pp 63–66

Mock MB, Bentivoglio L, Dorros G, Kent K, Myler R, Williams DO, Ringqvist I, Fisher L, Gillespie MJ, Mullin S (1980) NHLBI interim registry for PTCA. In: Proceedings of the workshop on percutaneous coronary angioplasty, Bethesda, June 1979. NIH Publ 80-2030, pp 67–76

Myler RK (1980) Clinical experience: San Francisco. In: Proceedings of the workshop on percutaneous coronary angioplasty, Bethesda, June 1979. NIH Publ 80-2030, pp 15–18

Schwartz CJ (1980) Basic experimental studies in PTCA. In: Proceedings of the workshop on percutaneous coronary angioplasty, Bethesda, June 1979. NIH Publ 80-2030, pp 175–177

Simpson J (1980) PTCA in the cadaver heart. In: Proceedings of the workshop on percutaneous coronary angioplasty, Bethesda, June 1979. NIH Publ 80-2030, pp 157–160

Smith HL (1980) Ethical considerations of PTCA. In: Proceedings of the workshop on percutaneous coronary angioplasty, Bethesda, June 1979. NIH Publ 80-2030, pp 189–192

Stertzer SH, Wallsh E, Bruno MS (1980) A preliminary summary of 56 cases from Lenox Hill hospital center, New York City, New York. In: Proceedings of the workshop on percutaneous coronary angioplasty, Bethesda, June 1979. NIH Publ 80-2030, pp 25–26

Hirzel HO, Nuesch K, Gruntzig AR, Horst W, Krayenbuhl HP (1980) Thallium-201 exercise scintigraphy after percutaneous transluminal angioplasty of coronary artery stenoses. Symposium on noninvasive cardiac diagnosis II. Med Clin North Am 64: 163–176 (March)

Hor G, Kanemoto N, Stande R, Maul FD, Klepzig H Jr, Kober G, Kaltenbach M (1980) Transluminale Angioplastik: Erfolgskontrolle durch Verfahren der Nuklearmedizin nach nicht-operativer Dilatation kritischer Koronararterienstenosen. Herz 56: 168–176

Mathias VK, Schlosser V, Reinke M (1980) Katheterrekanalisation eines Subklaviaverschlusses. ROEFO 132 (3): 346–347 (March)

Pasternak RC, Baughman KL, Fallon JT, Block PC (1980) Scanning electron microscopy after coronary transluminal angioplasty of normal canine coronary arteries. Am J Cardiol 45: 591–598 (March)

Elishu EH, Haire HM, Tew FT, Newton LW (1980) Control of malignant renovascular hypertension by percutaneous transluminal angioplasty and therapeutic renal embolization. AJR 134: 815–817 (April)

Martin EC, Diamon NG, Casarella WJ (1980) Percutaneous transluminal angioplasty in non-atherosclerotic disease. Radiology 135 (1): 27–33 (April)

Logan AG, Steinhardt MI (1980) Restoration of renal function by unilateral percutaneous transluminal dilatation of stenosed renal artery. Can Med Assoc J 122: 910–912 (April)

Mullins CE, Hesslein PS, Driscoll DJ (1980) Balloon dilatation of discrete pulmonary vein stenosis. Pediatr Cardiol 1 (4): 320

Sniderman KW, Sos TA, Sprayregen S, Saddekni S, Cheigh JS, Tapia L, Tellis V, Veith FJ (1980) Percutaneous transluminal angioplasty in renal transplant arterial stenosis for relief of hypertension. Radiology 135 (1): 23–26 (April)

Alpert JR, Ring EJ, Freiman DB, Oleaga JA, Gordon R, Berkowitz HD, Roberts B (1980) Treatment of stenosis of the iliac artery by balloon catheter dilation. Surg Gynecol Obstet 150 (4): 481–485 (May)

Athanasoulis CA (1980) Therapeutic applications of angiography. First of two parts. N Engl J Med 302 (20): 1117–1125 (May 15)

Athanasoulis CA (1980) Medical progress; therapeutic applications of angiography (second of two parts). N Engl J Med 302 (21): 1174–1179 (May 22)

Block PC (1980) Percutaneous transluminal coronary angioplasty. Primary Cardiol 6: 114–122 (May)

Cowley MJ, Vetrovec GW, Wolfgang TC, Hess ML (1980) Clinical considerations with percutaneous transluminal coronary angioplasty. Clin Res 28 (5): 807A

Grollman JH, Del Vicario M, Mittal AK (1980) Percutaneous transluminal abdominal aortic angioplasty. AJR 134: 1053–1054 (May)

Ingrisch H, Häzlin M (1980) Perkutane transluminale Angioplastik einer Stenose in einem aortorenalen Veneninterpositionstransplantat. ROEFO 133 (5): 493–495

Ingrisch H, Schatzl M, Hess H, Mietaschk A, Frey KW (1980) Microdensitometric controls for quantification of the results in percutaneous transluminal recanalization of the femoral artery. Ann Radiol 23 (4): 283–285 (May)

Kropelin T, Mathias K, Wimmer B, Kauffmann GW (1980) Was gibt es neues in der Röntgendiagnostik der Niere? Med Welt 22: 3–10 (May 29)

Kumpe DA, Kempczinski RF (1980) Percutaneous transluminal angioplasty in the selected management of proximal arterial occlusive disease of the lower extremities: a preliminary report. Surgery 87: 488–493 (May)

Lee C, Stein S (1980) Percutaneous transluminal angioplasty: interventional radiology. Conn Med 44 (4): 214–215 (May)

Alpert JR, Ring EJ, Freiman DB, Oleaga JA, Gordon R, Berkowitz HD, Roberts O (1980) Balloon dilation of iliac stenosis with distal arterial surgery. Arch Surg 115: 715–717 (June)

Castaneda-Zuniga WR, Formanek A, Tadavarthy M, Vlodaver Z, Edwards JE, Zollikofer C, Amplatz K (1980) The mechanism of balloon angioplasty. Radiology 135 (3): 565–571 (June)

Colapinto RF, Harries-Jones EP, Johnston KW (1980) Percutaneous transluminal dilatation and recanalization in the treatment of peripheral vascular disease. Radiology 135: 583–587 (June)

Colapinto RF (1980) Inadvertent percutaneous transluminal dilatation of a renal artery with a four year follow-up. Radiology 135: 605–606 (June)

Dotter CT (1980) Transluminal angioplasty: a long view. Radiology 135 (3): 561–564

Freeny PC, Beebe HG (1980) Transluminal angioplasty with the Grüntzig catheter. Bull Mason Clin 34: 57–63 (Summer)

Hamby RI, Katz S (1980) Percutaneous transluminal coronary angioplasty: Its potential impact on surgery for coronary artery disease. Cardiology 45: 1161–1165 (June)

Hudgins LB,Gold RE, Gregory AW (1980) Percutaneous transluminal angioplasty – an alternative treatment for renovascular hypertension. South Med J 73: 810–812 (June)

Kalman PG, Colapinto RF, Harries-Jones EP, Silver MD, Johnston KW (1980) Preliminary results of transluminal dilatation in the treatment of peripheral arterial occlusive disease. Surg Gynecol Obstet 150 (6): 865–868 (June)

Motarjeme A, Keifer JW, Zuska AJ (1980) Percutaneous transluminal angioplasty and case selection. Radiology 135: 573–581 (June)

Motarjeme A, Keifer JW, Zuska AJ (1980) Percutaneous transluminal angioplasty of the deep femoral artery. Radiology 135: 613–617 (June)

Sniderman KW, Sprayregen S, Sos TA, Saddekni S, Hilton S, Mollenkopf F, Soberman R, Cheigh JS, Tapia L, Stubenbord W, Tellis V, Veith FJ (1980) Percutaneous transluminal dilation in renal transplant arterial stenosis. Transplantation 30 (6): 440–444

Tegtmeyer CJ, Ayers CA, Wellons HA (1980) The axillary approach to percutaneous renal artery dilatation. Technical notes. Radiology 135: 775–776 (June)

Tegtmeyer DJ, Dyer R, Teates CD, Ayers CR, Carey RM, Wellons HA, Stanton LW (1980) Percutaneous transluminal dilatation of the renal arteries: the techniques and results. Radiology 135: 589–599 (June)

Schwarten DE, Yune Hym Klatte EC, Grim CE, Weinberger MH (1980) Clinical experience with percutaneous transluminal angioplasty (PTA) of stenotic renal arteries. Radiology 135: 601–604 (June)

Van Andel GJ (1980) Transluminal iliac angioplasty: long-term results. Radiology 135: 607–611 (June)

Yune HY (1980) Percutaneous transluminal angioplasty of stenotic renal arteries. Diagn Radiol 135: 603–604 (June)

Zarins CK, Lu CT, McDonnel AE, Whitehouse WM (1980) Limb salvage by percutaneous transluminal recanalization of the occluded superficial femoral artery. Surgery 87 (6): 701–708 (June)

Carr D, Quin RO, Hamilton DNH, Briggs JD, Junior BJR, Semple PF (1980) Transluminal dilatation of transplant renal artery stenosis (technical note). Br Med J 281: 196–197 (July 19)

Cecile JÜ, Louchart JC, Canler A, Lorek J (1980) Angioplastie endoluminale des arteres renales et des arteres peripheriques. Gaz Med Fr 87: 3061–3068 (July)

Nadalini V, Positano N, Bruttini G, Fassone M, Medica M, Fasce L (1980) Angioplastie transluminale de l'artere renale pour hypertension renovasculaire. J Urol (Paris) 86 (7): 559–562

Kalman PG, Hobbs BB, Colapinto RF, Fenton SSA, Johnston KW (1980) Percutaneous transluminal dilatation of a stenotic arteriovenous bovine graft. Dial Transplant 9: 747, 778 (August)

Yune HY, Klatte EC (1980) Circumferential tear of percutaneous transluminal angioplasty catheter balloon. AJR 135: 395–396 (August)

Greeff K, Kleinschmidt A, Kohler JA, Loose KE, Luderitz B, Luthy E, Spitzbarth H (1980) Perkutane Katheterrekanalisation (Dotter-Technik) bei peripherer arterieller Verschlußkrankheit – Einfluß von Thrombozytenaggregationshemmern auf die Rezidivhäufigkeit nach einem Jahr. Herz/Kreislaufforsch 12 (9): 383–386

Mathias K, Mittermayer CH, Ensinger H, Neff W (1980) Perkutane Katheterdilatation von Karotisstenosen. ROEFO 133: 258–261 (September)

Ring EH, Alpert JR, Freiman DB, Oleaga JA, Berkowitz H, Roberts B (1980) Early experience with percutaneous transluminal angioplasty using a vinyl balloon catheter. Ann Surg 192 (3): 438–442 (September)

Rich S (1980) Percutaneous transluminal angioplasty nonsurgical therapy of occlusive arterial disease. Postgrad Med 68: 217–224 (September)

Schwarten DE (1980) Percutaneous transluminal angioplasty of the renal artery. Cardiovasc Intervent Radiol 3: 197–206 (September)

Wall CA, Murray RE, Myler RK (1980) Transluminal angioplasty: Adjunct or gimmick? Am J Surg 140 (2): 228–230 (September)

Block PC (1980) Experimental coronary dilatation. Cleve Clin Q 47 (3): 231–234 (Fall)
Grüntzig A, Turina M (1980) Percutaneous transluminal coronary angioplasty; two years' experience. Cleve Clin Q 47 (3): 228–230 (Fall)
Kent K, Banka V, Bentivoglio L, Block P, Cowley M, Diamond G, Dorros G, Ellestad M, Faxon D, Fiedotin A, Goldberg S, Grüntzig A, Hamby M, Hirshfeld J, Kaltenbach M, Köber G, Lach R, Leatherman L, Lee G, Meyer J, Myler R, Ockene I, Robert E, Rosing D, Simpson J, Sosa J, Spring D, Stertzer S, Vliestra R, Walton J, Dilliams D, Fisher L, Gillespie M, Mullin S, Mock M (1980) Percutaneous transluminal coronary angioplasty (PTCA): update from NHLBI registry (Abstr). Circulation 62 [Suppl III]: 160 (October)
Klepzig H Jr, Scherer D, Kober G, Kaltenbach M, Maul FD, Kanemoto N, Standke R, Hor G (1980) Ergebnisse der transluminalen koronaren Angioplastie (TAP). Z Kardiol 69 (10): 701
Mathias K, Mitterman C, Eninger H, Neff W (1980) (GE) Percutaneous catheter dilatation of carotid stenoses: Animal experiments. ROEFO 133 (3): 258–261
Meakins JL (1980) Percutaneous transluminal dilatation for post-transplantation renal artery stenosis. CMA 123: 711–712 (October 18)
Myler RK (1980) Percutaneous transluminal coronary angioplasty. Cleve Clin Q 47 (3): 238–242 (Fall)
Pepine CJ, Margolis JR, Conti CR (1980) Transluminal coronary angioplasty. JAMA 244: 1966–1969 (October)
Salvador M, Chamontin B, Guittard J, Joffre F, Levade M (1980) Hypertension artérielle réno-vasculaire traitée avec succès par angioplastie trans-luminale percutanée. Nouv Presse Med 9 (36): 2657 (October)
Turina M (1980) Surgical management of complications. Cleve Clin Q 47 (3): 235–237 (Fall)
Abbott WM (1980) Percutaneous transluminal angioplasty: surgeon's view. AJR 135: 917–920 (November)
Abele JE (1980) Balloon catheters and transluminal dilatation: technical considerations. AJR 135: 901–906 (November)
Athanasoulis CA (1980) Percutaneous transluminal angioplasty: general principles. AJR 135: 893–900 (November)
Bachman DM, Kim RM (1980) Transluminal dilatation for subclavian steal syndrome. AJR 135: 995–996 (November)
Block PC (1980) Percutaneous transluminal coronary angioplasty. AJR 135: 955–959 (November)
Block PC, Fallon JT, Elmer D (1980) Experimental angioplasty: lessons from the laboratory. AJR 135: 907–912 (November)
Cope C (1980) Balloon dilatation of closed mesocaval shunts. AJR 135: 989–993 (November)
Effeney DJ, Ehrenfeld WK, Stoney RJ, Wylie EJ (1980) Why operate on carotid fibromuscular dysplasia? Arch Surg 115: 1261–1265 (November)
Fallon JT (1980) Pathology of arterial lesions amenable to percutaneous transluminal angioplasty. AJR 135: 913–916 (November)
Gordon RL, Horev G, Shifrin EG, Beer G, Katz S (1980) Early experience with balloon catheter angioplasty. Isr J Med S 16 (9–10): 686–691 (November)
Grable GS, Smith DC (1980) The use of the Simmons "sidewinder" catheter in percutaneous transluminal angioplasty of the renal arteries. Radiology 137: 541–543 (November)
Greenfield AJ (1980) Femoral, popliteal, and tibial arteries: percutaneous transluminal angioplasty. AJR 135: 927–935 (November)
Horvath L (1980) Percutaneous transluminal angioplasty: Importance of anticoagulant and fibrinolytic drugs. AJR 135: 951–954 (November)
Ingrisch H, Holzgrev H, Middeke M, Frey KW (1980) New developments in diagnosis and treatment of renovascular hypertension. Klin Wochenschr 58 (19): 1105–1115 (November)
Mathias K, Billmann P, Liebig R, Kropelin T, Thierfel K (1980) Treatment of renovascular hypertension by catheter dilatation. Radiologe 20 (10): 494–499 (November)
Motarjeme A, Keifer JW, Zuska AJ (1980) Percutaneous transluminal angioplasty of the iliac arteries: 66 experiences. AJR 135: 937–944 (November)
Novelline RA (1980) Percutaneous transluminal angioplasty: Newer applications. AJR 135: 983–988 (November)

Saddekni S, Sniderman KW, Hilton S, Sos TA (1980) Percutaneous transluminal angioplasty of nonatherosclerotic lesions. AJR 135: 975–982 (November)

Schwarten DE (1980) Transluminal angioplasty of renal artery stenosis: 70 experiences. AJR 135: 969–974 (November)

Slater EE (1980) Renal artery angioplasty versus surgery: A hypertensionologist's dilemma. AJR 135: 961–962 (November)

Sprayregen S, Sniderman KW, Sos TA, Vieux U, Singer A, Veith FJ (1980) Popliteal artery branches: percutaneous transluminal angioplasty. AJR 135: 945–950 (November)

Staiger J, Mathias K, Friederick H, Heiss HW, Konrad S, Spillner G (1980) Peripheral occlusive disease: Influence of platelets aggregation inhibitor on the one year patency rate after catheter dilatation therapy (Dotter). Herz/Kreislaufforsch 12 (9): 383–386 (November)

Sundt TM Jr, Smith HC, Campbell JK, Vlietstra RE, Cucchiara RF, Stanson AW (1980) Transluminal angioplasty for basilar artery stenosis. Mayo Clin Proc 55: 673–680 (November)

Waltman AC (1980) Percutaneous transluminal angioplasty: iliac and deep femoral arteries. AJR 135: 921–925

Rubinstein ZJ, Morag B, Itzchak A (1980) Interventional therapeutic procedures in radiology. Isr J Med Sci 16 (12): 831–842

Stertzer SH, Myler RK, Wallsh E, Bruno MS, DePasquale NP (1980) Dilation of obstructed coronaries by percutaneous transluminal angioplasty. J Cardiovasc Med 5: 1059 (December)

Tegtmeyer CJ, Wellons HA, Thompson RN (1980) Balloon dilatation of the abdominal aorta. JAMA 244 (23): 2636–2637 (December)

Carr D, Quin RO, Hamilton DN, Briggs JD, Junor BJR, Semple PF (1980) Transluminal dilatation of transplant renal artery stenosis (technical note). Br Med J 281: 196–197

Colapinto RF, Harries-Jones EP, Johnston KW (1980) Percutaneous transluminal angioplasty of peripheral vascular disease: a two-year experience. Cardiovasc Intervent Radiol 3: 213–218

Couch NP (1980) Percutaneous transluminal angioplasty: Cardiovasc Intervent Radiol 3: 219–221

Furrer J, Grüntzig A, Kugelmeier J, Goebel N (1980) Treatment of abdominal angina with percutaneous dilatation of an arteria mesenterica superior stenosis. Cardiovasc Intervent Radiol 3: 43–44

Horvath L, Dezso F, Ivan I, Paolini RM, Frigyes G, Istvan T (1980) A renovascularis hypertonia gyogyitasanak radiologiai midszere. Orv Hetil 121 (40): 2435–2439

Johnston KW, Colapinto RF, Harries-Jones EP, DeMorais D, Kalman PG, Baird RJ, Goldman BS, Key JA, Weisel RD (1980) Transluminal dilatation in the treatment of peripheral arterial occlusive disease. Can J Surg 23: 547–548

Krayenbuhl B (1980) Treatment of arterial occlusive diseases of the lower limbs (in French). Ther Umsch 37: 132, 136

Kerber CW, Cromwell LD, Loehden OL (1980) Catheter dilatation of proximal carotid stenosis during distal bifurcation endarterectomy. AJNR 1: 348–349

Lux E, Seybold D, Grosse-Vorholt R, Zeitler E, Gessler U (1980) Perkutane transluminale Katheterdilatation von Nierenarterien-Stenosen bei Patienten mit renovaskulärer Hypertonie. Fortschr Med 98 (16): 563–568

Mathias K, Billmann P, Liebig R, Kröpelin T, Thierfelder K (1980) Klinik und Praxis. Behandlung der renovaskulären Hypertonie mit der Katheterdilatation. Radiologe 20: 494–499

Mathias K, Mittermayer CH, Ensinger H, Neff W (1980) Perkutane Katheterdilatation von Karotisstenosen. Tierexperimentelle Untersuchungen. ROEFO 133: 257–261

Mandel SR, Jaques PF (1980) Salvage procedure of Thomas femoral shunts by balloon angioplasty. Surg Gynecol Obstet 151: 673–674

McCarthy S, Stein S (1980) Renovascular hypertension treated by percutaneous transluminal angioplasty. Conn Med 44: 788–779

McCook TA, Mills SR, Kirks DR, Heaston DK, Seigler HF, Malone RB, Osofsky SG (1980) Percutaneous transluminal renal artery angioplasty in a $3^1/_2$-year-old hypertensive girl. J Pediatr 97: 958–960

Mock MB, Levy RI (1980) Percutaneous transluminal coronary angioplasty. J Cardiovasc Med 5: 31

Mullan S, Duda EE, Patronas NJ (1980) Some examples balloon technology in neurosurgery. J Neurosurg 52:321–329

Schwarten DE (1980) Transluminal angioplasty of renal artery stenosis: 70 experiences. AJR 135:969–974

Scott RF, Imai H, Makita T, Thomas WA, Reiner JM (1980) Lining cell and intimal smooth muscle cell response and Evans blue staining in abdominal aorta of young swine after denudation by balloon catheter. Exp Mol Pathol 33:185–202

Uflacker R, Goldany MA, Constant S (1980) Resolution of mesenteric angina with percutaneous transluminal angioplasty of a superior mesenteric artery stenosis using a balloon catheter. Gastrointest Radiol 5:367–369

Valeix B, Chabrillat Y, Labrunie P, Jahjah F, Malmejac C, Jouven JC, Levy S, Gerard R (1980) L'angioplastie coronarienne technique, indications actuelles, resultats. Ann Cardiol Angeiol (Paris) 30:383–388

Van Andel GJ (1980) Arterial occlusion following angiography. Br J Radiol 53:747–753

Yune HY, Klatte EC, Grim CE, Weinberger MH (1980) Transluminal balloon dilatation of renal artery stenosis causing hypertension: 18 months' experience. Clin Sci 59:483s–485s

Zeitler E (1980) Percutaneous dilatation and recanalization of iliac and femoral arteries. Cardiovas Intervent Radiol 3:207–212

Zeitler E (1980) Percutaneous transluminal angioplasty: cooperation among specialities. Cardiovasc Intervent Radiol 3:221

Dotter CT (1980) Transluminal angioplasty. In: Foley WT (ed) Advances in the management of cardiovascular disease, vol 1. Yearbook Medical, Chicago, p 143

Katzen BT (1980) Intervention diagnostic and therapeutic procedures. Springer, Berlin Heidelberg New York

Myler RK (1980) Thallium-201 imaging, angiography and angioplasty. New England Nuclear, Boston

Roth F-J, Cappius G (1980) Die Angioplastie der in der Leiste gelegenen Arterienabschnitte. In: Müller-Wiefel H, Barras J-P, Enringer H, Krüger M (eds) Mirkozirkulation udn Blutrheologie. Witzstrock, Baden-Baden, pp 430–432

Grüntzig A (1981) Percutaneous transluminal angioplasty (Editorial). AJR 136:216–217 (January)

O'Mara CS, Neiman HL, Flinn WR, Herman RJ, Yao JST, Bergan JJ (1981) Hemodynamic assessment of transluminal angioplasty for lower extremity ischemia. Surgery 89 (1):106–117

Sos TA, Sniderman KW (1981) Percutaneous transluminal angioplasty. Semin Roentgenol 11 (1):26–41

Levade M, Joffre F, Railhac JJ, Sabatier JC, Putois (1981) Notre experience du traitement des stenoses des arteres iliaques angioplastie transluminale per-cutanee. J de Radiol 62 (2):134

White RI (1981) Selected techniques in interventional radiology. JAMA 245:741–744 (February 20)

Whiteside CI, Cardella CJ, Yeung H, Uldall PR, deVeber GA, Cook T (1981) Percutaneous transluminal dilatation for transplant renal artery stenosis. Kidney Int 19:395 (February)

Williams DO, Korr KS, Most AS (1981) Beneficial effect of percutaneous transluminal coronary angioplasty on coronary circulatory dnyamics. Clin Res 92 (2):250A

Bartlett JE, Pfieffer RP (1981) Percutaneous transluminal angioplasty. Mo Med 78 (3):123–125 (March)

Cowley MJ, Vetrovec GW, Wolfgang TC (1981) Efficacy of percutaneous transluminal coronary angioplasty: technique, patient selection, salutary results, limitations and complications. Am Heart J 101:272–280 (March)

Maynar M, Garcia-Pumarino JL, Salvador G, Rodriguez JE, Estevan MA, Diez-Valencia O, Gomez Martinez JLG, Seco YMA (1981) Angioplastia transluminal percutánea en extremidades inferiores. Radiologia 23:73–82 (March–April)

Schultz H, et al. (1981) Dilatation of vertebral artery stenosis. N Engl J Med 732 (March 19)

Berger SM, Gorfinkel HJ (1981) Candidates for transluminal coronary angioplasty. Am J Cardiol 48 (4):810

Goebel VN, Grüntzig A, Kugelmeier J, Turina M (1981) Koronarstenose bei Aortenisthmusstenose: Zweiseitige Therapie mit Dilatation und Resektion. ROEFO 135 (4):492–493

Lawrence PF, Miller FJ, Mineau DE (1981) Balloon catheter dilatation in patients with failing arteriovenous fistulas. Surgery 89 (4): 439–442

Moore T, Russell W, Parent A, Parker L, Smith R (1981) Nonsurgical treatment of "subclavian steal syndrome" with percutaneous transluminal angioplasty. Neurosurgery 9 (4): 466

Pinot JJ, Burelle H, Laroche JP, Mathieu P, Kasbarian M (1981) Angioplastie d'une stenose sous clavier gauche. Nouv Presse Med 10: 25 (April)

Spittell JA Jr (1981) Recognition and management of chronic atherosclerotic occlusive peripheral arterial disease. Mod Concepts Cardiovasc Dis 50 (4): 19–23 (April)

Klepzig H Jr, Scherer D, Kober G, Maul FD, Kanemoto N, Standke R, Hör G, Kaltenbach M (1981) Funktionsverbesserung nach transluminaler koronaler Angioplastik (TCA). Herz 6 (4): 252–258

Takabatake T, Yamamoto Y, Takemori Y, Maekawa M, Ohta H, Arai S, Nomura G, Hattori N (1981) Treatment of renovascular hypertension with percutaneous transluminal angioplasty. Jpn J Nephr 23 (4): 479–488

Tegtmeyer CJ, Bezirdjian DR (1981) Removing the stuck, ruptured angioplasty balloon catheter. Radiology 139: 231–232

Waller JL, Kaplan JA, King SB, Douglas JS, Craver JM (1981) Percutaneous transluminal coronary angioplasty: anesthesiologist's role. Anesth Analg, Cleve 60: 280–281 (April)

Barth KH, Brusilow SW, Kaufman SL, Ferry FT (1981) Percutaneous transluminal angioplasty of homograft renal artery stenosis in a 10 year old girl. Pediatrics 67 (5): 675–677

Cowley MJ, Block PC (1981) Percutaneous transluminal coronary angioplasty. Mod Concepts Cardiovasc Dis 50 (5): 25–29 (May)

Ferris EJ (1981) Why operate on carotid fibromuscular dysplasia? Radiology 139: 534 (May)

Ford WB, Wholey MH, Zikria EA, Somadana SR, Sullivan ME (1981) Percutaneous transluminal dilation of aortocoronary saphenous vein bypass grafts. Chest 79: 529–535 (May)

Goebel N (1981) Primary and follow-up angiographic results after percutaneous transluminal coronary angioplasty. Ann Radiol 24 (5): 349–352

Hasso AN et al. (1981) Fibromuscular dysplasia of the internal carotid artery: percutaneous transluminal angioplasty. AJR 136: 955–960 (May)

Joyce E (1981) Transluminal angioplasty: pro/con. Miami Med 51 (5): 9–11

Lowman BG, Queral LA, Holbrook WA, Estes JT, Bayly B (1981) The treatment of innominate artery stenosis by intraoperative transluminal angioplasty. Surgery 89 (5): 565–568 (May)

Madias NE, Ball JT, Millan VG (1981) Percutaneous transluminal renal angioplasty in the treatment of unilateral atherosclerotic renovascular hypertension. Am J Med 70: 1078–1083 (May)

Oleaga JA, Grossman RA, McLean GK, Rosen RJ, Freiman DB, Ring EJ (1981) Arteriovenous fistula of a segmental renal artery branch as a complication of percutaneous angioplasty. AJR 136: 988–989 (May)

Puijlaert CBAJ, Boomsma JHBB, Ruijs JHI, Oei HY, Franken AH, Koekstra A, Geyskes GG (1981) Dilatation des stenoses arterielles renales a l'aide d'un catheter a ballonnet. Ann Radiol 24 (5)

Rankin RN, Ulan RA, Keown PA, Stiller CR (1981) Percutaneous transluminal dilatation of transplant renal artery stenosis. Postgrad Med J 57: 300–303 (May)

Solt J, Rauth J, Horvath L (1981) Gezielte Dilatation benigner Oesophagusstenosen mit einem Ballonkatheter. Extracta Gastroenterologica 10 (5): 313–324

Valiestra RE, Holmes JR, Smith HC, Hartzler G, Orszulak TA (1981) Percutaneous transluminal coronary angioplasty. Mayo Clin Proc 56: 287–293 (May)

Zorn-Bopp VE, Ingrisch H, Mietaschk A, Frey KW (1981) Transluminale Gefäßdilatation der distalen Bauchaorta, der Arteria iliaca communis und externa. ROEFO 134: 471–500 (May)

Baxi R, Epstein HY, Abitbol C (1981) Percutaneous transluminal renal artery angioplasty in hypertension associated with neurofibromatosis. Radiology 139: 583–584 (June)

Cecile JP, Fournier A, Sorez JP, Louchart JC (1981) Diagnostik et traitement simple anodin et économique de l'hypertension artérielle réno-vasculaire (Angioplastie rénale). Ann Radiol (Paris) 24 (6): 508–514

Jacobson HG (1981) Diagnostic radiology; Interventional radiology. JAMA 245: 2220 (June 5)

Katafuchi T, Abe I, Kawasaki T, Muratani H, Omae T, Fukiyama K, Numaguchi Y (1981) A case of renovascular hypertension treated with percutaneous transluminal angioplasty. Jpn J Nephr 23 (6): 789–797

Katzen BT, Breda AV (1981) Low dose streptokinase in the treatment of arterial occlusions. AJR 136: 1171–1178

Legoff JJ, Doyon D (1981) L'angioplastie transluminale percutanee traitement non chirurgical des stenoses et occlusions vasculaires par des sondes a ballonnet. Nouv Presse Med 10 (26): 2197–2201 (June 13)

Lowman BG, Queral LA, Holbrook WA, Estes JT, Dagher FJ (1981) Transluminal angioplasty during vascular reconstructive procedures. Arch Surg 116: 829–832 (June)

Verstraete M, Vermylen J, Verhaeghe RH (1981) Peripheral arterial diseases. Clin Haematol 10: 669–689 (June)

Roberts B, Gertner MH, Ring EJ (1981) Balloon-catheter dilation as an adjunct to arterial surgery. Arch Surg 116: 809–812 (June)

Connolly JE, Kwaan JHM, McCart PM (1981) Complications after percutaneous transluminal angioplasty. Am J Surg 142: 60–66 (July)

Link DP, Foerster JM, Lantz Bo MT, Holcroft JW (1981) Assessment of peripheral blood flow in man by video dilution technique: a preliminary report. Invest Radiol 16: 298–304 (July–August)

Rosen RJ, McLean GK, Oleaga JA, Freiman DB, Ring EJ (1981) A new exchange guide wire for transluminal angioplasty. Radiology 140: 242–243 (July)

Williams DO, Riley RS, Singh AK, Gewirtz H, Most AS (1981) Evaluation of the role of coronary angioplasty in patients with unstable angina pectoris. Am Heart J 102 (1): 1–9 (July)

Block PC, Myler RK, Stertzer S, Fallon JT (1981) Morphology after transluminal angioplasty in human beings. N Engl J Med 305 (7): 382–385 (August 13)

Levy RI, Mock MB, Willman VL, Passamani ER, Frommer PL (1981) Percutaneous transluminal coronary angioplasty – a status report. N Engl J Med 305 (7): 399–400 (August 13)

Motarjeme A, Keifer JW, Zusaka AJ (1981) Percutaneous transluminal angioplasty of the vertebral arteries. Radiology 139 (3): 715–717 (June)

Neiman HL, Brandt TD, Greenberg M (1981) Percutaneous transluminal angioplasty: an angiographer's viewpoint. Arch Surg 116: 821–828 (June)

Mills NL, Doyle DP (1981) Does operative transluminal angioplasty extend the limits of coronary artery bypass surgery – A preliminary-report. Circulation [Suppl 4] 64: 193 (August)

Tegtmeyer CJ, Teates CD, Cringer N, Gandee RW, Ayers CR, Stoddard M, Wellons HA (1981) Percutaneous transluminal angioplasty in patients with renal artery stenosis. Radiology 140 (2): 323–330 (August)

Cicuto KP, McLean GK, Oleaga JA, Freiman DB, Grossman RA, Ring EJ (1981) Renal artery stenosis: anatomic classification for percutaneous transluminal angioplasty. AJR 137: 599–601 (September)

Corwin RD, Singh AK, Karlson KE (1981) Balloon dilatation of ductus arteriosus in a newborn with interrupted aortic arch and ventricular septal defect. Am Heart J 102 (3): 446–447 (September)

Kang HJ, Trethewey KL, Bauer J, Lee HT (1981) Percutaneous transluminal angioplasty in renal artery stenosis. Mo Med 78 (9): 582–588 (September)

Majeska JA, Munda R (1981) Hazard of percutaneous transluminal dilation in renal transplant arterial stenosis. Arch Surg 116: 1225–1226 (September)

Spiegel RM (1981) Percutaneous transluminal angioplasty. A comprehensive overview. Ariz Med 38 (9): 680–686 (September)

Bailey RR, Lewis GRJ, Maling TMJ (1981) Percutaneous transluminal angioplasty: successful cure of malignant hypertension. Dunedin NZ Med J 693: 256–257 (October 14)

Clouse ME, Tomashefski JF, Reinhold RE, Gostello P (1981) Mechanical effect of balloon angioplasty: case report with histology. AJR 137: 869–871 (October)

Dacie JE (1981) Percutaneous transluminal angioplasty. Br J Hosp Med 26 (4): 314–326 (October)

Grim CE, Luft FC, Yune HY, Klatte EC, Weinberger MH (1981) Percutaneous transluminal dilatation in the treatment of renal vascular hypertension. Ann Intern Med 95 (4): 489–442 (October)

Joffre F (1981) Percutaneous trans-luminal angioplasty – personal experience. Applications clinique de Rayons et des à utres et physiques de exploration et de traitment. J Radiol 62 (10): 514

LeVeen RF, Wolf GL (1981) New rabbit atherosclerosis model for the investigation of transluminal angioplasty. Invest Radiol 16: 426 (September–October)

Marco par J, Gouel Y, Fournial G, Alibelli MJ, Bernies M, Berthoumieu F, Bernadet P (1981) Angioplastie transluminale des coronaires: Resultats preliminaires. Arch Mal Coeur 74 (10): 1131–1141

Ring EJ, McLean GK (1981) Interventional radiology: principles and techniques. Little Brown, Boston (October)

Freiman DB, McLean GK, Oleaga JA, Ring EJ (1981) Percutaneous transluminal angioplasty. In: Ring EJ, McLean GK (eds) Interventional radiology: principles and techniques, chapt 2. Little Brown, Boston, pp 117–243

Zajko AB, McLean GK, Freiman DB, Oleaga JA, Ring EJ (1981) Percutaneous puncture of venous bypass grafts for transluminal angioplasty. AJR 137: 799–802 (October)

Castaneda-Zuniga WR, Amplatz K, Laerum F, Formanek A, Sibley R, Edwards J, Vlodaver A (1981) Mechanics of angioplasty: an experimental approach. Radiographics 1: 1–14 (November)

Fogarty TJ, Chin A, Shoor PM, Blair GL, Zimmerman JJ (1981) Adjunctive intraoperative arterial dilation: Simplified instrumentation technique. Arch Surg 116: 1391–1398 (November)

Freiman DB, Spence R, Gatenby R, Gertner M, Roberts B, Berkowitz HD, Ring EJ, Oleaga JA (1981) Transluminal angioplasty of the iliac and femoral arteries: follow-up results without anticoagulation. Radiology 141: 347–350 (November)

Grüntzig AR (1981) Percutaneous transluminal angioplasty in coronary occlusion. Hosp Pract 16: 129–136 (November)

Kumpe DA (1981) Percutaneous dilatation of an abdominal aortic stenosis: Three-balloon-catheter technique. Radiology 141: 536–538 (November)

Kupersmit MA (1981) Percutaneous transluminal angioplasty of the renal arteries. J of AOA 81 (3): 173–176 (November)

Lock JE, Niemi T, Einzig S, Amplatz K, Burke B, Bass JL (1981) Transvenous angioplasty of experimental branch pulmonary artery stenosis in newborn lambs. Circulation 64 (5): 886–892 (November)

Martin EC, Fankuchen EI, Karlson KB, Dolgin C, Collins RH, Voorhees AB Jr, Casarella WJ (1981) Angioplasty for femoral artery occlusion: comparison with surgery. AJR 137: 915–919 (November)

Martin EC, Mattern RF, Baer L, Fankuchen EI, Casarella WJ (1981) Renal angioplasty for hypertension: predictive factors for long term success. AJR 137: 921–924 (November)

Motarjeme A, Keifer JW, Zuska AJ (1981) Percutaneous transluminal angioplasty as a complement to surgery. Radiology 141: 341–346 (November)

McDonald WJ (1981) Renal artery stenosis causing hypertension: The current status of classical surgical therapy versus percutaneous transluminal dilatation. Am J Kidney Dis 1 (3): 185 (November)

Navarro-Lopez F, Urbano-Marquez A, Castaner A, Panes J, Botey A, Rozman YC (1981) Tratamiento de la hipertension vasculorrenal por dilatacion transluminal percutanea de la arteria renal estenotica. Med Clin (Barc) 77 (8): 333–337 (November)

Reilly DT, Wood RFM, Watkin EM (1981) Transplantation: attempted balloon catheter dilation of transplant renal artery stenosis and subsequent operative correction. Transplantation 32 (5): 444–445 (November)

Tegtmeyer CJ, Brown J, Ayers CA, Wellons HA, Stanton LW (1981) Percutaneous transluminal angioplasty for the treatment of renovascular hypertension. JAMA 246 (18): 2068–2070 (November)

Archie JP Jr (1981) Balloon catheter for dilatation and thrombectomy for acute aortoiliac occlusion. Cardiovasc Dis Bull Texas Heart Inst 8 (4): 546–549 (December)

Gutierrez OH, Izzo JL Jr, Burgener FA (1981) Transluminal recanalization of an occluded renal artery: Reversal of anuria in a patient with a solitary kidney. AJR 137: 1254–1256 (December)

Meier WL, Waller RM, Sones PJ Jr (1981) Budd-Chiari web treated by percutaneous transluminal angioplasty. AJR 137: 1257–1258 (December)

Mills SR, Wertman DE Jr, Grossman SH (1981) Renal cortical arteriovenous fistula complicating percutaneous renal angioplasty. AJR 137: 1251–1253 (December)

Saffitz JE, Totty WG, McClennan BL, Gilula LA (1981) Percutaneous transluminal angioplasty. Radiological-pathological correlation. Radiology 141: 651–654 (December)

Sos TA, Sniderman KW, Beinart C (1981) Grüntzig catheter with a 10-cm-long balloon. Radiology 141: 825–826 (December)

Angelini P, Leatherman L, Springer A, Krajcer Z, Lufschanowski R, Stamatiou E, Wagner E, Armburst C, Leachman R (1981) Early experience of transluminal coronary angioplasty (TCA) by the brachial artery (the Sones technique in transluminal angioplasty). Cathet Cardiovasc Diagn 7: 13–25

Bergan JJ (1981) Introduction to the symposium on transluminal angioplasty. Arch Surg 116: 804–805

Born ML, Gerlock AJ Jr, Goncharenko V, Hollifield JW, MacDonell RC Jr (1981) Radionuclide evaluation of renal artery dilatation. Cardiovasc Intervent Radiology 4: 177–182

Bredfeldt JE, Pingoud EG, Groszmann RJ, Tilson MD, Conn HO (1981) Balloon Dilatation of stenotic portacaval anastomosis. Hepatology 1: 448

Bret J (1981) Neuroradiology; Recanalization of Sylvian aqueduct. Eur J Radiol 1: 67–70

Cherrier par F, Booman F, Serruys PW, Cuilliere M, Danchin N, Reiber JHC (1981) L'angiographie coronaire quantitative: Application a l'evluation des angioplasties transluminales coronaires. Arch Mal Coeur 74 (12): 1377–1387

Colapinto RF, Harries-Jones EP, Johnston KW (1981) Percutaneous transluminal recanalization of complete iliac artery occlusions. Arch Surg 116: 277–281

Descotes J, Lyonnet D, Barral X, Brusz A, Pinet A (1981) La dilatation endoluminale arterielle, methode complementaire ou concurrente do l'entarterietomie iliaque? Chirurgie 107: 224–228

Dorros G, Spring DA (1981) A coronary pressure-recording and contrast-delivery system for percutaneous transluminal coronary angioplasty. Cathet Cardiovasc Diagn 7: 451–454

Ekelund L, Johnsson N, Lindstedt E, Stridbeck H, Lundquist SB (1981) Dilatation of experimental renal artery stenosis by balloon catheter. Acta Radiol Diagn 5: 561–569

Freudenberg H, Lichtlen PR, Engel HJ (1981) Zur transluminalen Angioplastie von Koronargefäßen; Analyse der wichtigsten Komplikationen aufgrund postmortaler Untersuchungen am menschlichen Herzen. Z Kardiol 70: 39–44

Funke-Volkers R, Weichert HC, Freundlieb O, Szy DAG, Strotges MW (1981) Veränderung der Nierenfunktion nach Eingriffen an den Nierenarterien unter besonderer Berücksichtigung der Methode nach Dotter. Radiologe 21: 574–577

Garrido E, Montoya J (1981) Transluminal dilatation of internal carotid artery in fibromuscular dysplasia: A preliminary report. Surg Neurol 16: 469–471

Grosse-Vorholt R, Groos G (1981) Komplizierter Verlauf einer perkutanen Gefäßrekanalisation. Radiologe 21: 84–86

Grüntzig A, Fischer M, Goebel N, Schlumpf M (1981) Percutaneous transluminal coronary angioplasty (PTCA). Ann Radiol 24: 377–379

Haft JI, Prasad PV, Manvar BN (1981) Incidence of potential candidates for percutaneous transluminal coronary angiography (PTCA) among patients with coronary disease. Clin Res 29: A 203

Hasso AN, Bird CR, Zinke DE, Thompson JR (1981) Fibromuscular dysplasia of the internal carotid artery: Percutaneous transluminal angioplasty. AJNR 2: 175–180

Humphries AL, Nesbit RR, Caruana RJ, Hutchins RS, Heimburger RA, Wray CH (1981) Thirty-six recommendations for vascular access operations. Am Surg 47: 145–151

Ingrisch H (1981) Diagnostik der Nierenarterien-Stenose durch Angiotomographie. Fortschr Med 99: 774

Kuhlmann U, Vetter W, Grüntzig A, Schneider E, Pouliadis G, Steurer J, Siegenthaler W (1981) Percutaneous transluminal dilatation of renal artery stenosis: 2 years' experience. Clinic Sci 61: 481–483

Lowman BG, Queral LA, Holbrook WA, Estes JT, Dagher FJ (1981) Transluminal angioplasty during vascular reconstructive procedures. Arch Surg 116: 829–832

Lyonnet D, Pinet A, Barral X, Descotes J (1981) Possibilities at limites de la dilatation endoluminale des stenoses arterielles. Lyon Chir 77 (1): 36–38

Mahler F, Probst P, Weidmann P, Krneta A (1981) Transluminal dilatation of renal artery stenoses due to atherosclerosis and fibromuscular dysplasia: early results and follow-up of twelve consecutive cases. Ann Radiol 24: 355–356

Mathias K, Struck E, Schindera F, Urbanyi B (1981) Percutaneous treatment of renovascular hypertension. Pediatr Radiol 11: 154–156

Mathias K (1981) Perkutane transluminale Katheterbehandlung supraaortaler Arterienobstruktionen. Angio 3: 47–50

Manly RJ, Belzer FO (1981) Spontaneous reversal of renal failure by renal artery recanalization. Arch Surg 116: 107–109

Medina M, Butt KMH, Gordon DH, Thanawala S, Solomon N (1981) A complication of percutaneous transluminal angioplasty in the transplanted kidney. Urol Radiol 3: 59–61

Meyer J, Messmer BJ, Reifferscheid M (1981) Präoperative Behandlung hochgradiger Koronarstenosen mit der Ballontechnik bei Patienten mit operablen Karzinomerkrankungen. Dtsch Med Wochenschr 106: 1366–1369

Olbert F, Weidinger P, Schlegl A, Teiner G, Hagmuller GW, Denck H (1981) Combined transluminal percutaneous dilation and surgical reconstruction of the iliac, femoral and popliteal arteries. Ann Radiol 24: 369–374

Paolini RM, Marcondes M, Widman A, Sabbaga E, Bernardes Silva H, Nissensweig I, De Almeida Magalhaes A (1981) Percutaneous transluminal angioplasty of renal artery stenosis. Acta Radiol [Diagn] (Stockh) 22: 571–575

Pierangeli LF (1981) La desobstruction endoluminale par voie percutanee des stenoses arterielles. Ann Radiol (Paris) 24: 170–177

Pinot JJ, Burelle H, Laroche JP, Branchereau A, Kasbarian M (1981) Angiographie par vole percutanée. Expérience personnelle. J Radiol 62: 526

Puel P, Vaislic C, Bouissou E, Boucays A, Moreau JP, Levade M, Boccalon H, Cerene A, Joffre F, Enjalbert A (1981) L'Angioplastie transluminale percutanee appliquee au traitement des arteriopathies des membres inferieurs (a propos de 24 patients). Rev Med Toulouse 17: 617–624

Puijlaert CBAJ, Boomsma JHB, Ruijs JHJ, Geyskes GG, Franken AH, Hoekstra A, Oei HY (1981) Transluminal renal artery dilatation in hypertension: technique, results, and complications in 60 cases. Urol Radiol 2: 201–210

Rentrop P (1981) Recanalization of coronary arteries in acute myocardial infarction. Ann Radiol 24: 357–359

Rutsch W, Schartl M, Mathey D, Kuck K, Merx W, Dorr R, Rentrop P, Blanke H (1981) Percutaneous transluminal coronary recanalization: Procedure, results and acute complications. Am Heart J 102: 1178

Schoop W (1981) Dilatation of pelvic artery stenoses. Ann Radiol 24: 375–376

Schuur KH, Vencken LM (1981) Arterial hypertension treated by angioplasty (Dotter), a serious complication. Diagn Imaging 50: 47–51

Schwarten DE (1981) Percutaneous transluminal renal angioplasty. Urol Radiol 2: 193–200

Shehadi W (1981) Percutaneous transluminal coronary angioplasty. Ann Radiol 24: 349–352

Spence RK, Freiman DB, Gatenby R, Hobbs CL, Barker CF, Berkowitz HD, Roberts B, McClean G, Oleaga J, Ring EJ (1981) Long-term results of transluminal angioplasty of the iliac and femoral arteries. Arch Surg 116: 1377–1386

Von Stößlein F, Bürger K, Wierny L, Widera R, (1981) Die Kombinationstherapie arteriosklerotischer Durchblutungsstörungen der unteren Extremität – perkutane transluminale Angioplastik und chirurgische Revaskularisation. Zentralbl Chir 106: 1521–1528

Turcotte JK, Lu CT, Zarins CK (1981) The role of transluminal angioplasty in limb salvage and claudication. J Surg Res 30: 428–434

Van Andel GJ (1981) Long-term results of iliac and femoral angioplasty. Ann Radiol 24: 365–368

Van Andel GJ (1981) Transluminal iliac artery dilatation: Technique of the Dotter procedure. Diagn Imaging 50: 32–42

Zeitler E, Grosse-Vorholt R, Richter EI, Saida Y (1981) Techniques of percutaneous transluminal angioplasty (PTA) and additional treatment of leg arteries. Ann Radiol 24: 361–364

Zühlke HV, Sörensen R, Häring R, Konradt J (1981) Die intraoperative offene transluminale Angioplastie (IOTA). Chirurg 52: 265–270

Brevers G, Scholl J-M, Chaitman BR, Dupras G, David P-R, Lesperance J, Bernard P, Val PG, Bourassa MG (1982) Interet de l'electrocardiogramme a l'effort et de la scintigraphie myocardique au thallium dans l'evaluation des patients referes pour angioplastie coronarienne transluminale percutanee. Union Med Can 111: 19–23 (January)

David PR, Bourassa MG, Lesperance J, Scholl JM, Crepeau J, Dyrda I, Hudon G, Chaitman BR, Dupras G, Pelletier C, Maille JG, Paquet E (1982) Angioplastie coronaire transluminale percutanee. Resultats initiaux chex nos premiers 110 patients. Union Med Can 111: 11–17 (January)

Hudon G, Goulet C (1982) Angioplastie transluminale percutanee: Principles et revue de la Litterature. Union Med Can 111: 3–10 (January)

Hudon G, Hebert Y, Goulet C, Lemarbre L, Pelletier C (1982) Dilatation et recanalisation arterielle des membres inferieurs par angioplastie transluminale percutanee. Union Med Can 111: 25–31 (January)

Lu C, Zarins CK, Yang C, Sottiurai V (1982) Long-segment arterial occlusion: percutaneous transluminal angioplasty. AJR 138: 119–122 (January)

Meyer J, Merx W, Dorr R, Lambertz H, Bethge C, Effert S (1982) Successful treatment of acute myocardial infarction shock by combined percutaneous transluminal coronary recanalization (PTCR) and percutaneous transluminal coronary angioplasty (PTCA). Am Heart J 103 (1): 132–134 (January)

Mitty HA, Gribetz ME (1982) The status of interventional uroradiology. J Urol 127: 2–9 (January)

Shaver RW, Soong J (1982) Angioplasty through aortofemoral graft: Use of catheter-introducer sheath. AJR 138: 168–169 (January)

Singer MI, Rowen M, Dorsey TJ (1982) Transluminal aortic balloon angioplasty for coarctation of the aorta in the newborn. Am Heart J 103 (1): 131–132 (January)

Sperling DR, Dorsey TD, Rowen M, Gazzaniga AB (1982) Percutaneous transluminal angioplasty of congenital coarctation of the aorta. Clin Res 30 (1): 112A

Barbaric ZL (1982) Percutaneous transluminal angioplasty of the renal artery. Urol Clin North Am 9: 169–175 (February)

Flanigan DP, Schuler JJ, Spigos DG, Lim LT (1982) Anatomic and hemodynamic evaluation of percutaneous transluminal angioplasty. Surg Gynecol Obstet 154: 181–185 (February)

Katz RJ, Leiboff RH, Aaron BL, Mills M, Wasserma AG, Ross AM (1982) Intra-operative retrograde balloon angioplasty of the left anterior descending coronary artery for reperfusion of jeopardized proximal branches. Circulation 66 (2): 30–34 (February)

Levin DC, Murray P, Harrington DP (1982) New curved catheter for renal angioplasty. AJR 138: 359–360 (February)

Lu C, Zarins CK, Yang C, Turcotte JK (1982) Percutaneous transluminal angioplasty for limb salvage. Radiology 142: 337–341 (February)

Mills NL, Doyle DP (1982) Does operative transluminal angioplasty extend the limits of coronary artery bypass surgery? A preliminary report. Circulation [Suppl 1] 66: 1–26–29 (February)

Scholl JM, Chaitman BR, David PR, Dupras G, Brevers G, Val PG, Crepeau J, Lesperance J, Bourassa MG (1982) Exercise electrocardiographiy and myocardial scintigraphy in the serial evaluation of the results of percutaneous transluminal coronary angioplasty. Circulation 66 (2): 380–389 (February)

Spring DA, Dorros G (1982) Dorros spring pressurizer an inflation device for use in transluminal angioplasty procedures. Cathet Cardiovasc Diagn 8 (2): 209–213

St. Louis EL, Provan JL, Gray RR, Grosman H, Ameli FM, Elliott DS (1982) Percutaneous transluminal angioplasty in peripheral vascular disease: a review. Can Fam Physician 28: 291–294 (February)

Gerard DF, Devin JB, Halasz NA, Collins GM (1982) Transplant renal artery thrombosis revascularization after $5^1/_2$ hours of ischemia. Arch Surg 117: 361 (March)

Hillman BJ, Ovitt TW, Capp MP, Prosnitz EH, Osborne RW Jr, Goldstone J, Zukoski CF, Malone JM (1982) The potential impact of digital video substraction angiography on screening for renovascular hypertension. Radiology 142: 577–579 (March)

Kukharch VV, Arabidze GG, Matveeva LS, Shpilkin VM, Kungurts VV, Khalchev VM, Kutsenko AI, Saveliev VY (1982) Transcutaneous intravascular balloon dilatation in patients with stenosis of the renal artery and arterial hypertension. Kardiologia 22 (3): 38

Kumpe DA, Jones DN (1982) Percutaneous transluminal angioplasty: radiologic viewpoint. Appl Radiol 11: 29–40 (March–April)

Mahler F, Probst P, Haertel M, Weidmann P, Krneta A (1982) Lasting improvement of renovascular hypertension by transluminal dilatation of atherosclerotic and nonatherosclerotic renal artery stenoses: a follow-up study. Circulation 65 (3): 611–617 (March)

Motarjeme A, Keifer JW, Zuska AJ (1982) Percutaneous transluminal angioplasty of the brachiocephalic arteries. AJR 138: 457–462 (March)

Nakada T, Yanagi S, Katayama T (1982) Successful treatment of renovascular hypertension with percutaneous transluminal angioplasty. J Urol 127: 526–527 (March)

Sniderman KW, Sos TA (1982) Percutaneous transluminal recanalization and dilation of totally occluded renal arteries. Radiology 124 (3): 607–610 (March)

Baxi RK (1982) A case report of percutaneous transluminal angioplasty following failure of femoro-popliteal venous bypass graft. Cardiovasc Intervent Radiol 5: 30–33

Bookstein JJ, Meser KM, Hougie C (1982) Coagulative interventions during angiography. Cardiovasc Intervent Radiol 5: 46–56

Cantelmo NL, LoGerfo FW (1982) A technique of angioplasty of the profunda and superficial femoral arteries. Surg Gynecol Obstet 154: 564–565 (April)

Cho KJ (1982) Renal angiography in renovascular hypertension. Urol Radiol 3: 213–218

Faxon DP, Weber VJ, Haudenschild C, Gottsman SB, McGovern WA, Ryan TJ (1982) Acute effects of transluminal angioplasty in three experimental models of atherosclerosis. Arteriosclerosis 2: 125–133 (April)

Goertz KK, Linshaw MA, Lee KR, Hermreck A, Mattioli L, Bailie MD (1982) Transluminal arterial dilation of a postsurgical stenosis of renal artery implant in a child with recurrent hypertension. Pediatrics 69: 489–491 (April)

Grüntzig A (1982) Results from coronary angioplasty and implications for the future. Am Heart J 103 (4): 779–783

Madias NE, Kwon OJ, Millan VG (1982) Percutaneous transluminal renal angioplasty, a potentially effective treatment for preservation of renal function. Arch Intern Med 142: 693–697 (April)

Ritter VH, Großmann K, Basche S, Heerklotz I, Schiffmann R, Schumann E (1982) Die perkutane transluminale Angioplastik (PTA) von Aortenbogenästen. ROEFO 4 (136): 365–370 (April)

Sos TA, Saddekni S, Sniderman KW, Weiner M, Beinart C, Pickering TG, Case DB, Vaughan ED Jr, Laragh JH (1982) Renal artery angioplasty: techniques and early results. Urol Radiol 3: 223–231

Berman HL, Martin MB (1982) A simplified method for antegrade sheath introduction into the common femoral artery. AJR 138: 973 (May)

Block PC, Elmer D, Fallon JT (1982) Release of atherosclerotic debris after transluminal angioplasty. Circulation 65: 950–952 (May)

Cumberland DC (1982) Percutaneous transluminal angioplasty – experience in balloon dilatation of peripheral, coronary and renal arteries. Br J Radiol 55: 330–337 (May)

Curry R, Johnston L (1982) Percutaneous transluminal angioplasty. Ulster Med J 51: 59–66 (May)

Glover JL, Bendick PJ, Dilley RS, Holden RW, Yune HY, Richmond BD, Klatte EC (1982) Efficacy of balloon catheter dilatation for lower extremity atherosclerosis. Surgery 91: 560–565 (May)

Laerum F, Vlodaver Z, Castaneda-Zuniga WR, Edwards JE, Amplatz K (1982) The mechanism of angioplasty: Dilatation of iliac cadaver arteries with intravascular pressure control. ROEFO 136 (5): 573–576

Lu C, Zarins CK, Yang C, Sottiurai V (1982) Approach to transluminal angioplasty in patients with groin scarring or vascular grafts. Radiology 143: 395–398 (May)

Madias NE (1982) Percutaneous transluminal renal angioplasty. Chest 81: 632–634 (May 5)

Stevens RK, Hyde GL, Loh FK (1982) Transluminal angioplasty (TLA) in occlusive vascular disease. J Ky Med Assoc 80(5): 278–282

Train JS, Mitty HA, Efremidis SC, Rabinowitz JG (1982) Visualization of a fine periluminal vascular network following transluminal angioplasty: possible demonstration of the vasa vasorum. Radiology 143 (2): 399–403 (May)

Castaneda-Zuniga WR, Lock JE, Vlodaver Z, Rusnak B, Rysavy JP, Herrera M, Amplatz K (1982) Transluminal dilatation of coarctation of the abdominal aorta. An experimental study in dogs. Radiology 143: 693–697 (June)

Jacobson HG (1982) Radiology: Interventional radiology. JAMA 247: 2220–2221 (June 4)

Lock JE, Castaneda-Zuniga WR, Bass JL, Foker JE, Amplatz K, Anderson RW (1982) Balloon dilatation of excised aortic coarctations. Radiology 143: 689–691 (June)

Maxwell DD, Mispireta LA (1982) Transfemoral renal artery embolectomy. Radiology 143: 653–654 (June)

Neiman HL, Bergan JJ, Yao JST, Brandt TD, Greenberg M, O'Mara CS (1982) Hemodynamic assessment of transluminal angioplasty for lower extremity ischemia. Radiology 143: 639–643 (June)

Roberts B (1982) Balloon angioplasty in the treatment of peripheral vascular disease. J Cardiovasc Surg (Torino) 23 (3): 225–228

Roberts B, Ring EJ (1982) Current status of percutaneous transluminal angioplasty. Surg Clin North Am 62: 357–372 (June)

Silverton NP, Elamin MS, Ionescu MI, Smith DR, Whitaker W (1982) Quantitative evaluation of the outcome of percutaneous transluminal coronary angioplasty (Abstr). Clin Sci 63 (3): P50

Tamura S, Sniderman KW, Beinart C, Thomas A (1982) Percutaneous transluminal angioplasty of the popliteal artery and its branches. Radiology 143: 645–648 (June)

Tegtmeyer CJ (1982) Percutaneous transluminal renal angioplasty. The evolution of a procedure (Editorial). Arch Intern Med 142: 1085–1086 (June)

Tegtmeyer CJ, Elson J, Glass TA, Ayers CR, Chevalier RL, Wellons HA Jr, Studdard WE Jr (1982) Percutaneous transluminal angioplasty: the treatment of choice for renovascular hypertension due to fibromuscular dysplasia. Radiology 143: 631–637 (June)

Al-Bassam MS, Farrell EM, Rubio PA (1982) Percutaneous transluminal coronary angioplasty in the treatment of unstable angina pectoris. Tex Med 78: 57–59 (July)

Belan A, Vesela M, Vanek I, Weiss K, Peregrin JH (1982) Percutaneous transluminal angioplasty of fibromuscular dysplasia of the internal carotid artery. Cardiovasc Intervent Radiol 5: 79–81 (July)

Castaneda-Zuniga WR, Laerum F, Rysavy J, Rusnak B, Amplatz K (1982) Paralysis of arteries by intraluminal balloon dilatation. An experimental study. Radiology 144: 75–76 (July)

Gerlock AJ, Regen DM, Shaff MI (1982) An examination of the physical characteristics leading to angioplasty balloon rupture. Radiology 144: 421–422 (July)

Haynes IG, Simon J, West RJ, Hamer JD (1982) Idiopathic retroperitoneal fibrosis with occlusion of the abdominal aorta treated by transluminal angioplasty (technical note). Br J Surg 69 (7): 423–433

Heeney DJ, Bookstein JJ, Carey PH, Rapoport S (1982) The role of para renal collaterals in assessing renal artery stenosis before and after percutaneous transluminal angioplasty. Cardiovasc Intervent Radiol 5: 71–78 (July)

Scully RE, Mark EJ, McNeely BU (1982) Case records of the Massachusetts General Hospital, case 29. N Engl J Med 307: 237–242 (July)

Smith DC, Durkos JL (1982) An improved ruptured-balloon retrieval set. Radiology 144: 430–431 (July)

Castaneda-Zuniga WR, Smith A, Kaye K, Rusnak, Herrera M, Miller R, Amplatz, Weens C, Ketchum D (1982) Transluminal angioplasty for treatment of vasculogenic impotence. AJR 139: 371–373 (August)

Golden DA, Ring EJ, McLean GK, Freiman DB (1982) Percutaneous transluminal angioplasty in the treatment of abdominal angina. AJR 139: 247–249 (August)

Katz RJ, Beiboff RH, Aaron BL, Mills M, Wasserman AG, Ross AM (1982) Intraoperative retrograde balloon angioplasty of the left anterior descending coronary artery for reperfusion of jeopardized proximal branches. Circulation 66: I-30–I-34 (August)

Mayer JH, Wills PJ (1982) A localization grid for percutaneous transluminal angioplasty. Radiology 144: 649–650 (August)

Picard JD, Frileux C, Nguyen M, Morere K, Olivier C (1982) Reflections on percutaneous recanalization of the left iliac vein. Chirurgie 108: 144–147 (August)
Ring EJ, Freiman DB, McLean GK, Schwarz W (1982) Percutaneous recanalization of common iliac artery occlusions: an unacceptable complication rate? AJR 139: 587–589 (September)
Waltman AC, Greenfield AJ, Novelline RA, Abbott WM, Brewster DC, Darling RC, Moncure AC, Ottinger LW, Athanasoulis CA (1982) Transluminal angioplasty of the iliac and femoropopliteal arteries. Arch Surg 117: 1218–1221 (September)
Etheregce SB, Mahony JR, Savdie E, Waugh RC, Sheil AGR (1982) Treatment of renal transplant artery stenosis by percutaneous transluminal dilatation. Clin Nephrol 17: 217–221
Harries J (1982) Interventional radiology – a new subspecialty. S Afr Med J 61 (16): 585–586
Ruckert RF, Brunner U (1982) Der segmentäre femoro-popliteale Verschluß. Langzeit-Ergebnisse nach offener Thrombendarterektomie. Helv Chir Acta 49: 85–89
Puijlaert CBAJ, Geyskes GG, Oej HY, Ruijs JHJ, Boomsma JHB, Wüstefeld PJ, Mali WPT (1982) Renal angioplasty in hypertension, technique, radiological and clinical results in 108 dilatations in 96 patients. In: Oliva L, Pires-Veiga JH (eds) Proceedings of the second international symposium on interventional radiology, Venice-Lido, 27 September 1981. Excerpta Medica, Amsterdam, pp 317–322 (International congress-series no 575)
Dotter CT (1983) Transluminal angioplasty. In: Abrams HL (ed) Angiography, 3rd edn. Little Brown, Boston
Dotter CT (1983) Transluminal angioplasty, method, indications and role in therapy. Proceedings of vascular surgery course, June 1982, Minneapolis. In: Delaney JP (ed) Advances in vascular surgery. Yearbook Med Publishers, Chicago, pp 143–149

Subject Index